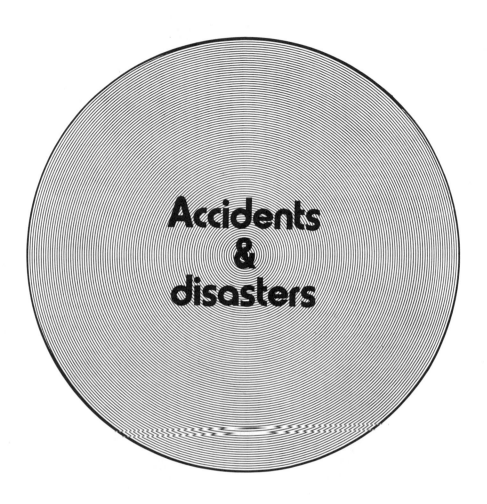

ALTON L. THYGERSON

Brigham Young University

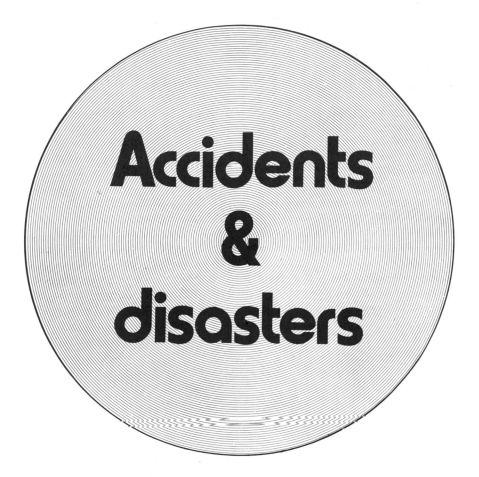

Accidents & disasters

CAUSES AND COUNTERMEASURES

Prentice-Hall, Inc., Englewood Cliffs, New Jersey

Library of Congress Cataloging in Publication Data

THYGERSON, ALTON L.
    Accidents and disasters.

    Includes the author's Safety (2nd ed.), which is
also published separately.
    Includes bibliographical references and index.
    1. Accidents—Prevention.   2. Accidents—United
States.   3. Safety education.   I. Thygerson,
Alton L.   Safety.   1976.   II. Title.
HV675.T526   614.8   75-38981
ISBN   0-13-000968-7

Printed in the United States of America

10   9   8   7   6   5   4   3

Part III is based on the Suggested Citizen Instructions contained in *Disaster Operations: A Handbook for Local Governments* by permission of the Defense Civil Preparedness Agency and *Disaster Preparedness: Report to the Congress* by permission of the Federal Disaster Assistance Administration.

Prentice-Hall International, Inc., *London*
Prentice-Hall of Australia Pty. Limited, *Sydney*
Prentice-Hall of Canada, Ltd., *Toronto*
Prentice-Hall of India Private Limited, *New Delhi*
Prentice-Hall of Southeast Asia Pte. Ltd., *Singapore*

Dedicated to my children—

sons, Scott, Michael, Steven, and Matthew
daughter, Whitney

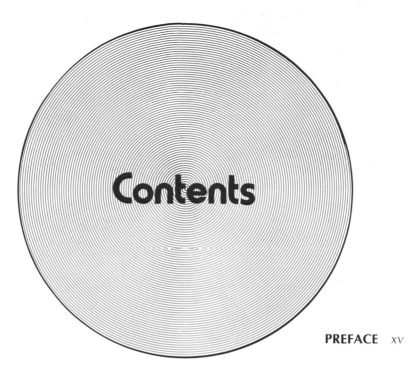

Contents

part III **DISASTERS**
Causes and Countermeasures

chapter 18

EARTHQUAKES *321*

chapter 19

LANDSLIDES *337*

chapter 20

TSUNAMIS *346*

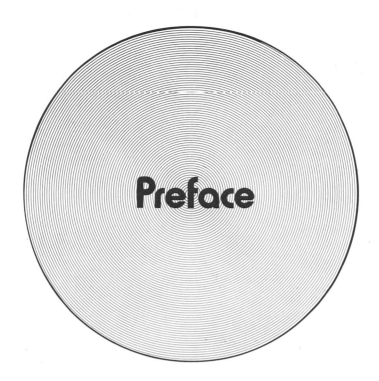

Preface

This book presents an account of the foundations of safety which I hope will be understandable and interesting to those with little previous knowledge of the subject. My intention has been to give the reader a better understanding of the safety, accident, and disaster fields. There will, of course, not be perfect agreement among safety authorities on which topics should and should not have been chosen for treatment.

An attempt has been made to relate the findings of research and medicine to the needs of the layman and the safety specialist. A large portion of the text is devoted to providing literature that might otherwise be difficult to obtain or understand because of the technical nature of the resources used and their usual inaccessibility.

Part I of the book deals extensively with the problems of defining the term "accident," exploring the concept of risk, analyzing accident proneness and scare techniques, presenting a framework for developing countermeasures based on epidemiology and other models, and offering a rationale for safety instruction. Parts II and III present causes and countermeasures for the major types of accidents and disasters.

The appendix offers the reader exposure to the consumer product hazards.

Special thanks go to my wife, Ardith, for her encouragement and patience throughout the research and writing of the book. For her typing skill and helpful suggestions I express recognition to my sister, Sherry

Littler. It is the author who must accept total responsibility for errors; corrections would be most gratefully accepted and appreciated.

A remark by Samuel Johnson impresses me with its truth: the best way to learn about a subject is to write a book.

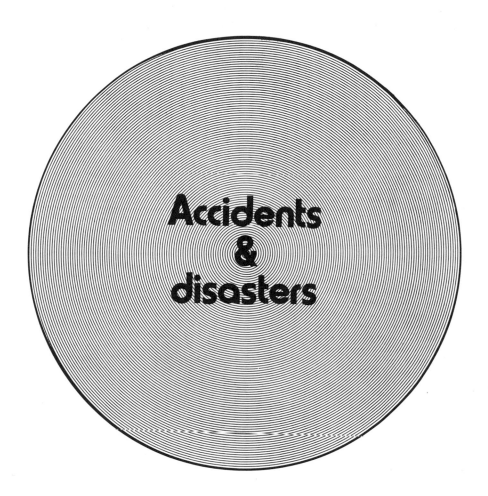

Accidents & disasters

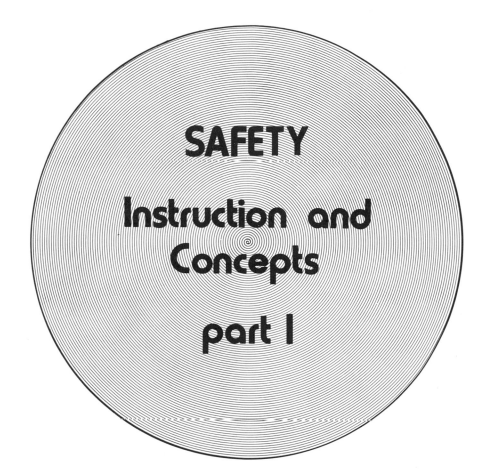

SAFETY

Instruction and Concepts

part I

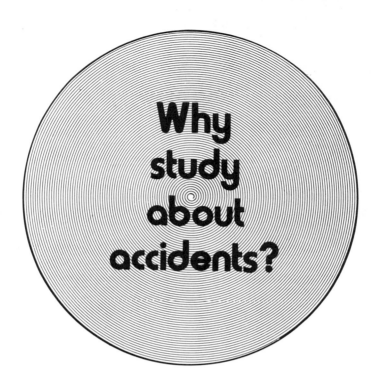

Why study about accidents?

1 The term *accident* is seldom used to describe unexpected injuries due to biological agents such as viruses and bacteria, but rather unexpected physical and chemical injuries to the body and other structures. The traditional concept of an accident gives no indication of causes or results. Although the term is retained in common usage, it is neither medically nor scientifically appropriate for most purposes.

If an accident is considered the end product of a sequence of acts or events which results in some "unanticipated" and "undesirable" consequence, it will be apparent that what is unanticipated and undesirable will vary with the interests of the individual. Medically, for example, accidents are a cause of death or injury. The accident itself is not of interest, but the fact that it produces an unhealthful condition. Emphasis is thus primarily on the consequence, and what is called an accident depends on whether injury follows. On the other hand, a legal point of view would emphasize the antecedent of the accident to determine liability.

It seems unlikely that an accident can be defined as a single, unitary concept, and a "range" definition rather than a "class" definition may be necessary. For example, three major characteristics have been suggested as criteria: (1) degree of expectedness—the less anticipated, the more the event may be classed as an accident; (2) degree of avoid-ability—the less the event could be avoided, the more the event can be classed as accidental; (3) degree of intention—the less the event in-volves deliberate action, the more likely the event is to be labeled an accident.[1]

This eliminates injury or damage as a part of the definition, and thus whether and why injury results becomes a separate question from why the accident occurred. This makes it possible to study a class of events quite independently from their consequences.

Scientists have questioned the common term *accident*. Gibson states:

The term "accident" . . . refers to a makeshift concept with a hodgepodge of legal, medical, and statistical overtones. . . . Defined as a harmful encounter with the environment, a danger not averted, an accident is . . . subject to pre-diction and control. But defined as an unpredictable event, it is by definition uncontrollable.

And he concludes,

The word should be discarded in scientific discussion.[2]

In a similar vein, Cantelli notes that "accidents . . . should perhaps better be called 'incidents,' all ascribable to some causative factor."[3]

Haddon concludes that the term *accident*

. . . is neither medically nor scientifically appropriate for most purposes, and that it is gradually being replaced by descriptions of the injuries themselves and the physical and chemical agents whose release is responsible for their occur-rence.[4]

As a partial solution for the difficulties arising from the use of the concept *accident*, Suchman suggests:

We cannot define accidents as a simple unitary concept; instead we must list a set of criteria for characterizing accidental events. . . . Thus, an accident may be defined as that group of events which involves a low level of unexpectedness, avoidability, and intention. . . . From this point of view, the definition of an event as an accident becomes a matter of setting up a cut-off point as to the degree of the unexpected, unavoidable, and unintentional that is required be-fore one is willing to accept an event as being an accident.[5]

It is doubtful, then, that any single definition would cover events called accidents. One definition might be, "An accident is a nondeliberate, unplanned event which may produce undesirable effects, and is preceded by unsafe, avoidable acts(s) and/or condition(s)." Let us examine the elements of this statement in detail.

Nondeliberate Acts

Nondeliberate acts include accidents (falls, drownings, etc.) and disasters (tornadoes, earthquakes, etc.). Deliberate acts include crime (assault, arson, etc.), wars, riots, and insurrections. It is important to differentiate between actions that are deliberate and those that are nondeliberate. Identification of causes and appropriate countermeasures differ according to the classification of an event. In other words, countermeasures for suicide and crime differ from those for drownings and poisoning.

An Unplanned Event

The definition of the word *accident* hinders accident prevention efforts. For instance, medical science has long emphasized the resultant damage of a disease rather than its "unexpectedness"; this emphasis has proved rather successful. To many, the word *accident* implies that something unexpected and unpleasant occurred and that: it could not be helped, but was an accident; it was inevitable and could have happened to anyone; it was unforeseen and thus uncontrollable; and it was not our responsibility and we are therefore not to be blamed. The idea of an unplanned or unpredictable occurrence implies an event which may be uncontrollable.

Undesirable Effects

Tobacco smoking was not a recognized problem as long as most people smoked. Only when a large number of people decided that tobacco smoking was harmful (after considering the evidence) and said, "Isn't it awful!" did smoking become a recognized problem. Awareness of a problem requires that we make a *value judgment*, a decision that the condition is "good" or "bad." A person's value judgment may define a condition as either undesirable, and therefore requiring change, or proper and acceptable. Consequently, what is called undesirable may vary from individual to individual, from situation to situation, even from culture to culture.

People in our society decide that accidents are unacceptable because they cause undesirable effects such as death, injury, and property damage. It should be noted that the ingestion of a polio virus or *bacillus botulinus* is not usually classified as an accident, whereas swallowing lye or an insecticide is. Such an inconsistency sets a definite limitation upon the definition of an accident. Undesirable or harmful effects are no longer the focal point in accident studies but now have minor significance in the investigation of accident causation. The resulting injuries are a consequence of the unplanned event and do not constitute the accident—they follow afterward. Thus, if Mike falls on top of Steve, who gets a tooth broken, Mike has the unplanned event and Steve the injury, but who has the accident? It is Mike and not Steve who is usually charged or credited on the accident reports.

Death, injury, or property damage—consequences of an unplanned event—do not in themselves constitute the accident, but are the results of it. The consequences are merely the last in a series of happenings, each of which contributes something to the accident. For example, if a driver falls asleep at the wheel but awakes in time to avoid a collision, the event is not recorded as an accident. A study of these near accidents, however, could furnish clues to accident causation. The events recorded as accidents—those involving death, injury, or property damage—represent a very small percentage of the total consequences of unplanned happenings. Additional undesirable effects include anger, fear, and embarrassment, which are often correlated with both accidents and near accidents.

All consequences of accidents are not negative or undesirable. For example, though a child is burned by touching a hot pan or pot, he learns very quickly that pans and pots can be hot and they can cause pain. Thus, this child avoids future contact with hot pans and pots or possibly even any hot object and is not burned again. This child's experience, though temporarily painful, has a long-term positive effect in regard to the avoidance of fire and hot objects.

Another example is the aftereffects of a disaster. Though human life may be taken, survivors learn that living in certain river bottoms in the spring of the year or being near a beach during a hurricane or tsunami has been disasterous and therefore should be avoided.

It is not suggested that everyone try to experience things in order to determine consequences. Rather, all people should gain from others' experiences. This is the basis for instruction and education—a shortcut to experience, but also an avoidance of events which may have negative effects upon health and life.

Avoidable Events

Until recently, everybody talked about the weather but nobody did anything about it. For instance, floods were simply a misfortune to be endured before the development of flood control. Now that we can exercise some control over the weather through new developments such as cloud-seeding and proper placement of dams, we see that a previously undesirable condition can be prevented. Similarly, an accident becomes a problem when we believe it can be avoided. Often the prevention of an accident can be determined only by trial and error. In the meantime, the accomplishments of accident prevention to date encourage us to try to avert the great loss of life and property and the many injuries that result from accidents.

We note a significant trend toward emphasis on prevention of further loss after the event called an accident, rather than on prevention of the accident. In the past, efforts to reduce accident losses have been made through such means as education, prohibitions, and licensing, which aim at accident prevention. Today, several authorities believe that more emphasis should be placed upon safeguards such as safety belts, steel-toed shoes, first aid, transportation of injured, and other after-the-accident countermeasures.

Accident avoidance for prevention has been criticized on the basis that it is too narrow and does not convey the idea of the basic problem (that of injuries) and of the desired end (reducing losses due to injuries). Some authorities show evidence that countermeasures to the injury problem should not be limited primarily to prevention of the initial event, but may involve any stage of the injury-producing process that can be effectively changed. The term suggested is "injury control" rather than "accident prevention or avoidance." This may appear to be an improvement, but it makes no distinction between accidental (nondeliberate) injury and deliberate injury (for example, crime). It would appear that property damage is not clearly identified either, since "injury" usually refers in most cases only to physical human body damage.

Unsafe Act(s) and/or Unsafe Condition(s)

A realistic appraisal of recent accident data clearly shows that *few* events labeled accidents really are accidents in that they are purely chance events. Like other events, accidents are caused and, therefore, can be controlled when their causes are identified and understood. Frequently, accidents are not unforeseeable, because most of them are not chance occurrences but rather reflect inefficiencies in the system.

Accidents occur because people make mistakes. The statement that "80 percent of accidents are *caused* by human beings" may be simplistic and require confirming research. Human error frequently underlies unsafe conditions such as poor design, construction, and maintenance; therefore, most accidents are still attributable to human error.

Arbous and Kerrich point out that:

. . . our attempts to oversimplify the accident-causing situation by seeking to subdivide it into "personal causes" and "environmental causes" tends to lead us nowhere. . . . Surely the essence of accident causation is the rather intricate interrelationship which exists between the individual and the environment and the influence of one cannot be appreciated without considering its interaction with the other.[6]

Finally, it should be mentioned that several authorities suggest that the term *accident* be discarded. They believe it more reasonable to classify the resultant injuries as electrical, chemical, mechanical, and the like. The misconceptions that accompany the term *accident* can also be avoided by this classification. In science if the cause of an event is known, that event is not an accident; most accident causes are known, but we still persist in calling them accidents. However, the word may be too deeply entrenched in the language to go out of use.

John J. Brownfain makes a discerning observation about defining accidents:

If we label all of life's unpleasant surprises as accidents, then we come to perceive ourselves as the playthings of fate and we cultivate a philosophy of carelessness and irresponsibility. On the other hand, if we look for causes and hold ourselves accountable for the mishaps in our lives, we become people of resource and confidence, increasingly able to control the direction of events. If these conclusions are as true as I think they are, it matters very much how we define the word accident.[7]

Definitions of Common Safety-Related Terms

Since definitions are important, some commonly used terms are defined below for the sake of clarity:

Safety — frequently defined as "freedom from hazards." Since it is practically impossible to eliminate all hazards completely, safety is a relative protection from exposure to hazards.

Hazard — a condition with the potential of causing injury, such as one involving fire, electricity, or chemicals.

Danger — expresses a relative exposure to a hazard. A hazard may be present, but there may be little danger because of the precautions taken. (For example, a person driving on a freeway is subject to the hazard of a fatal collision. When he wears a safety belt the danger is reduced, but it is still present if the belt is incorrectly worn or an object penetrates the automobile interior.)

Risk — an expression of possible loss; the chance of a loss. It is usually indicated by the probability of an accident happening.

Disaster — a major emergency affecting a large number of people. The Metropolitan Life Insurance Company labels those accidents that take five or more lives as catastrophes.[8] A disaster is a great, sudden misfortune resulting in loss of life, serious injury, or property loss. Strictly speaking, if such misfortune befalls even one person, it is a disaster. However, in current usage, the term is used to refer to a sudden occurrence that kills and injures relatively large numbers of persons. This is the sense in which the word "disaster" is used in this book. To be more specific, the *Statistical Bulletin* lists only those disasters resulting in the loss of 25 or more lives. *Accident Facts* (see page 90) compiles those disasters with 100 or more fatalities.

Accident — a nondeliberate, unplanned event which may produce undesirable effects, and is preceded by unsafe, avoidable act(s) and/or condition(s).

REASONS FOR STUDYING ABOUT ACCIDENTS

Awareness

Individuals should be aware of the main accident problems. Have you ever visited a place and then been surprised at how often you heard or read about that place afterward? The place had been mentioned just as frequently before you visited it, but you never noticed these comments until you were acquainted with it; thereafter, you found meaning in each reference because it related to something that had become familiar. Similarly, if we are aware of a particular accident problem we notice each reference to it in the newspaper, possibly take time to read a magazine article about it, or become more attentive when it comes up in conversation. In this way we constantly increase our knowledge of a problem and the validity of our judgments about it.

Factual Knowledge

An intelligent analysis must rest upon facts. It makes little sense to discuss an accident problem unless someone in the group knows what he or she is talking about. Although fact gathering will not solve any problem automatically, it is impossible to analyze a problem until the facts have been collected, organized, and interpreted.

Misconceptions about safety and accidents exist because all the facts may not be known or presented. Unfortunately, these misconceptions and myths persist yet, in spite of educational efforts. (See Figures 1–1 and 1–2.) As a self-check for misconceptions, see how well you perform on the test in Table 1–1.

Understanding the Science of Accident Prevention

It is valuable that we have a general understanding of how and why accidents occur, how people are affected by accidents, and how we can deal with them. This provides a frame of reference within which we can catalog data and study specific problems. If we have a thorough understanding of the science of accident prevention, we can intelligently organize and analyze data on any particular accident. In addition, this understanding enables us to interpret new data correctly and to keep up to date. Acci-

table 1–1   *Test on Safety Myths*

Which of the statements below are misconceptions in safety?

_____	1	Lightning never strikes twice in the same place.
_____	2	Red is the hunter's best clothing color.
_____	3	A silver spoon or silver coin will turn black after coming in contact with a poisonous mushroom.
_____	4	Boiling or soaking poisonous mushrooms in saltwater makes them safe.
_____	5	A rattlesnake gives warning before striking.
_____	6	The first procedure in saving a drowning person is to jump in the water.
_____	7	It is impossible to stay afloat in water for long with clothes on.
_____	8	If a boat overturns, you should swim to shore.
_____	9	A drowning person always comes up for air three times.
_____	10	Applying a tourniquet is the best way to stop bleeding.
_____	11	Put butter on a burn.
_____	12	Put beefsteak on a black eye or wound.
_____	13	Put a cold knife on a bump on the head.
_____	14	Rub snow on frostbite.
_____	15	The primary danger from leaking gas is asphyxiation.
_____	16	Coffee will help sober up a drunk.
_____	17	Smaller vehicles can stop in less time and distance than larger ones.
_____	18	Pumping the brakes helps stop a car more quickly on dry pavement.

Now turn to p. 11 for correct answers.

dent data often become obsolete and accident problems may change considerably within a few years. For example, there is a change in concern about motorcycle and snowmobile death and injury statistics and a decrease in concern about abandoned refrigerators and ultrathin plastic clothing covers as potential hazards. Yet, if the individual understands the science of accident prevention, he or she will not find it hard to interpret new data and understand new accident trends.

Our attitudes and values determine the meanings we find in the facts we observe. A study of some widespread fallacious attitudes toward accidents may help show why people react to facts so differently. Such a study may also help show why we may always have accident problems.

Listed below are some fallacious beliefs presented by authors Richardson, Hein, and Farnsworth:

1 The "other fellow" concept, whereby it is assumed that accidents happen to other people but won't happen to you.

2 The "your number's up" concept, whereby it is assumed that "when your number is up," you will get hurt and there is nothing you can do about it.

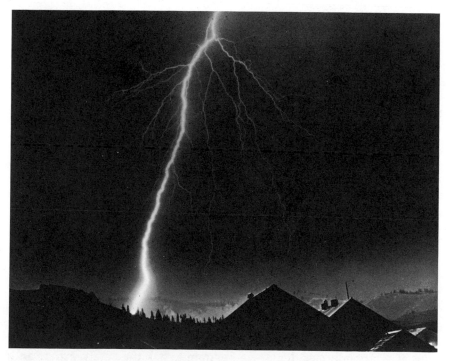

figure 1–1 Does lightning ever strike twice in the same place? Reproduced courtesy of the National Oceanic and Atmospheric Administration.

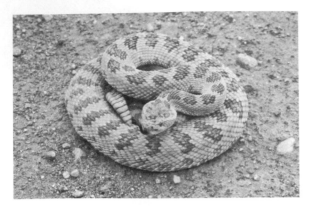

figure 1–2 Myths exist about the rattlesnake. The venom of bees, wasps, and hornets causes more deaths in the United States each year than are caused by the venom of a rattlesnake. Reproduced courtesy of the Utah Division of Fish and Game.

3   The "law of averages" concept, whereby accidents and injuries are shrugged off as due to inevitable statistical laws.

4   The "price of progress" concept, whereby accidents are rationalized as the inevitable price of scientific advancement.

5   The "spirit of '76" concept, whereby living dangerously is glorified and safety measures are regarded as sissy.

6   The "act of God" concept, whereby accidents are seen as divinely caused — for punishment or for some purpose unknown to us.[9]

A Sense of Perspective

Some people find the study of accidents upsetting. Just as people are frightened by all the diseases they find listed in a medical textbook, some individuals are disturbed by the great amount of expressed or implied criticism of our society that they find in a safety course. For others, awareness of imperfections which result in accidents may become an obsession. They are so distressed with the tragedy, suffering, and waste caused by an accident-plagued society that they fail to see more encouraging aspects of the total picture. We need a sense of perspective if we are to see without exaggeration or distortion.

Appreciation of the Proper Role of the Expert

Opinions are not equally valuable. If we want a useful opinion on why our head throbs or our car stalls, we ask the appropriate experts. However, as we ponder accidents, we hesitate to ask the safety expert and confidently announce our own opinions, perhaps after discussing the questions with others who know no more than we.

This contradiction stems from our failure to distinguish between *questions of knowledge* and *questions of value.* In questions of knowledge there are right and wrong answers, whereas in questions of value there are differences of opinion. The layman and the expert are equally qualified to answer questions of value, but they are not equally qualified to answer questions of knowledge. For instance, the question of whether leisure time should be used in viewing operas or football games is a matter of value. But the question of whether a four-phase driver education program is more or less effective than a two-phase driver education program requires expert knowledge to answer.

Stated in simple terms, *the role of the expert is not to tell people what they should want, but to tell them how they may best get what they want.* Even experts are not infallible; all may be wrong on a given issue. When experts disagree, any one answer should not be considered positive or final. Experts in safety agree that accidents are caused and do not "just happen"; the layman who feels an accident was an event which could not have been avoided reveals his ignorance.

In the field of safety, the function of the expert is to provide accurate descriptions and analyses of accidents and to show laymen what consequences may follow each countermeasure proposal. However, experts have met with limited success when they attempted to tell people what would be best for them in a given situation. It usually takes a near-accident, an accident, or even a tragedy before people become sufficiently concerned and motivated to take overt action.

The task of the individual is to learn how to recognize an expert and guide his own thinking by expert knowledge rather than by guesswork.

Answers to the Test on Safety Myths — All answers are false.

NOTES

[1]Edward A. Suchman, "A Conceptual Analysis of the Accident Phenomenon," *Social Problems,* August 1961, pp. 241–53.

[2]J. J. Gibson, "The Contribution of Experimental Psychology to the Formulation of the Problem of Safety: A Brief for Basic Research," in *Behavioral Approaches to Accident Research,* ed. H. H. Jacobs et al. (New York: Association for the Aid of Crippled Children, 1961), pp. 77–89.

[3]E. J. Cantelli, "A Philosophy for Accident Prevention," *Traffic Engineer,* May 1965, p. 44.

[4]William Haddon, Jr., "The Prevention of Accidents," in *Preventive Medicine,* ed. Duncan W. Clark and Brian MacMahon (Boston: Little, Brown and Company, 1967), p. 592.

[5]Suchman, "A Conceptual Analysis of the Accident Phenomenon," p. 243.

[6]A. G. Arbous and J. E. Kerrich, "Accident Statistics and the Concept of Accident Proneness," *Biometrics,* July 1951, p. 340.

[7]John J. Brownfain, "When Is an Accident Not an Accident?" *Journal of the American Society of Safety Engineers,* September 1962, p. 20.

[8]Metropolitan Life Insurance Company, *Statistical Bulletin* (New York: Metropolitan Life Insurance Company, January 1975), p. 6.

[9]Reprinted from Charles E. Richardson, Fred V. Hein, and Dana L. Farnsworth, *Living* (Glenview, Ill.: Scott, Foresman and Company, 1975), pp. 339–40.

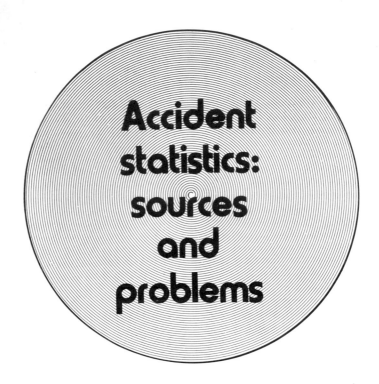

Accident
statistics:
sources
and
problems

2 The first decennial census was taken in the United States in 1790. However, it was not until after the turn of the twentieth century that accident data were collected systematically.

ACCIDENT FACTS

Issued annually by the National Safety Council, *Accident Facts* now constitutes a most reliable source of nationwide frequency for all types of accidents reported in the United States.[1] In addition to presenting annual reports on the four principal classes of accidents, *Accident Facts* presents data on rates and trends; hence this compendium is an available source for evaluating the relative efficiency of accident-prevention agencies. The National Safety Council has been aided in the collection and interpretation of accident data by many organizations, companies, and individuals.

OTHER SOURCES OF ACCIDENT STATISTICS

Except for statistical studies made by individual investigators which are usually limited to small samples of accident victims, the large-scale gathering of statistical data is necessarily a task of the government. At present, there are several sources available for accident statistics:

1. *Law Enforcement Agencies.* Officials involved in the investigation of accidents include municipal and state police and a wide variety of sheriffs, constables, and special peace officers.

2. *Legislative Committees.* In recent years, state and national legislatures have made increasing use of their broad investigatory powers for the exploration of problems pertaining to accidents. Congressional hearings involving highway safety and consumer product safety have gained national attention.

3. *Insurance Companies.* The Metropolitan Life Insurance Company publishes a monthly publication entitled *Statistical Bulletin*. Almost every issue contains data and information pertinent to accident problems. Insurance records usually have too little information to be really valuable. They are usually hard to retrieve because they are generally inaccessible to the public.

4. *National Center for Health Statistics.* This federal agency conducts the National Health Survey. Surveys are made of a preselected household sample of the entire population. Based upon the survey, an annual accidental injury total is estimated. Details of the place, nature, severity, and sources of personal injury occurring in the two weeks prior to the interview are gathered. Accidents are included but are a relatively small portion of the survey. Its weakness is that it does not get enough information.

5. *The National Electronic Injury Surveillance System* (NEISS) is a computerized system yielding statistically valid, nationally representative accidental injury data from selected hospital emergency rooms located throughout the United States. Over 100 hospitals are included and physicians' offices are incorporated to broaden its scope of coverage.

6. *The National Highway Traffic Safety Administration* has a traffic accident record program. Most states have traffic records of accidents, and until recently these records were sorted and tallied by hand. The volume of data, plus the need for rapid retrieval, requires the use of the most advanced computers. Although a few reports have become available, most of the information has not.

7. *State Agencies.* Organizations such as state departments of vital statistics, highway departments, and safety councils frequently collect, analyze, and distribute information on the incidence of accidents in their particular geographical areas.

8. *Community Agencies.* Selected agencies in some towns and cities also gather accident data. In addition, these agencies may serve as collecting agencies for state organizations.

9. *Other.* Data may be collected by other organizations for their own use. An elementary school or a university department of physical education may realize the need for accident reporting as an aid to accident

prevention. Industry, business, and government often tabulate information concerning the frequency of accidents within their respective jurisdictions.

The problems with many of these sources are: (1) information incomplete, (2) reporting of only severe types, (3) information not easily available or not made public, (4) inaccuracies, and (5) variations in definition of accident and/or injury.

PROBLEMS OF STATISTICAL ANALYSIS

Statistics play an important role in accident prevention. The reason statistics are not used more is probably because of what some call a "statistical neurosis."

An early statistician coined a phrase that has since been repeated to generations: "It's not that the figures lie—it's that the liars figure." Although deceptive figures do appear in accident statistics, it is probable that the largest number of statistical studies are compiled by those desiring to inform rather than misinform. Nevertheless, a statistic that misleads through honest error can be just as confusing as one that is deliberately constructed to misrepresent. In the following paragraphs we will discuss several sources of error found in accident statistics; these may be divided into the following groups: sources of error in *collection, presentation,* and *interpretation.*

Sources of Error in the Collection of Accident Statistics

Deliberate Suppression.   There are several forms of suppression. One can be attributed to administrative self-protection rather than to darker motives. Keeping the accident rate down is a perennial concern of administrators. Frequently, a slightly injured worker is immediately returned to the job to keep the factory record spotless, although the injured worker should be home after the accident resting from the shock and caring for his injury.

Only a few accident statistic errors in collection result from distortions introduced deliberately or negligently. Most of these errors are either partly or totally unavoidable because there are certain problems peculiar to data gathering. The following sources of error are highly difficult or impossible to eradicate.

Failure to Complain.   Since an accident is not known until someone reports it, any statistic that purports to represent the total number of any type of accident that has taken place is necessarily an informed guess based on the addition of an estimated number of *unreported* accidents of the same category. Certain types of accidents tend to be reported with much greater accuracy than others. For example, deaths resulting from motor-vehicle operation are usually reported quite accurately because there are legal requirements to make such reports and great value is placed upon human life. However, motor-vehicle accidents causing less than $100 worth of damage may go unnoticed and even unreported as a result of legal stipulations and $100 deductible insurance coverage which may not require the reporting of small accidents. Even reports of damage costs may be totally in error since most estimated costs are quite subjective in nature.

Geographical Variations in the Definition of Certain Accidents.   There is one obstacle hindering a uniform system of accident reporting which will not be overcome until all jurisdictions employ similar definitions for classifying accidents. For example, different definitions yield different statistics. In Belgium a person is considered a highway fatality only if he dies at the accident scene. In France an interval between injury and death that would still permit such a classification is three days, 24 hours in Spain, thirty days in Britain, and a year in the United States, Canada, and Mexico.

Differences in the Reporting of Accidents Within the Same Area.   An administrator has his biases. If a relative of his or a person with high status has an accident, the administrator may never report it in order to keep a record clear of any blemish that might hinder future promotions and advancements for that person.

William E. Tarrants reported at a National Safety Congress:

A mid-western manufacturing plant with a fairly stable injury frequency rate decided to hire a full-time safety engineer to see if this rate could be cut down. Within a short time after the safety engineer was hired, the injury frequency rate nearly doubled. Should we conclude that the safety engineer caused these accidents and quickly fire him? A closer look revealed that the safety engineer instituted a new accident investigation and reporting system which produced more reports of disabling injuries, thus increasing the frequency rate.[2]

Lack of Uniformity in Collecting and Recording Techniques.   Tallying the number of known accidents is a considerably more complicated process than it would seem to be. Conceivably, reports from rural areas reveal a lower rate of actual accident occurrence than do reports from urban areas. A motor-vehicle accident is usually witnessed, whereas there may be no witnesses to a home accident involving minor cuts or burns, making accurate reporting more difficult.

Sources of Error in the Presentation of Accident Statistics

When we consider statistical data there is probably no assertion more misleading than the frequently heard statement: "The figures speak for themselves." Because long columns of figures convey an impression of factuality, it is essential to discuss the more common misunderstandings that arise from faulty presentation of data.

Misleading Use of Simple Sums Rather than Rates.   The fact that Town *A* records 50 motor-vehicle deaths as compared with 100 reported by Town *B* does not necessarily mean that Town *B* is twice as accident-ridden as Town *A*. The reverse may be true. If Town *B* has four times the population of Town *A*, the reverse *is* true. Total accident figures do not become meaningful until they are transformed into *rates* (ratios or percentages) based on the total population under consideration. Similarly, this principle applies to changes in the incidence of accidents. Town *C*, in 1980, may report twice as many accidents as it did in 1960—yet its population may have doubled during this period. If this is true, then the accident rate remains the same.

Misleading Use of Averages and Percentages.   The precaution of translating simple sums into averages and percentages does not assure the proper presentation of data; these measures can be as misleading as the raw totals. Consider the following statement: "The average number of accidents per family in the Lakeview residential area is three per year." This statement gives the impression that each family living in the Lakeview residential area has about the same number of accidents each year. This assumption may not be correct at all. A count reveals that five families live in the area. Three households report one accident, whereas the fourth family reports two accidents that year. The fifth family has a total of ten among its members. Thus the "average" figure obtained by adding the total number of accidents and dividing by five is mathematically accurate but misleading.

As the illustration demonstrates, an *average* is meaningless without information about the variation of the measures that compose it. The importance of this principle is further illustrated by an example taken from *Accident Facts*. In one year the following rates for traffic deaths were revealed for cities with populations over 1,000,000 (see Table 2–1).

On the basis of these figures we could assert that it is safer to drive a

table 2–1   *Motor-Vehicle Traffic Deaths per 100,000 Population for 1973 for Selected U.S. Cities*

Los Angeles	13.7
Chicago	9.5
Detroit	14.7
New York	10.4
Philadelphia	11.1
Houston	15.8

source: Reprinted from National Safety Council, *Accident Facts* (Chicago: National Safety Council, 1974, p. 65, by permission of the Council.

motor vehicle in Chicago than in Detroit. However, caution is still urged since a death rate based upon mileage rather than population might indicate the reverse.

Pitfalls of Graphic Presentations.   For some readers, long columns of figures are not only impressing but downright intimidating. For this reason statisticians and publicists often present their findings graphically or pictorially. Although this method presents material in quick, easy-to-comprehend form, it can also mislead the reader.

Sources of Error in the Interpretation of Accident Statistics

The "Self-Evident" Conclusion.   Disraeli, Mark Twain, and others have observed that there are three kinds of lies — plain lies, damned lies, and statistics. This humorous statement implies that statistics can be manipulated to support any point of view. The use of statistics, however, should not be completely dismissed, for statistics mislead and confuse only when one does not know how to interpret them. There are elaborate formulas for determining the significance and reliability of a statistic, [3] but this text offers some simple tests which the reader can apply.

In his informative and amusing book *How to Lie with Statistics*, Darrel Huff points out a number of statistical tricks.[4] He calls attention to biased samples, meaningless averages, purposeful omissions, apple and peach comparisons, illogical correlations, the *post hoc, propter hoc* fallacy (this happened after that, therefore that caused this), the cut-off graph, the deceptive map, and the two-dimensional picture to express three-dimensional facts.

If you want to analyze a statistical statement, advises Huff, ask these questions: Who says so? How does he know? What's missing? Did somebody change the subject? Does it all make sense? He cites, among scores of amusing examples, the statement that "four times more fatalities occur on the highways at 7 P.M. than at 7 A.M." Huff says that people fail to realize that more people are killed in the evening than in the morning simply because more people are on the highways at that hour to be killed. Another amusing example of nonsense statistics is found in Table 2–2.

Huff points out that many a statistic is "false on its face." "It gets by," he says, "only because the magic of numbers brings about a suspension of common sense." Huff's moral is plain: BEWARE! He characterizes the unfortunate acceptance and utilization of statistical information as follows:

The secret language of statistics, so appealing in a fact-minded culture, is employed to sensationalize, inflate, confuse, and oversimplify. Statistical methods and statistical terms are necessary in reporting the mass data of social and economic trends, business conditions, "opinion" polls, the census. But without writers who use the words with honesty and understanding and readers who know what they mean, the result can only be semantic nonsense.

table 2–2 *Pickles Will Kill You*

Pickles will kill you: Every pickle you eat brings you nearer to death. Amazingly the "thinking man" has failed to grasp the terrifying significance of the term "in a pickle." Although leading horticulturists have long known that Cucumis sativus possesses an indehiscent pepo, the pickle industry continues to expand.

Pickles are associated with all the major diseases of the body. Eating them breeds wars and communism. They can be related to most airline tragedies. Auto accidents are caused by pickles. There exists a positive relationship between crime waves and consumption of this fruit of the cucurbit family. For example:

Nearly all sick people have eaten pickles. The effects are obviously cumulative.

99.9% of all people who die from cancer have eaten pickles.

100% of all soldiers have eaten pickles.

96.8% of all communist sympathizers have eaten pickles.

99.9% of all the people involved in air and auto accidents ate pickles within 14 days preceding the accident.

93.1% of juvenile delinquents come from homes where pickles are served frequently.

Evidence points to the long-term effects of pickle eating:

Of the people born in 1839 who later dined on pickles, there has been a 100% mortality.

All pickle-eaters born between 1849 and 1859 have wrinkled skin, have lost most of their teeth, have brittle bones and failing eyesight — if the ills of eating pickles haven't already caused their death.

Even more convincing is the report of a noted team of medical experts: rats force-fed with 20 pounds of pickles per day for 30 days developed bulging abdomens. Their appetites for WHOLESOME FOOD were destroyed.

In spite of all the evidence, pickle-growers and packers continue to spread their evil. More than 120,000 acres of fertile soil are devoted to growing pickles. Our per capita yearly consumption is nearly four pounds.

Eat orchid petal soup. Practically no one has as many problems from eating orchid petal soup as they do from eating pickles.

In popular writing on scientific matters the abused statistic is almost crowding out the picture of the white-jacketed hero laboring overtime without time-and-a-half in an ill-lit laboratory. Like the "little dash of powder, little pot of paint," statistics are making many an important fact "look like what she ain't." A well-wrapped statistic is better than Hitler's "big lie"; it misleads, yet it cannot be pinned on you.[5]

The field of safety and accident prevention is replete with figures, statistics, numbers, and ratios. There is little literature available regarding the proper use of accident statistics. William Tarrants, at a National Safety Congress, presented information which he felt was pertinent for the safety educator:

During World War II about 375 thousand people were killed in the United States by accidents and about 408 thousand were killed in the armed forces. From these figures, it has been argued that it was not much more dangerous to be overseas in the armed forces than to be at home. A more meaningful comparison, however, would consider rates of the same age groups. This comparison would reflect adversely on the safety of the armed forces during the war—in fact, the armed forces death rate (about 12 per thousand men per year) was 15 to 20 times as high, per person per year, as the over-all civilian death rate from accidents (about 0.7 per thousand per year).

The same fallacy is noted in the widely publicized statistical appraisal which states that "Sometime during the Korean War we passed a grim milestone. One day an American soldier fell in battle. He was the 1,000,000th American soldier to die in our wars since the nation was born. A few months later the 1,000,000th American perished in a modern highway traffic accident. [*Author's note:* The 2,000,000th traffic fatality probably occurred sometime in January 1974.] Our wars go back to 1776. The traffic figure starts with 1900." The article concludes that "war is dangerous business but getting from one place to another by automobile is even more dangerous." Again, we should consider rates, not numbers, and comparisons should also consider the same age groups.

Peacetime versions of the same fallacy are also common. We often hear that "off-the-job activities are more dangerous than places of work, since more accidents occur off-the-job" or that "The bedroom is the most hazardous room in the home since more injuries occur in the bedroom than any other room." Here again the originators fail to consider differences in quantity of exposure, type of exposure, age, and other influencing factors.[6]

The Confusion of Correlation with Cause.   In chapter 5 "causes" of accidents will be discussed in detail. A favorite method of searching for "causes" is to hunt for statistical associations. It is often claimed, without real justification, that there are associations and correlations between contributing factors and accidents. Individuals often have diffi-

table 2–3 *When Does a Percentage Indicate A Statistical Association?*

if:	we need to know:	before trying to decide:
50% of fatal accidents involve drinking drivers.	What percent of all driving is done by drinking drivers?	Whether drinking drivers contribute more or less than their share of fatal accidents.
50% of injuries to boys in the first three school grades are due to lack of knowledge.	What percent of all boys of similar age lack safety knowledge?	Whether lack of knowledge is associated with school injuries to boys.
30% of fatal accidents involve vehicles being driven too fast.	What percent of all driving is done beyond the speed limit?	Whether driving too fast is correlated with fatal accidents.
300% as many deaths occur off the job as on the job.	What percent of time is spent both on the job and off the job?	Whether a worker is safer at work than elsewhere.

culty contrasting the association of these factors with the total situation; illustrations are given in Table 2–3 to help them overcome this difficulty. The central point is that a genuine association exists *only* when two things appear together *either more frequently or less frequently than would normally be expected.*

NOTES

[1] *Accident Facts* may be obtained from the National Safety Council, 425 North Michigan Avenue, Chicago, Illinois 60611, for a nominal fee.

[2] WILLIAM E. TARRANTS, "Removing the Blind Spot in Safety Education Teacher Preparation," *School and College Safety*, National Safety Congress Transactions (Chicago: National Safety Council, 1965), p. 107.

[3] For more information see N. M. Downie and R. W. Heath, *Basic Statistical Methods* (New York: Harper & Row, 1970), and John T. Roscoe, *Fundamental Research Statistics* (New York: Holt, Rinehart and Winston, Inc., 1969).

[4] DARRELL HUFF, *How to Lie with Statistics* (New York: W. W. Norton and Company, 1954).

[5] Ibid., pp. 8–9.

[6] TARRANTS, "Removing the Blind Spot in Safety Education," pp. 107–8.

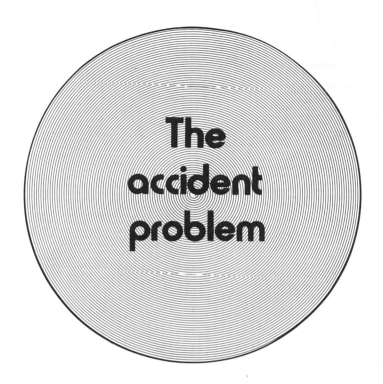

The
accident
problem

THE EXTENT OF ACCIDENT OCCURRENCE

3 Reading statistics can be quite dull. Reading accident statistics may be repulsive and gory as well. However, accident statistics of any kind tell us only where and how accidents happened, but not why. Let us consider some general accident statistics.

Every year in this country approximately 115,000 accidental deaths are reported by the National Safety Council. This averages out to one death every five minutes.[1] Over 11 million injuries are reported annually. Disabling injuries are not reported on a nationwide basis, therefore the total numbers of injuries are estimates and should not be compared from year to year. However, the number of work injuries tabulated tends to be quite accurate because there is good reporting and an established definition of a disabling injury. In contrast, the total number of nondisabling injuries treated at home, in doctors' offices, or in emergency hospital rooms is unknown.

Table 3–1 ranks accidents with other major causes of death. The tragedy of the high accidental death loss is that trauma kills thousands who otherwise could expect to live long and productive lives, whereas those afflicted with heart disease, cancer, stroke, and many chronic diseases usually live an overprotected existence and die late in life.

The human suffering and financial loss from preventable accidental

table 3–1   *Accidents vs. Other Causes of Death*

1	Heart disease
2	Cancer
3	Stroke (cerebrovascular disease)
4	Accidents
5	Pneumonia
6	Diabetes mellitus
7	Arteriosclerosis
8	Cirrhosis of liver
9	Suicide
10	Homicide
11	Congenital anomalies

source: National Safety Council, *Accident Facts,* 1974, p. 9.

death constitute a public health problem second only to the ravages of ancient plagues or world wars. In making comparisons of fatal accidents with war, it must be kept in mind that nearly everyone is exposed to accidents, but relatively few are exposed to war deaths. Perhaps for a more effective army we should follow the suggestion of a TV comedian who proposed sending our drivers to fight our wars since they are more prolific killers. The point is that we are very much concerned about war and its effects, but to be unconcerned about a domestic problem which causes as much or even more damage betrays a paradox in human thought and values.

One in four Americans are annually injured enough to require medical attention or activity restriction for at least one day. Accidents cause more deaths each year than all infectious diseases combined. Although accidental deaths were reduced by over 30 percent during the past 75 years, accidental death rates have increased 5–10 percent during the past decade.

The accident picture in the United States is grim; yet it is fair to assume that without organized safety efforts and safety education, America's accident record would be even more shocking than it is. Following heart disease, cancer, and stroke, accidents are the fourth principal cause of death in the United States. Accidents are the leading cause of death among those persons aged one to 38 years.[2]

We often think of accidents only when they are catastrophes because these events make newspaper headlines. From a statistical point of view, a catastrophe is an accident in which five or more lives are lost.[3] It is significant that a very small percentage of accident catastrophes occur as a result of natural forces such as floods, hurricanes, tornadoes, and earthquakes (see Figure 3–1). Rather, the majority of newspaper headline catastrophes are caused by some kind of human failure which

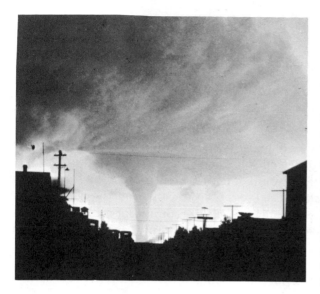

figure 3–1 Tornadoes occur in many parts of the world and in all 50 states. They are the most violent type of weather condition; however, the hurricane is the most destructive. Reproduced courtesy of the National Oceanic and Atmospheric Administration.

results in airplane crashes, mine cave-ins, explosions, and the like. However, the record of national catastrophes reveals that relatively few lives are lost in this way when contrasted with the total number of deaths resulting from other types of unspectacular, unpublished accidents.

WORTH OF A HUMAN LIFE

What value is to be placed on a human life? How can we determine its worth? Two things will give some indication of the value of human life: (1) what these lives have cost up to this point—the labor, material, and struggle that has gone into their creation and development; and (2) the effective use to which they can be put—the benefits that result from productivity and contribution to society.

How much is a human life worth? All people have worth. Almost everyone recognizes a moral obligation to minimize the loss of life—most religions and philosophies are based upon the tenets that human life has worth and life is worth living.

The value of life often is measured in terms of money—how much is a company or a parent willing to pay to protect those under their stewardship from accidental death. For example, a parent may place a great deal of emphasis on safety by purchasing and using infant car safety seats and appliances with UL ratings, and by discarding hot-water vaporizers in favor of "cool mist" vaporizers. Another parent may take none of these precautions.

There are several ways to recover the loss of a human life: (1) *legal limitations*—several states (Colorado—$20,000, Kansas—$25,000, and Illinois—$30,000) have set limits on the amount a traffic accident victim's dependents can collect for his death. (2) *Replacement costs*—a productive life is a loss and must be replaced. The military services have identified for the various military ranks the worth (in dollars) in case of a loss. Legally (in a court of law) a man or woman with no dependents would probably not be compensated for as much as a person with a family. (3) *Insurance claims*—the amount of insurance is collected in the event of a death. (4) *Accumulated assets*—often appearing in the news media are listings of the richest people in a particular country or in the world. Income tax collecting agencies (federal, state, county) appraise the worth of individual holdings at various times (e.g., probate court, bankruptcy, real estate values, etc.). Too often, we wrongly judge and evaluate a human's worth by his material possessions rather than other standards.

SURVEYS OF ACCIDENTS AMONG THE GENERAL PUBLIC

The National Health Survey, conducted by the National Center for Health Statistics, is a survey of households to collect information on the number of injuries sustained by household members during the two weeks prior to the survey interview. (It should be noted that other health information is also surveyed.) The total number of injuries is then estimated for the entire United States based upon these findings from approximately 40,000 households. We realize that differences in definition produce different injury totals when we compare the results of the National Health Survey with the totals presented by the National Safety Council.

An examination of accident injury data gathered from the general population suggests the following conclusions:

1   Estimates of the number of accidents based solely on the data of deaths or reported injuries are incomplete.

2   Data derived from these sources point out the need for a standard accident definition and reporting system.

The question of definition—and *who does the defining*—is a crucial one. For example, one may never detect or report the housewife who burns her fingers. This type of incident occurs commonly in daily living and illustrates how large numbers of accidents remain unknown.

Regardless of the error and incompleteness of accident data, we can conclude that there is definitely an immense loss from accidents.

THE ANATOMY OF ACCIDENTS IN THE UNITED STATES

The accidents reported in *Accident Facts* are categorized into nine separate types and four principal classes. In view of the differing definitions of accidents used by various agencies, this categorization represents an impressive achievement; without it and the National Health Survey an overall estimate or source of accident rates would not exist. Because of its importance in providing standarized definitions of accident types, an adaptation of the categorization found in *Accident Facts* is provided in Table 3–2.

Accident Facts lists the principal classes of accidents as motor-vehicle, work, home, and public. Table 3–3 defines each of the four classes. Each

---

table 3–2   *Types of Accidents*

all accidents   The term "accidents" includes most deaths and injuries from violence; but specifically excludes homicides, committed and attempted suicides, and deaths and injuries in war operations.

motor-vehicle accidents   Includes those accidents involving mechanically or electrically powered highway-transport vehicles in motion (except those on rails), both on and off the highway or street.

falls   Includes falls from one level to another or on the same level, except falls in or from railway-, road-, water-, or air-transport vehicles, or those occurring in cataclysms.

drowning   Includes all drownings (work and nonwork) in boat accidents and those resulting from swimming, playing in the water, or falling in. Excludes drownings in floods and other cataclysms.

fires, burns, and accidents associated with fires   Includes those accidents from fires, burns, and from injuries in conflagrations—such as asphyxiation, falls, and being struck by falling objects. Excludes burns from hot objects or liquids.

firearms   Includes firearm accidents in recreational activities or on home premises and a small number (less than 3 percent) from explosions of dynamite, bombs, grenades, etc. Excludes accidents in war operations.

poisoning by solids and liquids   Includes those accidents resulting from medicines, as well as from commonly recognized poisons. Mushroom and shellfish poisoning are included, but poisoning from spoiled foods—botulism, etc.—is classified as disease.

machinery accidents   Includes those accidents involving all types of machinery. Nearly half occur on farms in the course of work; of these, approximately three-fourths involve tractors. About one-third occur in industry. Five percent occur in the home.

poisoning by gases and vapors   Principally carbon monoxide due to incomplete combustion, involving cooking stoves, heating equipment, and standing motor vehicles. Excludes accidents in conflagrations, or associated with transport vehicles in motion.

all other types   Most important types included are: inhalation or ingestion of food or other objects, mechanical suffocation, air transportation, blow by falling object, electric current, railroad, excessive heat or cold, cataclysm.

source: Adapted from the National Safety Council, *Accident Facts* (Chicago: National Safety Council, 1974), pp. 6–7, by permission of the Council.

table 3–3   *Classes of Accidents*

motor vehicle   Includes those accidents involving mechanically or electrically powered highway-transport vehicles in motion (except those on rails), both on and off the highway or street.

work   Includes those accidents which arise out of and in the course of gainful work, except that (1) work injuries to domestic servants, and (2) injuries occurring in connection with farm chores, are classified as home injuries.

home   Includes those accidents in the home and on home premises to occupants, guests, and trespassers. Also includes domestic servants but excludes other persons working on home premises.

public   Includes those accidents in public places or places used in a public way, not involving motor vehicles. Most sports and recreation deaths are included. Excludes accidents in the course of employment.

source: Adapted from National Safety Council, *Accident Facts* (Chicago: National Safety Council, 1974), pp. 42, 72, 80, 97, by permission of the Council.

class is then subdivided into accident types. For example, public accident types are listed below:

1   Falls

2   Drowning

3   Firearms

4   Fires, burns, and deaths associated with fires

5   Air transport

6   Water transport

7   Railroad

8   Other transport

9   All other public accidents

ESTIMATES OF THE COST OF ACCIDENTS

Reliable estimates of the overall cost per annum of accidents in the United States are difficult to make, and those who have investigated the problem will probably conclude that even approximate figures would be inaccurate.

We can compare accident costs to an iceberg—only a small portion appears above water that we can actually see and measure. The indirect and hidden costs form the rest of the iceberg, the part below water that is not easily measured. As in the iceberg, hidden costs of accidents are not visible on the surface but they are there just the same. Examples of hidden costs are among those listed in Table 3–4.

table 3–4   *Some Social and Economic Consequences of Accidents*

	social		economic
1	Grief over the loss of loved ones	1	Costs of rescue equipment required
2	Loss of public confidence	2	Accident investigation and reporting
3	Loss of prestige	3	Fees for legal actions
4	Deterioration of morale	4	Time of personnel involved in rescue
5	Denial of education	5	Medical fees (doctors, hospitals, etc.)
6	Lack of guidance for children	6	Disability costs of personnel badly injured
7	Psychological effects of a change in standard of living	7	Replacement cost of property damaged or lost
8	Psychic damages affecting behavior	8	Slowdown in operations while accident causes are determined and corrective actions taken
9	Embarrassment	9	Loss of income
10	Lost pride	10	Loss of earning capability
11	Inconvenience	11	Rehabilitation costs for those who have lost limbs, mental abilities, or physical skills
12	Adversely affected interpersonal relationships (anger, resentment, etc.)	12	Funeral expenses for those killed
		13	Pensions for injured persons or for dependents of those killed
		14	Training costs and lower output of replacements
		15	Production loss for employer

THE GEOGRAPHICAL DISTRIBUTION OF ACCIDENTS IN THE UNITED STATES

Regional Accident Rates

Rates of reported accidents vary widely from one region to another. In accidental death rates, the Middle Atlantic region ranks lowest. The Rocky Mountain region has the highest rate of accidental deaths. Various explanations could be offered for these wide variations, but they would probably still not account for all the variations found.

Rural-Urban Variations

Accident death rates tend consistently to increase with greater density of population. The difference in rates between the most densely populated and the least densely populated communities is sizable.

Rural Accident Rates

For reporting purposes, *Accident Facts* classifies areas with less than 5000 inhabitants as "rural." Because they are incomplete or not tabulated, reports from rural areas probably reveal a lower rate of actual accident occurrence than do reports from urban areas.

INTERPRETING RURAL-URBAN ACCIDENT DISTRIBUTION

The apparently consistent relationship between population density and accidental death rates leads us to conclude that the higher the population concentration, the higher the accident rate (see Figure 3–2). When the urban centers are grouped in descending order of size, the accident rate decreases. Difficulties arise, however, with this general explanation:

1 Urban centers of similar size but in different regions of the country show great variation in their accident rates.
2 Even within the same geographical region, the rates do not always decline according to declining size of population.

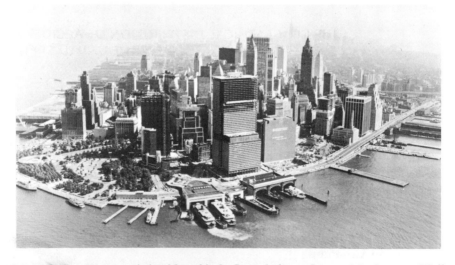

figure 3–2 A view of the New York City skyline—Lower Manhattan (Wall Street). Accident death rates tend to increase with population density. Reproduced courtesy of the New York Convention and Visitors Bureau; photo by Allen Green taken from a Hel-Aire Copter.

3   Among cities the same size and within the same region, there are often significant variations in accident rates which can only be accounted for in terms of factors specific to the particular cities.

The last explanation brings us closer to the core of the accident problem in urban environments.

GENERAL CHARACTERISTICS OF THE ACCIDENT VICTIM

The "typical" accident victim exists only as a vague abstraction created from statistical figures. Nevertheless, statistics enable us to say:

1   Most accident victims are males. After the first year of life, males have more accidents than females, at all age levels.

2   Most accident victims are young. Accidents are the leading cause of death for persons aged one to 38 years; however, the rate for accidental deaths is highest for those under one and over 65 years of age.

3   Most accident victims reside in an urban center; the Rocky Mountain region of the United States has the highest accident rate. This discrepancy is explained by the fact that most Rocky Mountain region residents are urban dwellers.

4   Most accidental deaths occur in a motor vehicle, but most injuries occur in the home. This is explained by the excessive energy involved in larger amounts in motor-vehicle accidents.

5   Most accidents happen to the victim in a cyclical manner, reaching peaks in frequency on a certain day and at a particular time in the year.

As was discussed in chapter 2, finding a way to make facts talk without having them say more than they actually do presents a real problem.

SOCIAL AND ECONOMIC CONSEQUENCES OF ACCIDENTS

Accidents produce consequences of grave importance in terms of death, injury, and property damage. Table 3–4 presents in brief form some social and economic implications of accidents.

We should consider the serious consequences of accidents in terms of their disruptive effects on the home, on the family, and on employment. The notions of "life years lost" and "working years lost" are helpful in gauging the magnitude of the accident problem. Table 3–5 shows us that back in 1945, accidental deaths were responsible for a greater loss of working years in the country than were deaths from those diseases listed.

table 3–5   *Estimated Number of Working Years Lost in the U.S. in 1945 As a Result of Death from Various Causes*

cause of death	working years lost (thousands)	percentage of total deaths
Accidents	1980	12.6
Heart disease	1892	12.0
Pneumonia	1274	8.1
Cancer	1155	7.3
Tuberculosis	1144	7.3
Nephritis (kidney disease)	484	3.1
Cerebrovascular disease	465	3.0

source: Reprinted from "The Unsleeping Dragon," *World Health,* The Magazine of the World Health Organization, June 1967, p. 7, by permission of the World Health Organization.

NOTES

[1] National Safety Council, *Accident Facts* (Chicago: National Safety Council, 1974), p. 11.

[2] All statistical references in this book are from the National Safety Council publication, *Accident Facts,* 1974.

[3] Metropolitan Life Insurance Company, *Statistical Bulletin* (New York: Metropolitan Life Insurance Company, January 1975), p. 6.

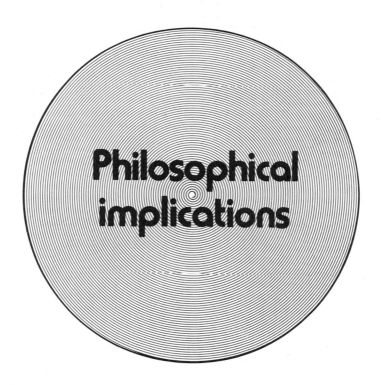

Philosophical implications

4 The types of accident problems discussed in this book fall into two main categories: those caused by natural forces and those that are the result of man's action. Both can result in suffering or death. Examples of those accidents that occur from natural causes are: a fatal shipwreck caused by a storm; death in the (frozen) north by freezing because of insufficient food and clothing; a hurricane that causes death from flooding and other damage; a tidal wave that strikes the West Coast causing death to hundreds; death from a grizzly bear attack on hikers in Yellowstone National Park; death from a rattlesnake bite in southern Texas.

Many justify these natural calamities by maintaining that they impel us to overcome them, and teach us how to live in the world. For example, the tornado teaches us to build storm cellars for protection and to set up weather observation points for advance warning. The tidal wave that struck the Hawaiian Islands a few years ago caused great devastation of life and property and taught the Hawaiians certain lessons; now when tidal waves strike the Islands, very few, if any, lives are lost. Men, then, are forced by circumstances to devise ways of signaling the danger before it arrives.

Certainly, one of the most universal and perplexing problems facing mankind is the existence of suffering. Is suffering a punishment for laws broken? Do the innocent suffer with the guilty? Can man grow through suffering? Is suffering necessary for greatness? (Most great men have suffered.)

Great works of literature often give us insight into the purpose of suffering and death in life. For example, we see suffering in the Book of Job in the Bible, and the suggestion of growth through suffering in the life of Hester Prynne in Hawthorne's *Scarlet Letter.* "The Lament" by Anton Chekhov presents two universal human qualities: the need to share sorrow and the difficulty of finding anyone sympathetic with whom to share it. Luigi Pirandello's "War" is a story of the struggle between the mind's ability to reason away sorrow and the emotions' tendency to burst forth beyond the control of reason. "Compensation" by Ralph Waldo Emerson makes some profound explorations into suffering. Emerson tells us that in every triumph there is defeat, and in every defeat triumph; in every gain there is loss, and in every loss gain; in every pleasure there is pain, and in every pain pleasure; and all experiences of success and failure, health and sickness, happiness and sorrow balance themselves out, which he calls "compensation." William Wordsworth's poem "Michael" depicts the developing greatness of his central character through his suffering—which dignifies him.

The experience of death comes to every man, for sooner or later we all must die. This experience affects us in two ways: (1) we die young and bring sorrow to family and friends, or (2) we live long and feel sorrow as family and friends die. Man's reactions to death are well portrayed in works by poets, dramatists, and novelists, such as Hemingway's *For Whom the Bell Tolls* or Miller's *Death of a Salesman.* "The Death of a Dauphin" by Alphonse Daudet, for example, shows us the universality of death, whereas poems like Edward FitzGerald's translation of "The Rubaiyat of Omar Khayyam," James Thomson's "The City of Dreadful Night," and Robinson Jeffers's "May–June 1940" reflect a negative attitude toward death. Poems expressing positive views are William Shakespeare's "Sonnet 146," John Donne's "Death Be Not Proud," William Wordsworth's "We Are Seven," as well as "Prospice" and "Rabbi Ben Ezra" by Robert Browning.

The second type of problem consists of those accidents that are the direct result of man's behavior. Three factors seem to explain suffering caused by human behavior:

1. We have made great scientific advancements because we can rely on the basic law and order of our physical world—two and two always make four and not five. The solar system moves in mathematically correct orbits, enabling us to land a man on the moon (see Figure 4–1). The earth's gravitational pull determines that what we throw into the air must be pulled back to the earth; this always happens—even though the object might be a car that plunges off a mountain road taking the occupants to their deaths.

2. Man is a free agent. He is prevented from doing what he wants because there are limits set upon him by the environment in which he lives, as well as by various social circumstances and limitations of the physical body. Being a free agent, however, means that he can do what he pleases, but will suffer the consequences of his actions — good or bad.

3. What one person does may vitally affect his neighbors because human lives are intermingled. When automobile accident insurance premiums rise, the owner of a car with no accident record becomes alarmed. After all, he is paying for others' accidents. Thus, other people's behavior affects him. When an automobile crosses through the freeway median guardrail and crashes into another car, killing its occupants, it is obvious that others have been affected by this stranger's actions and behavior.

Dying and death are events from which none of us escape. We can postpone death, gain reprieves from it, but ultimately we must die. Many people react to these statements by feeling there is something morbid in thinking about death. They comment, "I'm interested in life,

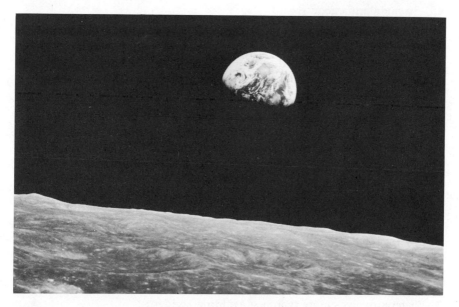

figure 4–1   This view of the rising earth greeted astronauts of Apollo 8 as they came from behind the moon (the sunset terminator bisects Africa). Reproduced courtesy of the National Aeronautics and Space Administration.

not death." Is this not a form of ostrich behavior to avoid one of the essential realities of life?

The critical question is not the dichotomy of life and death but rather how each one of us reacts to the knowledge that death is inevitable. Throughout man's history, the concept of death has been at the core of our religious and philosophical thought and thus affects our outlook toward daily living.

Contradictions arise about the existence of death. Death is viewed by some as a "wall," the ultimate personal disaster, whereas others regard death as a "doorway," a point in time on the way to eternity. However, while we are living, we should do all we can to preserve our lives.

REASONS FOR SAFETY

In the previous section we examined ideas pertaining to suffering and death which attempt to soften the "sting of death." Several reasons for avoiding accidents which produce injury and death are:

1 To avoid pain.
2 To avoid inconvenience.
3 To avoid material loss.
4 To maintain a good record.
5 To protect life.
6 To preserve talent (see Table 4–1).
7 To avoid other social and economic consequences (see Table 3–4).

The period of greatest achievement for artists, authors, scientists, and scholars averages just under 50 years of age, reports Robert Thorndike. Sorenson supports Thorndike's "masterpiece age" by reporting that most scholars and scientists do their best work at about 50 years of age with a variance within ten-year periods before and after 50.[1]

SUMMARY OF BASIC "CORE" BELIEFS

Today most safety educators and specialists are in agreement with the following basic statements:

1 Safety is not an end in itself; it is just a means to a more productive life. "Safety First" is a poor slogan.
2 Safety involves more than just avoiding accidents.
3 Safety is a relative thing and is extremely difficult to define. It varies from day to day, which implies that a person is at different levels of safety every day of his life.

4   Safety is a many-sided subject which draws upon interdisciplinary fields for its approach and content.

5   Accidents are caused and thus are preventable.

6   There are no such things as chance and luck. Luck and chance are names for unrecognized causes.

7   Human life has value and should be preserved.

8   Life at its best is taking risks for things "worthwhile."

9   Safety education reduces the risks in living.

table 4–1   *Missing Contributions*

What does society lose by the premature impairment or death of genius? Can society ever measure that intangible potential that was never realized? What might the world have gained by improving the vitality and length of life of persons with great abilities?

name	partial contributions or identification	age at death	approximate number of years lost
Louis Braille	Devised braille system of reading for the blind	43	27
John M. Burnham	Designer of the submarines Nautilus, Seawolf, and Skate	40	30
Edwin J. Cohn	Medical research authority (gamma globulin, etc.)	59	11
Stephen Crane	Journalist, novelist, poet	29	41
Guy de Maupassant	Writer of almost 300 short stories and novels	43	27
Enrico Fermi	Nuclear physicist	53	17
Eugene Gardner	Atomic physicist	37	33
John C. Glover	A.A.U. 100-yard swimming champion, 1955	22	48
Joseph G. Hamilton	Pioneer in atomic medicine	49	21
Thomas J. "Stonewall" Jackson	Military leader	39	31
John Keats	Poet	26	44
Joseph W. Kennedy	Discoverer of plutonium	40	30
Edward Arthur Milne	One of the world's great mathematicians	54	16
Wolfgang Amadeus Mozart	One of the world's renowned composers	35	35
Takashi Nagai	Medical and radiation scientist	43	27
Edgar Allen Poe	Author and poet	39	31
Raphael	Painter	37	33
Edward R. Stettinius	Diplomat and Secretary of State	49	21
Robert Louis Stevenson	Novelist	44	26
Johann Strauss (the elder)	Composer of more than 150 of the world's most beautiful waltzes	45	25
Henry David Thoreau	Author and naturalist	45	25

lost in this group alone: 599 years of genius in given fields.

source: Data courtesy of O.E. Byrd, Stanford University; Dick Hayden, from an unpublished manuscript.

RISK

Risk is a natural occurrence in life. From an optimistic point of view, life is an adventure and man is continually pushing into new endeavors which are frequently dangerous (see Figure 4–2). For example, exhilarating leisure-time activities such as mountain climbing, motorcycling, parachuting, scuba diving, and snowmobiling are probably adventuresome enough to attract thousands of participants annually. Yet, in the opinion of other thousands of nonparticipants, the sports enthusiasts of these activities are labeled daredevils or even "crazy."

Throughout history men and women have had to take risks, starting in early childhood when competent parents teach us what objects and actions are unsafe and how to avoid being hurt by them. Later we travel safely to school because of parental teaching and discipline and school patrols. Laws and regulatory devices enforce our protection more and more as we become older. But the most constant discipline becomes that which we impose on ourselves.

We learn good or bad risk taking, or perhaps overcautious or foolhardy risk taking. If you cross a downtown main street and observe traffic regulations and stay alert, you are taking a necessary risk, with

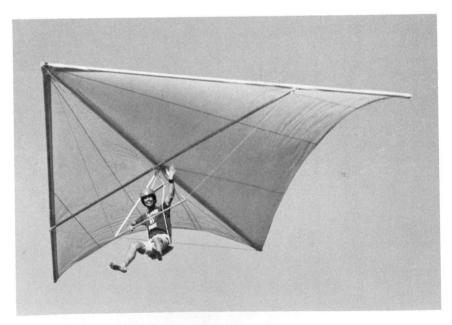

figure 4–2 What may be risky for some may not be for others. Reproduced courtesy of Dan Poynter.

proper safety precautions. If you crowd the change in traffic lights and ignore both pedestrian and vehicular traffic, you have engaged in bad risk taking. If you timidly refuse to cross at all, you won't accomplish much during the day. If you ignore the traffic signals, rush out into a stream of traffic, and with the imagined skill of a toreador, defy all oncoming cars and cleverly evade one after another until you reach the opposite curb, you are guilty of foolhardy risk taking. Good risk taking may be the most important individual, personal precaution against accidents.

In the stories we read about great men, safety is seldom mentioned except as a timid virtue almost akin to cowardice. So the impression is that the great men of history—the leaders, heroes, adventurers—plunged into danger with a reckless disregard for personal safety. If a deeper look is taken into history, a less distorted portrait of the hero would be found. Each hero had three things in common:

Each had a burning desire to reach a goal.

Each accepted risk only for a good reason.

Each planned carefully to avoid the accidents that would mean failure.

The folklore that glorifies the boldness of a hero often hides the fact that he succeeded only because he stayed alive, and he stayed alive only because he was skillful, trained, and prudent.

Hundreds of men tried to reach the North Pole and failed. Accidents—unforeseen events—denied them success, so their names are covered with dust in the pages of history. But Robert Peary succeeded, and his name became a household word. He reached his goal because he knew that only preventive planning for every foreseeable emergency could make a reality of his dream.

Thus, safety becomes a positive force, not a negative one. The early slogan "Safety First" made safety sound unattractive because it seemed to put safety ahead of every other consideration in human affairs. Safety asks for a worthwhile goal that gives purpose to risk. Safety is a means to an end.

Risk taking is influenced by an evaluation of the odds—is there enough potential gain to assume the hazard? Among the "rewards" for successful risk taking are saving time, gaining status, experiencing a thrill, satisfying our egos, eliminating a hazard, meeting a challenge, gaining a skill, receiving a cash reward, meeting a dare, and performing necessary functions.

The degree of risk may vary with time and situation; some are personal, some involve other people.

Risk is a relative thing. What may be risky to one person may be an everyday event to another. The margin of safety varies from person to person and even changes for the same person at different times and in different locations. In some risk-taking activities the margin of safety is the same for all. For example, in sky diving or mountain climbing, risk is obviously relative to the skill and experience of the participant—less skill increases the hazard. However, in Russian roulette with a six-chamber revolver and only one bullet, the margin of safety is the same for all participants—there are no experts.

Most societies have their risk takers. Whether they be Vikings or astronauts, they have received a hero's reward in victory. Sports such as bullfighting, boxing, sports car and motorcycle racing, ice hockey, football, surfing, mountain climbing, sky diving, scuba diving, and snow skiing all involve risk. Contemporary "heroes" are among the participants in these sport activities but have spent many hours learning ways to minimize the hazards. The idea of risk can be illustrated by judging the degree of risk involved in specific types of activities (see Table 4–2) and then comparing your evaluations with those of a friend.

Thus, risk is an expression of possible loss and is in the area of probability of which the next section treats.

PROBABILITY

"It is probable that . . . "; "The chances are . . . "; "It's likely . . . ." These three expressions are very common in everyday conversation. We use them whenever we talk about something that we are not certain will happen. Yet, all of us must make decisions about the probable outcome of future events before they occur. Every day we make decisions based to some extent on guesswork. Should I buy gasoline now, or do I have enough in the tank to get me home? Considering the traffic at this hour, which street will be quicker, University or Center? Am I likely to be home by 6:00? What are the chances that dinner will be ready? Decisions in such instances are based largely on guesswork.

What guesswork means is that life is in reality a risky business. Risk is the essence of living. Everything and everybody in the world is exposed to the daily risk of loss from injury, damage, or destruction.

It would be wonderful if we could measure the certainty or uncertainty of future events. Then we could reduce the risk involved in making decisions. On the question "Considering the traffic at this hour, which street will be quicker, University or Center?"—if you've driven on University and Center streets before, and did this under varying traffic conditions, then your guess will be better than mine for I've never driven there. Or consider this verse: Red sky at night, sailor's

table 4–2   *Risk-Taking Questionnaire*

part I: individual risk

Below are behaviors which involve some degree of risk for any individual who engages in them. Mark in the left-hand column the average degree of risk you believe an individual runs when he engages in each behavior.

degree of risk: 0 = no risk   1 = low risk   2 = average risk
                      3 = moderate risk   4 = high risk

_____ 1	driving a car	_____
_____ 2	drag racing	_____
_____ 3	driving a motorcycle	_____
_____ 4	playing football	_____
_____ 5	swimming alone	_____
_____ 6	sky diving	_____
_____ 7	scuba diving	_____
_____ 8	surfing	_____
_____ 9	snowmobiling	_____
_____ 10	mountain climbing	_____
_____ 11	snow skiing	_____
_____ 12	bullfighting	_____
_____ 13	flying in a plane	_____
_____ 14	deer hunting	_____
_____ 15	trampolining without spotters	_____
_____ 16	taking another person's prescription drug	_____
_____ 17	climbing a ladder	_____
_____ 18	lighting fireworks	_____
_____ 19	swallowing large slices of meat	_____
_____ 20	not using safety belts	_____
_____ 21	drinking alcohol and driving	_____
_____ 22	living on a fault where previous earthquakes have happened	_____
_____ 23	living in the "tornado belt"	_____
_____ 24	working in an underground coal mine	_____
_____ 25	riding a bicycle on a street	_____

Place an A for the most risky behavior on the above list; a B for the second most risky behavior; and a C for the third most risky behavior.

part II: social risk

The same behaviors are to be used again. For each, estimate the degree of risk that society encounters on the average when individuals engage in such behaviors (above and beyond the direct risk to the individual). Use the same scale. Place responses in the right-hand column.

delight; red sky in the morning, sailors take warning. Suppose you and I observe a red sky in the evening. If I know this verse and you don't, I am more likely to predict good weather tomorrow than you are.

Another example: You remember reading somewhere that traffic fatalities over the four-day Christmas holiday in a recent year amounted to 700 deaths, compared with 700 deaths the year before and 650 deaths two years before. Your guess as to this year's figure will be closer to what actually occurs than will the guess of someone who does not know these figures.

In other words, a knowledge of past events will improve our chances of guessing the outcome of future events with success. Sometimes we feel so sure of our correctness in guessing the outcome of future events that we assign numbers to our "guesstimates": the likelihood is nine out of ten she'll be late. Chances are 50–50 that the school will win the basketball game. There's a 25 percent chance of getting my lost wallet back. These are all examples of assigning numbers to chance or probability.

Mathematicians have a way of assigning numbers to events that involve a degree of chance or risk. This branch of mathematics is called probability.

A knowledge of probability theory has tremendous use in everyday life. For example, have you ever: Seen a building on fire? Seen an automobile accident? Seen results of a tornado or hurricane? Been injured? If you are average, you probably answered yes to two or three.

Thus, the term *risk* is an expression of possible loss. When a person takes a risk, he has entered a dangerous (hazardous) situation.

Risk has been calculated for several activities. Refer to Figure 3–1 to see the riskiness of drinking alcohol and driving.

Risk determination and prediction have been used by insurance companies for hundreds of years.

A variation of "Murphy's Law" comes into play regarding the assessment of a hazard: No matter how difficult it is to have an injury, a way will be found.

TYPES OF RISK TAKERS

The concept of risk taking has been little examined in the safety literature. The following risk takers can be identified.

Risk takers include those who know about the danger but may not be aware of its presence. These people take an attitude of accepting the consequences of their risk taking but believe that there is little chance for injury.

Another group includes those who could recognize a hazard but are not thinking about it. These people may be required to make quick decisions under stress. Decisions made in such circumstances have the problem of emotionally based errors.

Probably the most well known type of risk taker is the one who deliberately enters a dangerous situation after appraising the hazard and deciding that the odds on not being injured favor him.

Another class consists of those who are ignorant of risks involved in a hazard and enter a hazardous situation and may or may not escape injury.

Then there are those who know about the dangers in a hazard but believe they are personally invulnerable to danger.

Sometimes risks must be taken to avoid a hazard. "Act or be acted upon," Brigham Young exhorted the Mormons who were headed west to begin a new life in what is now Utah. It is a choice that all of us face every day of our lives. To act, to really live, is to take risks. To be acted upon is to relinquish not only responsibility but also control. Intelligent risk assessment involves, first, defining goals — is attaining it of value? or worth the danger? Then, estimate the odds against achieving it. Get all the facts.

David Klein believes that there are three separate groups involved in risk taking:

The first group consists of people who work or live with a primitive, unsophisticated, or unautomated technology. Construction workers, miners, and lumbermen are examples in the industrial sector; the poor, who live with space heaters, lead paint, high traffic density, and other hazards, are examples in the domestic sector. . . . Today, as both the work and the home environment become technologically more sophisticated, this group is smaller and its fatality rate is lower.

The second group consists of workers whose jobs have been so routinized that they are forced to seek autonomy and high personal achievement by taking recreational risks. The size of this group is growing as our society becomes increasingly bureaucratized and our technology increasingly complex — and this is reflected in the rising rate for recreational fatalities.

There is a third group, not heretofore mentioned, that is probably far more conspicuous than its actual size would justify. It consists of individuals who have been socialized to so high a need for achievement and control over the environment that they are chronically dissatisfied with their current achievements, no matter how noteworthy, and are constantly seeking new challenges, both in occupation and in recreation. We are all familiar with this type — with the successful scientist who enters politics, who flies his own aircraft, who competes in sports-car races, and so forth.[2]

ISSUES IN SAFETY

There are differing points of view with regard to specific topics and concerns in safety. These issues should be studied because they:

1   Need resolving or answering.
2   Are seldom found in textbooks because they are recent.
3   Can and do affect people.
4   Are interesting and provocative.

Listed below are some controversial issues related to safety:

1   The school safety patrol.
2   Driver and traffic safety education — is it effective in reducing accidents?
3   Firearm and ammunition registration.
4   Small vs. large cars — which are safer?
5   Football, boxing, and javelin throwing in the high schools.
6   Required safety equipment in automobiles (e.g., safety belts).
7   Required motorcycle helmet laws.
8   Alcohol tests and implied consent laws.
9   The use of snowmobiles.
10   Synthetic football-playing surfaces.
11   High-rise or standard style bicycles.

Certainly this textbook will not attempt to resolve the above issues or any others. However, the reader will recall from chapter 1 the difference between knowledge judgments and value judgments which will aid him in answering questions with regard to the problem of accidents and safety.

A high regard for safety competes occasionally with time, status and group pressures, personality shortcomings, courage, adventure, and other factors. A concern for safety enables us to choose between experiences that are unproductive, absurd, and even stupid, and those that enrich our lives, making them interesting and worthwhile. Our aim should be safety *for* rather than safety *from* — safety *for* an effective and productive life. Safety *from* has its place for the young child who does not know what is safe or unsafe and needs an adult or another responsible person to guide and direct his actions.

NOTES

[1]HAROLD S. DIEHL AND WILLARD DALRYMPLE, *Healthful Living* (New York: McGraw-Hill Book Company, 1973), pp. 4–5.

[2]DAVID KLEIN, "Some Social Characteristics of Accident Victims," *Traffic Safety*, April 1974, p. 35.

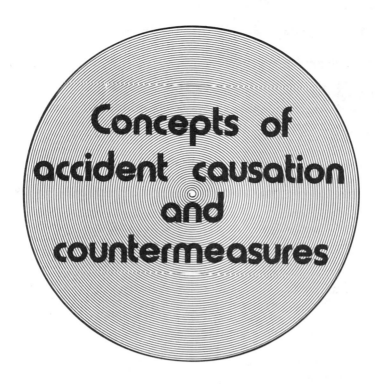

Concepts of accident causation and countermeasures

MULTIPLE CAUSE CONCEPT

5   Accidents generally result from a combination of closely interwoven factors. Let us consider these factors in detail.

Each of the factors which contributes to an accident is *a* cause, whereas *the* cause is the combination of these factors, each of which is necessary but none of which is sufficient by itself. A *factor* is any condition or action accompanying an accident whether it contributes to the accident or not. A contributing *cause* is a factor without which the accident would not have happened. Therefore, a cause is always a factor, but a factor is not always a cause.[1] Each cause, if it truly contributes to an accident, is an equally important factor in that accident, but could be identified as being distant, intermediate, or immediate in its relation to the accident.

The accident victim may "get away with" violations for years because all the other essential ingredients for an accident were not present. However, this does not guarantee that an accident would not occur the first time a violation is committed.

Too often the event directly preceding an accident is labeled the cause. The multiple cause concept refutes this.

There is the need to view accidents as a gradually developing sequence of multiple events, rather than solely in terms of the immediate, last factor, emergency situation.

Heinrich Domino Theory

The sequence of events or factors that contribute to an accident has been described in a number of ways. Heinrich said that people, not things, cause accidents:

The occurrence of an injury invariably results from a completed sequence of factors, the last one of these being the injury itself. The accident which caused the injury is in turn invariably caused or permitted directly by the unsafe act of a person and/or mechanical or physical hazard.[2]

Heinrich described the sequence as a series of events that

. . . occur in a fixed and logical order. One is dependent on another, thus constituting a chain that may be compared with a row of dominoes placed on end and in such alignment in relation to one another that the fall of the first domino precipitates the fall of the entire row. An accident is merely one link in the chain.

If this series is interrupted by the elimination of even one of the several factors that comprise it, the injury cannot possibly occur.[3]

The steps or the dominoes are: (1) ancestry or social environment, (2) fault of a person, (3) unsafe act or condition, (4) accident, and (5) injury. Petersen raises the question, when an act and/or a condition that "caused" the accident is identified, how many other causes are not mentioned? All realize that there are many factors or causes of an accident. The idea of multiple causation is that these factors come together to cause an accident. Thus, an investigation of an accident should identify as many as possible of the causes rather than one act and/or one condition.

Petersen contrasts the domino theory with the multiple causation theory:

We shall look at a common accident: a man falls off a stepladder. If we investigate this accident under our present investigation forms we are asked to identify one act and/or one condition:

The unsafe act: Climbing a defective ladder

The unsafe condition: A defective ladder

The correction: Getting rid of the defective ladder

This would be typical of a supervisor's investigation of this accident under the domino theory.

Let us look at the same accident in terms of multiple causation. Multiple causation asks what are some of the contributing factors surrounding this incident? We might ask:

1   Why was the defective ladder not found in normal inspection?
2   Why did the supervisor allow its use?
3   Didn't the injured employee know he shouldn't use it?
4   Was he properly trained?
5   Was he reminded?
6   Did supervision examine the job first?

The answers to these and other questions would lead to these kinds of corrections:

1   An improved inspection procedure
2   Improved training
3   A better definition of responsibilities
4   Pre-job planning by supervisors

Our narrow interpretation of the domino theory has put blinders on us and has severely limited us in finding and dealing with root causes in accidents.[4]

One example of an attempt to show the multifactorial background of an accident is the "Dynamics of Home Accidents" developed by the National Safety Council's Home Safety Conference (see Figure 5–1).

EPIDEMIOLOGY OF ACCIDENTS

"Epidemic" literally means "in or among people" and thus "common to, or affecting at the same time, many in a community." Formerly, epidemiology was defined as the medical science dealing with epidemics. It was most often found in public health programs that dealt with infectious and communicable diseases. However, heart disease, cancer, and accidents have also been studied by the epidemiologist. The epidemiological approach to accident prevention has received much attention in recent literature. John Gordon (probably the first to use the epidemiological approach to the accident problem) and others emphasize the importance of viewing accidents as a public health problem because they play an increasingly significant role as a cause of death.[5] They also stress the fact that this problem should be treated in the same way, with the same methods used in the epidemiological approach to other public health problems.

Some examples of questions that require epidemiologic study of human populations are:

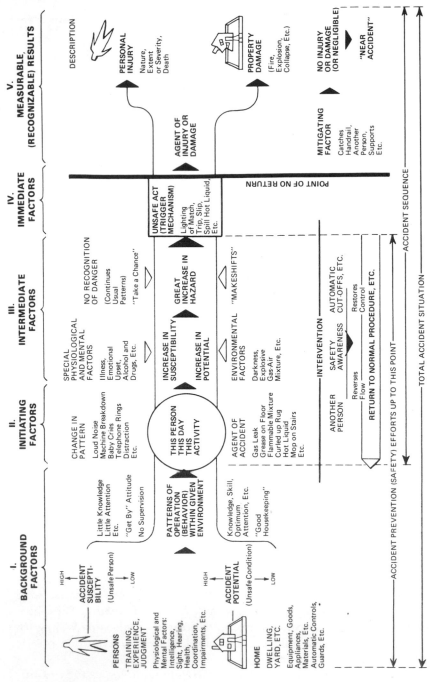

figure 5-1 The dynamics of home accidents. Source: National Safety Council, *Journal of Safety Research*, June 1973.

Why are we seeing an increase in public accidents these days?

How can the drinking driver accident problem best be prevented?

When can we expect the next increase in traffic accidents?

Why are bicycles causing such an injury problem?

Are countermeasures against accidents working?

Already discussed is the concept that more than one factor contributes to an accident's occurrence. For example, a traffic accident fatality is not caused merely by speeding or drinking alcohol. Not everyone driving too fast for conditions or exceeding the speed limit or drinking alcohol becomes an accident victim. Other factors can usually be identified which clearly contribute to the accident. These factors include being late to an appointment, a fight with one's spouse, and a host of other factors.

Epidemiologists have organized in various ways the complex multifactorial process leading to accidents and sometimes resulting in undesirable effects. (See chapter 1 for an elaboration on what an accident is.) One useful way to view the causation of some accidents is in terms of the agent, the environment, and the host (human).

Agent factors are not always obvious. Work by Haddon has led to an understanding that the agent in injury events is physical energy in its various forms (mechanical, chemical, thermal, radiation, electrical), and that most of the previously identified agents were simply carriers of the energy. It is important to distinguish between the actual injury-producing agents (e.g., mechanical and thermal energy) and their carriers (e.g., bullet, boiling water, dogs, and knives). Refer to Tables 5–1 and 5–2 for the types of energy involved and typical resultant injuries.

Haddon elaborates on the carriers of energy:

Energy that may reach the body, and the substances which may interfere with its normal function, are usually carried by inanimate objects or living organisms. These correspond to the "vehicles" and "vectors" of infectious diseases. Thus, electric lines are vehicles of electricity, hot rivets are vehicles of thermal energy, poison containers are vehicles of their contents, and moving objects are vehicles of mechanical energy. Similarly, poisonous plants and animals are vectors of their toxins, and animals which injure by tearing and crushing are vectors of mechanical energy. This concept is a useful one, since many preventive measures must be directed against the vehicles and vectors rather than against the physical and chemical agents that they transmit.[6]

Thus, vectors are "animate or living organisms," while vehicles are "inanimate or nonliving objects."

table 5–1 *Illustrations of Class I Injuries Caused by Delivery of Energy in Excess of Local or Whole-Body Injury Thresholds*

type of energy delivered	primary injury produced	examples and comments
Mechanical	Displacement, tearing, breaking, and crushing, predominantly at tissue and organ levels of body organization	Injuries resulting from the impact of moving objects such as bullets, hypodermic needles, knives, and falling objects; and from the impact of the moving body with relatively stationary structures, as in falls and plane and auto crashes. The specific result depends on the location and manner in which the resultant forces are exerted. The majority of injuries are in this group.
Thermal	Inflammation, coagulation, charring, and incineration at all levels of body organization	First-, second-, and third-degree burns. The specific result depends on the location and manner in which the energy is dissipated.
Electrical	Interference with neuromuscular function and coagulation, charring, and incineration at all levels of body organization	Electrocution, burns. Interference with neural function as in electroshock therapy. The specific result depends on the location and manner in which the energy is dissipated.
Ionizing radiation	Disruption of cellular and subcellular components and function	Reactor accidents, therapeutic and diagnostic irradiation, misuse of isotopes, effects of fallout. The specific result depends on the location and manner in which the energy is dissipated.
Chemical	Generally specific for each substance or group	Includes injuries due to animal and plant toxins, chemical burns, as from KOH, Br_2, F_2, and H_2SO_4, and the less gross and highly varied injuries produced by most elements and compounds when given in sufficient doses.

source: William Haddon, Jr., "The Prevention of Accidents," in *Preventive Medicine*, ed. Duncan W. Clark and Brian MacMahon (Boston: Little, Brown and Company, 1967), p. 593.

table 5–2   *Illustrations of Class II Injuries Caused by Interference with Normal Local or Whole-Body Energy Exchange*

type of energy exchange interfered with	types of injury or derangement produced	examples and comments
Oxygen utilization	Physiological impairment, tissue or whole-body death	Whole-body: suffocation by mechanical means. For example, by drowning, strangulation, and CO and HCN poisoning. Local: "vascular accidents." These also involve more than mere O_2 deprivation, since waste and nutrient exchange are also blocked.
Thermal	Physiological impairment, tissue or whole-body death	Injuries resulting from failure of body thermoregulation; frostbite; and death by freezing.

source: William Haddon, Jr., "The Prevention of Accidents," in *Preventive Medicine*, ed. Duncan W. Clark and Brian MacMahon (Boston: Little, Brown and Company, 1967), p. 594.

Changing the carrier is a good countermeasure. For example, if you have a biting dog, the dog bite results from excessive mechanical energy (the agent), but the easiest countermeasure may be simply to chain the dog (the vector or carrier).

DESCRIPTIVE EPIDEMIOLOGY

Descriptive studies usually involve the determination of the incidence, prevalence, and mortality rates for accidents in large population groups, according to basic group characteristics such as age, sex, and geographic area. In this way the general distribution of injuries in the population is described.

The major characteristics of interest in descriptive epidemiology may be the categories of person (host), place (environment), and time (environment).

At first glance the goal of describing injury occurrence in this way may seem trivial and not worthy of the efforts of scientists. However, such studies are of importance and can serve the following purposes:

1   To focus national attention on an accidental injury problem.

2   To identify what types of persons (e.g., young or old, male or female) are most likely to be affected by a certain type of injury, to determine where and when the injuries will occur, and to measure long-range trends.

3   To aid in the planning of injury care facilities and priorities for countermeasures (e.g., number of ambulances needed for traffic injuries, placement of poison control centers and burn centers).

4   To identify clues to accident etiology and serve as a basis for further studies needed.

Person

Human factors constitute a great concern. Characteristics studied include age, sex, marital status, socioeconomic status, and physical condition.

Age.   Age is one of the most important factors in accident occurrence. Some accidents occur almost exclusively in one particular age group, such as home fall fatalities. Other accidents occur over a much wider age span but tend to be more prevalent at certain ages than others.

The time of life at which an accident predominates is influenced by such factors as the degree of exposure to the agent at various ages and variations in susceptibility with age. The influence of age-related exposure is illustrated by lead poisoning, which is most prevalent in children.

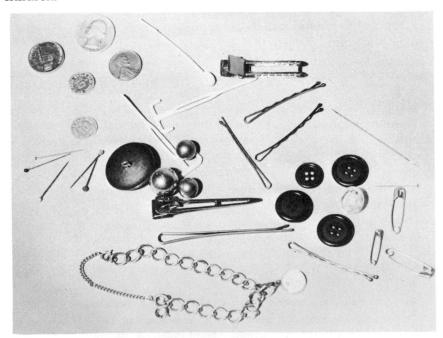

figure 5–2   Things children swallow. These are "agents of injury." Reproduced courtesy of New York State *Health News,* a monthly publication of the New York State Department of Health; photo by M. Dixson.

Many injuries, such as in fatally injured adult pedestrians, show a progressive increase in prevalence with increasing age. It is tempting to regard an accident with this age pattern as being due merely to aging itself. It should be remembered, however, that increasing age also marks the passage of time, during which the body is exposed to the effects of environmental influences.

Current Age Tabulations. The tabulation of death rates in relation to age at one particular time, as in Table 5–3, is known as a current, or cross-sectional, presentation. This shows death rates as they are occurring simultaneously in different age groups; thus, different people are involved in each age group.

Sex.   Some injuries occur more frequently in males, others more frequently in females. If sex-linked inheritance can be excluded, a sex difference in injury incidence initially brings to mind the possibility of hormonal or reproductive factors that either predispose or protect. For example, menstruation is a significant factor affecting women's susceptibility to accidents.

But men and women differ in many other ways, including habits, social relationships, environmental exposures, and other aspects of day-to-day living. The higher male prevalence of traffic fatalities is at least partly related to the fact that, on the average, men drive automobiles more than women.

Sex differences in injury occurrence are important descriptive findings and often suggest avenues for further research. Such differences need explaining.

Marital status is another important descriptive variable. Married persons have lower mortality rates than single persons. The unmarried have been shown to be more often involved in fatal traffic accidents than the married, and ski injuries are overwhelmingly found among the unmarried.

Socioeconomic Status.   Some epidemiologists categorize socioeconomic status as an environmental factor. This factor can be and usually is measured by the occupation or income of the family head, by his or her educational level, or by residence, in terms of the value of the home or dwelling unit.

Low socioeconomic status appears to be related to lead poisoning, snowmobile injuries, and adult pedestrian deaths. On the other hand, drownings involving power boats and yachts, injuries or deaths related

table 5–3   *Leading Causes of All Deaths by Age*

	death rate*		death rate*
all ages	943	**25 to 44 years**	232
Heart disease	361	**Accidents**	**50**
Cancer	162	Motor-vehicle	28
Stroke**	102	Drowning	3
Accidents	**56**	Falls	2
Motor-vehicle	27	Fires, burns	2
Falls	8	Other	15
Drowning	4	Heart disease	38
Fires, burns	3	Cancer	37
Other	14	**45 to 64 years**	1,139
under 1 year	2,127	Heart disease	421
Anoxia	569	Cancer	288
Congenital anomalies	321	Stroke**	74
Complications of preg-		**Accidents**	**58**
nancy and childbirth	298	Motor-vehicle	26
Immaturity	249	Falls	7
Pneumonia	177	Fires, burns	4
Accidents	**65**	Drowning	3
Ingestion of food, object	20	Other	18
Mech. suffocation	16	Cirrhosis of liver	43
Motor-vehicle	10	Pneumonia	24
Fires, burns	4	**65 to 74 years**	3,568
Falls	4	Heart disease	1,552
Other	11	Cancer	751
1 to 4 years	85	Stroke**	383
Accidents	**32**	Diabetes mellitus	92
Motor-vehicle	12	**Accidents**	**85**
Drowning	6	Motor-vehicle	33
Fires, burns	5	Falls	20
Falls	2	Fires, burns	8
Ingestion of food, object	1	Surg. complications	7
Other	6	Other	17
Congenital anomalies	10	Pneumonia	83
Cancer	8	Emphysema	68
5 to 14 years	41	**75 years and over**	9,706
Accidents	**20**	Heart disease	4,538
Motor-vehicle	10	Stroke**	1,610
Drowning	4	Cancer	1,205
Fires,burns	1	Pneumonia	360
Other	5	Arteriosclerosis	334
Cancer	6	**Accidents**	**220**
Congenital anomalies	2	Falls	124
15 to 24 years	127	Motor-vehicle	42
Accidents	**68**	Fires, burns	14
Motor-vehicle	47	Surg. complications	13
Drowning	7	Ingestion of food, object	4
Poison (solid, liquid)	3	Other	23
Firearms	2	Diabetes mellitus	196
Other	9	Emphysema	96
Homicide	12		
Suicide	9		

source: Deaths are for 1970, latest official figures from National Center for Health Statistics, Health Services and Mental Health Administration, U.S. Department of Health, Education and Welfare. From National Safety Council, *Accident Facts*, 1974, p. 8.

*Deaths per 100,000 population in each age group. Rates are averages for age groups, not individual ages.

**Cerebrovascular disease.

to private airplane crashes, and ski injuries are most often found among the high socioeconomic status groups.

Physical Condition.   Although alcohol is among the most important human factors known to be related to severe injury and death, other drugs are becoming more frequently involved. The intoxicated have difficulty in escaping from a hazard (fire or submerged automobile) or an obstruction that impedes those giving medical attention and treatment. Chronic health problems such as diabetes, epilepsy, and heart disease may also induce an accident. Over-exertion and fatigue reduce the attention, sensory acuity, and reaction time of any individual.

Place

Where accidents and injuries occur is a matter of great importance. Comparison of injury and death rates in different places may provide obvious clues to causation or serve as a stimulus to further fruitful investigation. The places of concern may be as large as a continent or as small as a room in a home. Examples of descriptive findings presented are international comparisons and comparisons of regions within the United States.

International Comparisons.   Because of the problems regarding the validity of mortality statistics (attributable to definition problems), it is difficult to take seriously small differences among nations in accident mortality rates (see Table 5–4). However, it is also difficult to explain away very large differences (e.g., where the death rate is in one country two or three times as large as the death rate in another). Large differences are impressive when both countries are known to have reasonably good vital statistics systems.

Comparisons of Regions Within Countries.   The availability of mortality statistics for states in the United States has permitted the discovery of interesting place-to-place variations in accidental death occurrence. Differences in mortality rates between urban and rural areas are a common finding. The higher mortality from traffic accidents in rural than in urban areas is consistent with the fact that faster driving occurs in rural areas, and it is the speed of the vehicle which is a major factor in death causation.

Geographic variation within the United States is quite distinctive, which suggests that climate or other factors may be involved (see Figure 5–3). For example, there is the finding in the United States of generally higher mortality rates for accidents in the mountain regions. While hypotheses abound, to date no one has convincingly explained this geographic distribution of fatal accidents.

table 5–4   *Accidental Death Rates by Nation*

nation	rate*	nation	rate*
Paraguay	18.2	Venezuela	46.3
Dominican Republic	18.3	Denmark	47.0
Philippines	25.0	Italy	47.3
Thailand	27.3	Poland	48.0
Cuba	32.0	Ecuador	50.2
England, Wales	33.5	Norway	51.6
Salvador	34.6	Australia	53.3
Spain	36.1	Portugal	54.3
Yugoslavia	37.3	New Zealand	54.8
Puerto Rico	37.4	Hungary	55.3
Costa Rica	38.5	East Germany	55.9
Greece	38.9	**United States**	**56.2**
Panama	38.9	Czechoslovakia	58.6
Japan	39.7	Canada	58.7
Sweden	42.4	West Germany	62.7
Ireland	42.5	Switzerland	63.0
Peru	42.9	Finland	64.8
Netherlands	43.2	Belgium	66.1
Bulgaria	43.6	Iceland	67.4
Scotland	44.5	Luxemburg	67.7
N. Ireland	44.9	Honduras	69.7
Taiwan	45.1	France	77.2
Uruguay	45.1	Austria	81.9
Israel	46.1		

source: World Health Organization, United Nations. Based on official reports of the nations.

*Per 100,000 population.

Areas Within a City.   When studying accidental injuries within a city, it is often desirable to plot the occurrence of such injuries in each census tract, since information about other characteristics of persons in each tract is available.

Lead poisoning and traffic accidents in cities have been mapped according to location and with results showing definite geographic distribution.

Time

The pattern of injury occurrence in time is often an extremely informative descriptive characteristic. A great variety of time trends may be found in the literature; these involve simple increases or decreases of injury incidence, or more complex combinations of these changes in time.

Short-Term Increases and Decreases in Injury Incidence.   Short-term changes are those increases or decreases in injury incidence that

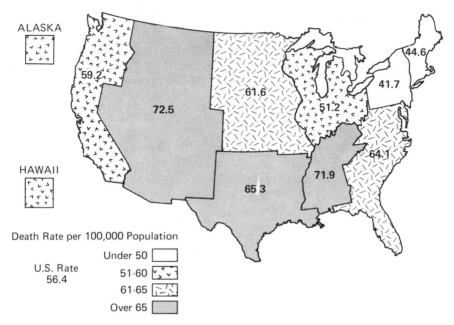

figure 5–3 Accident mortality by geographic division, United States, 1970.
Source: *Statistical Bulletin,* September 1974.

are measured in hours, days, weeks, or months. For example, two-thirds of all drownings occur in the afternoon or early evening, and about 40 percent occur on Saturdays and Sundays. July is the peak month, with more than half occurring in the summer months June through August.

Epidemics.   An epidemic, or outbreak, is the occurrence of an injury type in members of a defined population clearly in excess of the number of cases normally found in that population. Thus, the spectacular, short-term increases (some lasting several years) of injuries associated with backyard trampolines, go-carts, water skier's kites, abandoned refrigerators, and ultrathin plastic bags were suddenly major nationwide, accidental death problems.

Recurrent or Periodic Time Trends.   The incidence of certain accidental injuries shows regular recurring increases and decreases. This regular pattern exhibits cycles. Many cycles occur annually and represent variation in injury occurrence. Seasonal variation is a well-known characteristic for drownings, which occur mainly during the summer months, whereas carbon monoxide poisoning is most prevalent during the winter months while people are spending large amounts of time enclosed in automobiles and buildings.

Shorter-term periodic variations have also been observed. For example, death rates from automobile accidents show weekly cycles with the highest rates occurring on weekends, especially Saturdays. To date there are no available statistics on the number of passenger-miles driven on each day of the week. Thus it is not possible to state whether the weekend increase in deaths is due merely to an increased exposure of the population to the moving automobile or whether the risk of death per passenger-mile actually increases, possibly because of such factors as more reckless driving or more alcohol consumption on weekends.

Long-Term Trends. Some accidental deaths exhibit a progressive increase or decrease in occurrence that is manifested over years or decades.

Figure 5–4 shows the death rates of accidents from 1910 to 1973. A marked decrease in mortality from all accidents has occurred, representing about a 30 percent decrease. This decrease is believed to be due largely to a greater concern for safety. Rather than going back to 1910, it is suggested that only the past ten years should be considered. If this is the case, then a 3 percent increase has taken place in accidental death rates.

A marked long-term increase in public non-motor-vehicle accidents has occurred during the past decade. This increase is believed to be due to the availability of more leisure time and the invention of new recreational equipment (hang-gliders, motor boats, etc.), all of which leads to increased recreational activity.

INVESTIGATIVE EPIDEMIOLOGY

Investigative epidemiology is used to develop specific data related to the causes of the injury which would then point to feasible countermeasures. Whereas descriptive epidemiology identifies the accident

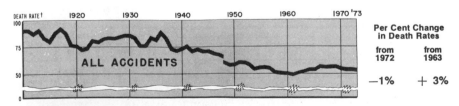

figure 5–4 Trends in accidental death rates. Source: National Safety Council, *Accident Facts,* 1974.

problem, investigative epidemiology gives the specifics on causation.

Investigative injury epidemiology was started in the U.S. Public Health Service during the 1960s. Complex interactions among the host, the environment, and the agent are disclosed. The investigations are conducted by a team of experts. These "multidisciplinary teams" involve a variety of professionals: medical/paramedical, social/behavioral, and physical/environmental personnel, engineers, statisticians, attorneys, and clerks. Nurses, pathologists, toxicologists, psychologists, sociologists, and physical therapists have provided the types of skills needed. The effort is a definite teamwork approach, which overcomes the failings of an individual specialist.

Investigations made include: (1) studies of a single type of injury where a small number of cases can provide clues, (2) identification of the specific environmental factors that may be hazards, (3) evaluation of the results of injury prevention programs, and (4) studies using experimental and control groups.

Marland of the U.S. Public Health Service says this about the value of investigative epidemiology:

The most important characteristic of investigative epidemiologic data is its specificity. When provided with the specific facts of injury-producing events, those persons responsible for injury control can develop an equally specific countermeasure. By the same token, those responsible for implementing the countermeasure are confident in their actions—be it redesign of a product, a local building code, a state law or an educational program. These programs became successful because their specificity is related to the injury just as surely as a cause and effect.[7]

Investigative Epidemiology Example.[8]   Here is the routine account one would have read of a crash that actually took place:

There was a 2-car crash last night on the Jones Expressway.

John X, driving a late model sedan, was speeding at 60 mph in the posted 40 mph zone when he hit William Z who was trying to turn left onto Beech Street. In the crash, which spun both cars some distance from the intersection, Mr. Z and his passenger, Marie W., were thrown from their car, and Mr. Z is in City Hospital in critical condition from stomach injuries.

Digging deeper into the account turns up quite a few different facts. The following is a summary of the findings by a multidisciplinary accident investigation team from the University of Miami. Sponsored by federal research funds, this team is typical of those being launched across the nation in a new in-depth approach to the real story behind crashes. The teams typically consist of engineers, physicians, psychiatrists, highway experts, and behavioral scientists.

John X was driving a "muscle car" (vehicle #1) which he had bought just two days before. A little less than a half mile from the accident scene, X, aged 21, stopped at a red light. Showing off the new car to his passenger, a buddy of the same age, X made a "drag start" coming out of the light. His wheels spun on pavement wet from rain which had fallen earlier. As he approached the intersection with Beech Street, he was traveling 60 mph in the posted 40 mph zone.

The second car, a luxury sedan, began to turn as it reached the intersection, into the path of the first car. At the time, X, driving in the right lane, froze when he became aware of the situation but he did apply the brakes. He went into a skid. Reacting to the skid sounds, Mr. Z, the driver of vehicle #2, attempted evasive action by turning farther to his left. (This point was borne out by initial damage contact as determined by the investigators.) John X could have taken evasive action by moving into the unoccupied parking lane to his right, but did not.

When the two vehicles crashed, car #1 had skidded 60 feet with one set of wheels, and 50 with the other, as indicated by the uneven lengths of skid marks on the pavement noticed by the investigators.

The forces of the impact produced violent counterclockwise rotation of car #2, and sideways linear motion of #1, resulting in a second impact contact by #2 with the left side of #1. At this point, the right front door of car #2 sprang open, and the occupants were ejected.

Car #2, without a driver, continued to spin while car #1 moved sideways for about 15 feet where it struck a sign that was at the edge of the road. The sign penetrated the vehicle roof and invaded the passenger compartment. However, car #1 continued to move and next struck a wooden power pole, also on the roadside. Meanwhile, the occupants of car #2, who had been ejected, bounced and rolled along the road, coming to rest alongside car #1.

In the final position, car #2 was about 95 feet from the initial crash point, and car #1 had traveled about 50 feet, yet all of this took no more than three seconds.

The driver of car #1, John X, had just had a fight with his wife. His physical condition before the crash was good. Injuries received: minor brain concussion, resulting in loss of consciousness for a short period of time; bruise over front of right arm; long, deep cut on back of his left elbow; and prolonged pain in left knee and shoulder. Although his car was equipped with lap belts and shoulder harnesses, as required by federal standards, John X and his passenger did not use them. Fortunately, the passenger braced himself prior to the impact and received only minor abrasions and leg pains.

The driver of car #2, William Z, a 54-year-old former bus and truck driver, had been visiting the home of Marie W, whom he had dated for nearly a year. After having two mixed drinks, the couple decided to go for a ride. According to the account Z gave the investigators during interviews, the mood in the car was calm and friendly. For some unspecified reason, Z decided to turn and proceeded slowly across the highway and into the path of X.

Neither Z nor his passenger was wearing the available lap belts, which would have prevented their ejection. While being ejected, Z sustained a laceration, bone deep and 10 centimeters in length, caused by the impact with the right roof rail. While sliding across the pavement, he sustained numerous abrasions about the head. He was taken, unconscious, to the local hospital. He regained consciousness the next morning, complaining of pain generally all over his body. On the third day, he was operated on for abdominal complaints, and a rupture of the duodenum was closed, but he did not improve, dying on the tenth day after the accident.

An autopsy was performed which revealed a .5 centimeter deep vital contusion on the right side of the brain. Although the immediate cause of death was peritonitis from the ulcerations of the stomach, this was directly related in turn to the brain damage. It is a well-known medical fact that people who suffer any head trauma may develop acute stress ulcers in the stomach which may perforate, as happened in this case.

Further digging by the investigators produced important facts about the two drivers' past records. John X, the driver of car #1, had been involved in a similar accident while in the military. At that time he had also frozen. His license had been revoked later for another offense. He characterized himself as a "defensive driver"—which in his code included slowing down or blocking anyone trying to pass or "tailgate" him.

As to the driver of car #2, William Z, his local traffic record included two previous violations for improper turning, both in the two years preceding the fatal crash. He also had been arrested for speeding on one occasion and for lane straddling on another.

The investigators concluded that 11 factors were instrumental in causing either the crash or the injuries:

1   Driver #1 was speeding.
2   Driver #2 failed to yield right of way and turned improperly.

3   Occupants chose not to wear safety belts, resulting in excessive injuries and death to William Z.

4   Right front door of car #2 sprang open on impact, allowing a path of ejection for occupants.

5   Lack of energy absorption in roof and presence of rail caused head injuries to occupants of car #2.

6   Damp pavement reduced coefficient of friction, allowing greater energy transferral between vehicles and objects.

7   Power pole and street sign were too near the road.

8   Driver education and reexamination after record of driving failures were lacking.

9   Braking pattern of two-day old car #1 was bad.

10   Speed and direction at impact exacerbated injury and damage levels.

11   Live power lines on road hampered assistance to injured.

The investigators ended their in-depth report with several recommendations for new legislation and regulation:

A. *Inspection.* The uneven braking pattern of car #1, delivered from the dealer only two days before the crash, raises the question of permitting ten days to elapse from delivery to state inspection. (There is also the possibility that the brakes contained a safety-related defect which should have been spotted and corrected.)

B. *Driver reexamination.* The previous record of John X, combined with the fact that he took no evasive action although other lanes were available to him, shows both a lack of proper driver training and reexamination.

C. *Accident reporting.* The report prepared by the authorities in this case was seriously inaccurate, both as to facts and conclusions. Increased training in new accident investigation and uniform reporting methods is needed.

D. *Safety belt legislation.* Proper use of available safety belts should be mandatory. At least, legislation should provide that failure to wear belts is contributory negligence in personal injury suits and that no damages or reduced damages can be recovered for personal injury by a party who fails to use belts.

The incomplete routine report which preceded the accident investigation just recounted is typical. The dilemma faced by highway safety leaders is the need for action in the face of a data base that is inadequate, inaccurate, and nonuniform. The development of effective safety measures for reducing the tragic crash losses sustained daily on our roads is vitally dependent upon complete data concerning the basic elements contributing to cause and effect of accidents.

A compelling need exists for the collection and analysis of data to measure accurately the exposure of drivers, vehicles, and environment across the entire highway traffic system. The data, beyond being accurate and sufficient in number, must be collected in a manner to identify statistically the major contributors to accident and injury severity and to isolate the changes needed in these elements.

The danger is that measures regarding both vehicle design and driver behavior will be espoused on the basis of myths or inaccurate accounts of crashes, such as the one first made of the accident described above. The sophisticated investigation recounted above demonstrates the vast number of complex factors behind crashes which have lain hidden for so many years.

Efforts, fortunately, are improving this situation. A new crash investigation system has been put in effect by the National Highway Traffic Safety Administration which is national in scope and which incorporates sophisticated techniques, procedures, and instrumentation. This new national system would have different layers, beginning at local communities with routine investigation by police and other authorities and culminating in the multidisciplinary team approach utilized by Miami University in the case which was cited above. The idea is for the mass of data to be collected in the routine investigation with a few selected accidents being given the in-depth treatment. In both cases, methods and procedures will reflect up-to-date methods and concepts. In particular, it must be stressed that all accident investigations should seek causes for the injuries as well as causes for the crash, looking into all phases of the crash—before, during, and after impact—and all aspects of the scene—vehicle, driver, and environment.

Accurate and in-depth accident investigation of the kind performed by multidisciplinary teams has another important objective besides pointing to new safety standards. Such work also can validate the efficacy of existing standards and regulations.

Obstacles to Acquiring Crash Data

The multidisciplinary accident investigation teams have been encountering serious problems in obtaining information from people in the crashes they investigate. Witnesses or parties to the accident are often reluctant to divulge information or to make vehicles available for detailed inspection. Despite the stated intention of the investigators to develop the data for research purposes only, parties confuse investigators with those seeking to bring legal actions against them or to involve them in such actions, both civil and criminal. As a result, people refuse access to information because they fear they will be harmed or embarrassed in some later legal action.

SYSTEMS SAFETY APPROACH

The engineering techniques of systems analysis have also been proposed for the solution of safety problems. In its emphasis on the interaction of man, machines, and environment, this approach is quite similar to the epidemiological one.

Too many well-written explanations of the systems safety approach have been published for this writer to elaborate further. Suffice it to define systems safety for the uninitiated with the hope that he or she will investigate further. Systems safety analysis is a logical, step-by-step method of examining situations with accident potential. It helps identify causes that could be overlooked if a less detailed method were used. Human, mechanical, and environmental factors are placed in an orderly, related schematic, inducing a logical thought process which leaves little to chance. It is a challenging and satisfying creative brainstorming approach.

While the systems safety approach has been highly successful in regard to the safe operations of some very complex systems, many problems yet remain in quantifying the influence of the human as an element in the system.

A system is an orderly arrangement of components which are interrelated and which act and interact to perform some task or function in a particular environment. The main points to keep in mind are that a system is defined in terms of a task or function, and that the components of a system are interrelated, that is, each part affects the others. Examples of systems are aircraft, production lines, and transportation.

No matter which method of analysis is used, it is important to have a model of the system. Most models take the form of a diagram showing all the components. This makes it easier to grasp the interrelationships and simplifies tracing the effects of malfunctions.

The systems approach to safety can help to change safety from an art to a science by classifying much of our knowledge. It can change the application of safety from piecemeal problem solving to a safety-designed operation. We can apply the question "What can happen if this component fails?" to the various elements of the systems and come up with adequate safety answers before the accident occurs, instead of after the damage has been done.

ETIOLOGY (CAUSES) AND COUNTERMEASURES

Dr. William Haddon, Jr., introduced a conceptual model for the U.S. Government's program to curtail traffic accident losses. The strategy or

concept which he has long propagated is to reduce losses due to inj
rather than merely to prevent injuries. Haddon states that even when an
accident cannot be prevented, there are many ways to prevent or reduce
the frequency and severity of injuries which result from an accident.

Haddon suggests approaching the problem of reducing injuries by
considering the three major phases that determine the final outcomes.
These three phases are shown in Table 5–5 with examples of countermeasures related to crashes, burns, electrocutions, poisonings, and
drownings.

The *first phase*, or pre-event phase, consists of many factors which
determine whether or not an accident will take place. Elements that
cause people and physical and/or chemical forces to move into undesirable interaction are included here. For example, probably the most important human factor in the pre-event phase is alcohol intoxication in
almost all accident types.

In the past, the emphasis in accident prevention has been on human
behavior and attempts to change it. Accidents are usually regarded as
someone's fault, rather than as a failure that could have been prevented
by some change in the system. For example, if a boy, while cutting the
grass with a power rotary lawn mower, ejects from the mower a stone
which cuts a bystander, the resulting injury (the cut from the stone) is
likely to be blamed on the boy operating the mower, rather than being
attributed to the fact that a rotary mower many times will have no protective device to avert the ejection of stones and debris. Such devices
are now required, but are often taken off.

Thus, the mower can contribute to the initiation of the accident, either by placing excessive demands or restrictions on the operator, or
through mechanical inadequacies or failure. For example, in automobile
crashes, steering, tire, and brake failures sometimes initiate crashes but
seldom are searched for after the crash.

Other pre-event countermeasures relate to the environment, and
there the principle of separation plays an important role. For example,
children can be separated from cleaning agents containing caustic ingredients through the use of child-resistant containers and by storing
containers in locked compartments out of reach of children.

The *second phase*, or event phase, begins when physical and/or chemical forces exert themselves unfavorably upon people and/or property.
Countermeasures preventing harmful effects even when excessive energy (mechanical, chemical, thermal, etc.) is contacted are part of this
second phase. Examples of event phase countermeasures for motor vehicle accidents include "packaging people" for crashes through the use
of safety belts, padded dashes, and collapsible steering wheel columns.

table 5–5 *Examples of Tactics for Reducing Injury Losses*

type of event	pre-event phase	event phase	post-event phase
impacts (e.g., from falls)	Alcoholism programs Handrails on stairs	Fire nets Padding on floors Football helmets	Trained ambulance crews Well-equipped ambulances Pneumatic splints
exposure to heat	Child-proof matches Eliminating floor heaters Venting explosive gases	Flame-retardant clothing Reducing surface temperature of heaters and stoves Sprinkler systems in buildings	Burn centers Skin grafting Rehabilitation
exposure to electricity	Covered electric outlets Insulation on electric handtools and wiring	Circuit breakers Fuses	Cardiopulmonary resuscitation Equipment and training
ingestion of poison	Child-proof medicine containers Separation of CO from passenger compartments of autos	Making cleaning agents inert or less caustic Packing poisons in small, nonlethal amounts	Poison information centers Detoxification centers
immersion in water	Fences around swimming pools Draining ponds	Life jackets Training to tread water or swim	Lifesaving training Teaching mouth-to-mouth resuscitation techniques to general population

source: Susan P. Baker and William Haddon, Jr., "Reducing Injuries and Their Results: The Scientific Approach," *The Milbank Memorial Fund Quarterly/Health and Society,* Fall 1974.

Non-traffic examples are boxing gloves, safety shoes, hard hats, helmets, lead x-ray shields, nets for acrobats, and gloves for laborers.

This second phase is to soften contact regardless of the cause. Stressing this phase follows the idea that because accidents will happen, let's protect humans and property the best we can. Tradition, on the other hand, has stressed the pre-event phase rather than the event phase.

The *third phase,* or post-event phase, involves salvaging people and/or property after contact with excessive energy (mechanical, chemical, thermal, etc.) has taken place. Early detection of aircraft crashes through transducers that start broadcasting a special signal at the time of a crash is an example of the third phase, as are fire detection systems (heat or smoke), SOS and MAYDAY signals, and the use of forest fire lookout towers.

In case of serious injury it is important to provide expert medical care as quickly as possible. Transportation for the injured, trained ambulance personnel, and emergency room staffs are appropriate countermeasures which are a part of this phase.

CHOOSING COUNTERMEASURES

Several considerations should be kept in mind when selecting countermeasures to reduce injuries. For example, economic considerations are important. The oft-heard statement that "it's worth it, if it saves just one life" is not true if, for the same amount of money or other resources, more than one life can be saved.

A television campaign in the United States that would have cost about seven million dollars if presented nationally was carefully evaluated in a community with dual television cables. Viewers on one cable saw a variety of high-quality, professionally prepared television messages designed to encourage people to wear safety belts. The evaluation revealed that the TV messages, although shown many times, did not increase safety belt usage.

Haddon considers that "passive" protection, whenever feasible, is preferable to "active" protection. "Passive" protection refers to measures that do not require individual cooperation in order to be effective. It should be noted that air bags (a passive restraint) still require safety belts (an active restraint).

Haddon further believes that countermeasures should not be determined by the relative importance of contributing factors. He states that priority should be given to measures that will be most effective in reducing injury losses.

Success requires a mixture of countermeasures from pre-event,

event, and post-event phases, with their choice and emphasis based on what each can do to reduce losses due to injuries. Some examples of this would be: using a net for an acrobat rather than urging him to "perform safely" and not to fall; placing thermal insulation on the handles of household pots, pans, and electric irons rather than telling users never to touch them with their bare hands; putting shoes on children rather than cautioning them not to stub their toes. These are illustrations of countermeasures being placed on a phase other than the pre-event phase.

The following poem shows the importance of stressing one phase over another in reducing injuries:

the parable of the dangerous cliff

> Twas a dangerous cliff, as they freely confessed,
>   Though to walk near its crest was so pleasant;
> But over its terrible edge there had slipped
>   A duke, and full many a peasant.
> The people said something would have to be done,
>   But their projects did not at all tally.
> Some said, "Put a fence 'round the edge of the cliff;"
>   Some, "An ambulance down in the valley."
>
> The lament of the crowd was profound and was loud,
>   As their hearts overflowed with their pity;
> But the cry for the ambulance carried the day
>   As it spread through the neighboring city.
> A collection was made, to accumulate aid,
>   And the dwellers in highway and alley
> Gave dollars or cents—not to furnish a fence—
>   But an ambulance down in the valley.
>
> "For the cliff is all right if you're careful," they said;
>   "And if folks ever slip and are dropping,
> It isn't the slipping that hurts them so much
>   As the shock down below—when they're stopping."
> So for years (we have heard), as these mishaps occurred
>   Quick forth would the rescuers sally,
> To pick up the victims who fell from the cliff
>   With the ambulance down in the valley.
>
> Said one, to his plea, "It's a marvel to me
>   That you'd give so much greater attention
> To repairing results than to curing the cause;
>   You had much better aim at prevention.
> For the mischief, of course, should be stopped at its source,

Come, neighbors and friends, let us rally.
It is far better sense to rely on a fence
  Than an ambulance down in the valley."

"He is wrong in his head," the majority said;
  "He would end all our earnest endeavor.
He's a man who would shirk this responsible work,
  But we will support it forever.
Aren't we picking up all, just as fast as they fall,
  And giving them care liberally?
A superfluous fence is of no consequence,
  If the ambulance works in the valley."

The story looks queer as we've written it here,
  But things oft occur that are stranger.
More humane, we assert, than to succor the hurt,
  Is the plan of removing the danger.
The best possible course is to safeguard the source;
  Attend to things rationally.
Yes, build up the fence and let us dispense
  With the ambulance down in the valley.[9]

Dr. Haddon and a colleague, Dr. Robert Brenner, put the three phases (pre-event, event, post-event) and the three epidemiological factors (human, agent, environment) together in a matrix which provides great practical and theoretical utility in categorizing countermeasure options.

In Table 5–6, the role of alcohol as a factor in crash initiation is a pre-event human matter. The resistance of the properly packaged human body to the forces of impact is a crash-human element. Table 5–7 shows drowning countermeasures.

The use of such a matrix stressing loss reduction rather than accident prevention provides a scientific approach when used with understanding. It should be clear, however, that this type of matrix still encompasses accident prevention efforts.

Tables 5–8 and 5–9 give an example of contributing factors and their countermeasures for one accident type — discarded or abandoned refrigerators. Not all of the contributing factors or countermeasures are given. Remember that this framework can be applied to most accident types.

EVALUATING HAZARDS AND COUNTERMEASURES

A frequently encountered problem is that of determining the seriousness of a known hazard and deciding on the commensurate resources to correct the hazard. A formula for calculating the risk due to a hazard is

table 5–6   *Countermeasures. Accident Type: Motor-Vehicle.*

Phases / Factors	Pre-event	Event	Post Event
Host	Driver education	Driver "packaging"	Proper first aid and emergency care of bleeding
Agent	Automobile safety inspection of brakes, tires, etc.	Collapsible steering wheel to avoid impaling or crushing driver's chest	Accessible and low cost of vehicle-damage repair
Environment	Adequate signs and signals	Breakaway posts and sign poles	Emergency telephones and adequate emergency systems

source: Adapted from William Haddon, Jr., "A Logical Framework for Categorizing Highway Safety Phenomena and Activity," *Journal of Trauma,* March 1972, by permission of the author.

presented in this section. It quantitatively evaluates the potential severity of a hazardous situation. It is not implied in any way that a cost, no matter how great, is not worthwhile if it will prevent an accident and save a human life.

The hazard evaluation method as developed and reported by William

table 5–7   *Countermeasures. Accident Type: Drownings.*

Phases / Factors	Pre-event	Event	Post Event
Host	Swimming instruction	Life jackets	Visible swimwear
Agent	No swimming pool	Shallow pool	Underwater lights
Environment	Barriers and fences	Lifelines	Rescue systems

source: Adapted from Park E. Dietz and Susan P. Baker, "Drowning Epidemiology and Prevention," *American Journal of Public Health*, April 1974.

Fine provides a means of quantifying, in a risk score (R), the seriousness of a hazard situation.[10] The risk score comprises the following factors: potential consequences (C), exposure (E), and probability of occurrence (P). Consequences are divided by severity into six classes ranging from continuous or often daily (10) to remotely possible (0.5). Probabil-

table 5–8 *Contributing Factors. Accident Type: Discarded or Abandoned Refrigerators.*

Phases / Factors	Pre-event	Event	Post Event
Host (human)	Children are attracted to "playthings"—refrigerator becomes a hiding place, playhouse, and/or jail	Inability for human to exist in oxygen deficit environment for 5-10 minutes	Oxygen deficit by victims
Agent	Refrigerators can contain a child or several children (one case reported that 5 children suffocated together.)	Children are trapped in a sealed, "airtight" heavily insulated compartment	Child not visible unless the refrigerator door is open
Environment	Refrigerators are abandoned in remote areas (i.e., junkyards) or are temporarily in disuse (as in empty apartments or those in the process of defrosting)	Abandoned refrigerators are usually in remote areas away from people who might observe children playing in or around them	Difficulty in locating the missing child by searchers

ity also has six classes with respective values, from most likely (10) to almost impossible (0.1). The product of the three factors, $R = C \times E \times P$, is an arbitrary risk score that can be used to compare two or more hazardous situations. This technique represents a useful method for identifying major hazards before an accident occurs. Causal factors with high

table 5–9 *Countermeasures. Accident Type:*
Discarded or Abandoned Refrigerators.

Phases Factors	Pre-event	Event	Post Event
Host (human)	Tell children to stay away from discarded refrigerators because they are not "playthings" and they can kill	If a child is missing, a first place to look is in refrigerators	Resuscitation training for parents and older children
Agent	Manufacturers install permanent trays in refrigerators which don't allow room for children to crawl into them	Manufacturers install an interior wall section which a child's force can puncture to allow ventilation	Escape worthiness, (i.e., door can be opened from within by a force of 5 pounds)
Environment	Imposed penalties for discarding refrigerators without removing hinges and door	Manufacturers install an alerting device which would indicate occupancy and use (light or buzzer)	A first place to look for missing children is in refrigerators

severity but very low frequency can be detected quickly by these methods, whereas a large data base and a long time period would be necessary to detect them statistically.

To calculate the risk of a hazardous situation, Fine provides a formula which gives a numerical evaluation to the urgency for remedial attention to the hazard.

calculating a risk score

Use of the formula can be demonstrated by using the following example: A quarter-mile stretch of two-lane road is used by both vehicles and pedestrians departing or entering the grounds of a plant. There is no sidewalk, so pedestrians frequently walk in the road, especially when the grass is wet or snow covered. There is little hazard to pedestrians when all the traffic is going in one direction only. The hazard occurs, however, when vehicles are going in both directions and passing by each other. The vehicles require the entire width of the road, and pedestrians must then walk on the grass alongside the road. An accidental fatality could occur if a pedestrian steps into the road, or remains in the road at a point where two vehicles are passing.

Three steps are required to determine a risk score for this situation. One must list the accident sequence of events that could result in the undesired consequences, select the value for each element in the formula, and perform the actual calculation.

The accident sequence might involve the following seven events.

1   It is a wet or snowy day, making the grass along the road wet and uninviting to walk on.

2   At quitting time, a line of vehicles and some pedestrians are leaving the grounds, using this road.

3   One pedestrian walks on the right side of this road and he is oblivious to the traffic.

4   Although traffic is "one way" out at this time, one vehicle comes from the opposite direction causing the outgoing traffic line to move to the right edge of the road.

5   The pedestrian on the right side of the road fails to observe the vehicles, and he remains on the road.

6   The driver of one vehicle fails to notice the pedestrian and strikes him from the rear.

7   The pedestrian is killed.

Given the above series of events, the components of the formula are supplied below. The consequence is a fatality; therefore, C = 25 [see Table 5–10]. In relation to exposure, the hazard-event is the pedestrian remaining in the road and having an attitude of disregard. This type of person appears occasionally. Therefore, E = 3. Factor 2 [in Table 5–10] gives the approximate frequency of occurrence.

The probability of all events of the accident sequence following the hazard-event is "conceivably possible, although it has not happened in many years. . . ." The probability (P) is equal to 0.5.

The third step involves substitution of values into the formula and the performing of the simple arithmetic.

$$R = C \times E \times P = 25 \times 3 \times 0.5 = 37.5$$

table 5–10 *Ratings for Risk Calculation and Cost Justification*

factor	classification	rating
1 Consequences (Most probable result of the potential accident)	Catastrophe; numerous fatalities; damage over $1,000,000; major disruption of activities.	100
	Multiple fatalities; damage $400,000 to $1,000,000.	50
	Fatality; damage $100,000 to $500,000.	25
	Extremely serious injury (amputation, permanent disability); damage $1,000 to $100,000.	15
	Disabling injury; damage up to $1,000.	5
	Minor cuts, bruises, bumps; minor damage.	1
2 Exposure (The frequency of occurrence of the hazard-event)	Hazard-event occurs:	
	Continuously (or many times daily).	10
	Frequently (approx. once daily).	6
	Occasionally (from once per week to once per month).	3
	Unusually (from once per month to once per year).	2
	Rarely (it has been known to occur).	1
	Remotely possible (not known to have occurred).	0.5
3 Probability (Likelihood that accident sequence will follow to completion)	Complete accident sequence:	
	Is the most likely and expected result if the hazard-event takes place.	10
	Is quite possible, not unusual, has an even 50/50 chance.	6
	Would be an unusual sequence or coincidence.	3
	Has never happened after many years of exposure, but is conceivably possible.	0.5
	Practically impossible sequence (has never happened).	0.1
4 Cost factor (Estimated dollar cost of proposed corrective action)	Over $50,000	10
	$25,000 to $50,000	6
	$10,000 to $25,000	4
	$1,000 to $10,000	3
	$100 to $1,000	2
	$25.00 to $100	1
	Under $25.00	0.5
5 Degree of correction (Degree to which hazard will be reduced)	Hazard positively eliminated 100%	1
	Hazard reduced at least 75%	2
	Hazard reduced by 50% to 75%	3
	Hazard reduced by 25% to 50%	4
	Slight effect on hazard (less than 25%)	6

source: William T. Fine, "Mathematical Evaluation for Controlling Hazards," *Journal of Safety Research*, December 1971.

Referring to Table 5–11 will reveal immediacy of action which should be taken to prevent an accident.

cost justification

Once a hazard has been recognized, appropriate corrective action must be planned and its cost estimated. A slight expansion of the formula used to determine risk scores can be used to measure "justification"; i.e., to determine if the estimated cost is justified. The formula is:

$$J = \frac{C \times E \times P}{CF \times DC}$$

C, E, and P refer to consequences, exposure, and probability as before; CF and DC refer to cost factor and degree of correction. The cost factor is a measure of the estimated dollar cost of the proposed corrective action. Factor 4 in Table 5–11 gives the values and their respective ratings. The degree of correction is an estimate of the degree to which the proposed corrective action will eliminate or alleviate the hazard, forestall the hazard-event, or interrupt the accident sequence. The estimate will be based on experience and knowledge of the activity concerned. The classification and the associated rating appear in Table 5–11 as Factor 5. They range from slight effect on the hazard to total elimination (100%).

When the required values are obtained, they are placed in the formula to determine the numerical value of a countermeasure's justification score. For any justification score of 10 or more, the expenditure will be considered justified. For a score less than 10, the cost of the contemplated corrective action is not justified. . . .

example of justification score

. . . A possible corrective action to reduce the risk involving the pedestrian and vehicle hazard would be the construction of a sidewalk alongside the road. The estimated cost is $1500. The J formula is then used to determine whether this

table 5–11   *Risk Score Summary and Action Sheet*

risk score	action
1500 ↑ 200	Immediate correction required. Activity should be discontinued until hazard is reduced.
199 ↑ 90	Urgent. Requires attention as soon as possible.
89 ↑ 0	Hazard should be eliminated without delay, but situation is not an emergency.

source: William T. Fine, "Mathematical Evaluation for Controlling Hazards," *Journal of Safety Research*, December 1971.

expenditure is justified. The C, E, and P components are given in the earlier discussion as 25, 3, and 0.5, respectively. Since the estimated cost is $1500, CF = 3. The degree of correction accomplished by building a parallel sidewalk is judged to be at least 75% but not 100%; therefore, DC = 2. (See Table 5–11, Factor 5). The calculations then are:

$$J = \frac{25 \times 3 \times 0.5}{3 \times 2} = \frac{37.5}{6} = 6.25$$

Since J is less than 10, the conclusion is that the cost is not justified. . . [11]

This formula could be applied to many personal situations, such as whether or not to cover an irrigation ditch, replace or repair a worn-out car, or fence a swimming pool. Although such calculations and conclusions are justified from a managerial viewpoint, a philosophical view would suggest that any cost, no matter how great, is worthwhile if it will prevent an accident and save a human life.

ACCIDENT PRONENESS

There is a difference between accident repetitiveness and accident proneness. Accident repetitiveness refers to the fact that some have more accidents than others. Accident proneness explains why a person may have more accidents than others or is an accident repeater. Several authorities list personality traits characteristic of the accident-prone. However, research indicates that there is no such thing as one type of accident-prone person. Rather, each individual develops a range of behavior; some of the behavior is unsafe, which makes that person more susceptible to accidents. Data show that there are such people, but their number is small and their contribution to the total accident problem is slight.

Almost all people have accidents. When a person has difficulty adjusting to the environment, he is referred to as temporarily accident prone or accident susceptible. However, if one is susceptible, it does not mean an accident will inevitably occur.

Accident proneness as a cause of accidents is based on the assumption that certain individuals have had more than their share of accidents, and that these individuals had characteristics which were stable and enduring over extended periods of time.

A major problem in the accident prone concept is that people who have accidents in one period of time are not necessarily those who have accidents in the next time period. Still, the fact remains that some people do have more accidents than others. Most people know of others who display bandages, casts, and contusions on a continuing basis as evidence of their accidents. The accident prone concept should not be confused with those people who enter hazardous situations (e.g., the traveling salesman who drives 50,000 miles per year). These high risk individuals will tend to have more accidents because the opportunities are greater or the exposure is greater.

Frederick McGuire offers a typology of accident prone individuals.[12] Type I accident proneness is short-term and has two subtypes: crisis reactions and reactions to transient conditions. In the crisis reaction type, the individual is in a stressful situation (e.g., the student who worried about low grades or the father who is concerned about financial burdens). When the crisis is resolved, the individual returns to a state of better adjustment and is no longer accident prone. The period of time involved may last from several weeks to several months.

Individuals who are reacting to transient conditions have stable personalities but may be under the influence of pressures which make them accident prone. For example, a person recovering from an infectious disease may be tired or a person over-exerting himself on the job may feel fatigued. Tiredness and fatigue in these cases may be a contributing factor to an accident.

McGuire's Type II accident prone individual involves relatively constant and long-term pressures stemming largely from internal sources. Three subtypes to long-term proneness are character conditions, intra-psychic conditions, and physical conditions.

Character traits are stable and are identified by the behaviors which characterize a particular person. Therefore, character traits which are exhibited as asocial or anti-social behavior would be displayed by law breaking (e.g., running stop signs, ignoring speed limits). Certainly, an individual can change his character as he or she matures with age, education, marriage, or responsibility.

Intra-psychic conditions are extremely varied. Symptoms such as depression, heightened irritability, tension, and compulsions, may predispose an accident. Not all neurotic or psychotic persons are accident prone. Conditions of this category may last from several months to many years.

Physical conditions (e.g., failing eyesight, senility, untreated diabetes) may impair a person's ability to perform safely.

These types may overlap or combine to produce an accident prone individual. McGuire's concepts are not new, but through the realization that accident proneness does exist in some people for short periods of time and in others for long periods of time, and is predictable, comes the concept that accidents which are behaviorally caused may be avoided if appropriate countermeasures are used for those individuals.

Everybody, at some time in his life, is accident prone. When a person is in this state an accident may not always occur, but it is more likely to occur.

BEHAVIORAL MODEL (IPDE) FOR ACCIDENT PREVENTION

Analyses of human behavior which identify specific tasks (e.g., automobile and motorcycle driving) is a relatively new endeavor. On the basis of these task analyses, a model for classifying human functions has been developed. Although researchers have classified these functions differently, their analyses appear to agree in substance. It is contended that this model may be applied in the modification of human behavior whether the behavior involves automobile driving, swimming, or any other activity which may involve risk. Refer to Table 5–12 for illustrations in four different activities.

The four functions of the model are to:

1   *identify* the relevant cues (I).
2   *predict* their consequences (P).
3   *decide* upon a course of action (D).
4   *execute* the decision (E).

The first human function in this model is to acquire a complete and accurate picture of the environment in order to *identify* (I) any critical objects or changes which may require offsetting actions. Some may prefer to use "perceive" instead of "identify."

After an individual identifies the position of important elements (cues) in the environment and their relationship to each other, the individual must project and *predict* (P) possible future relationships and outcomes. Some may prefer to use "judge," "evaluate," or "access" instead of "predict." Nevertheless, an evaluation of a hazard occurs in this phase.

The third human function is to formulate a course of action with the intent to execute it. This is called the *decision-making* (D) function. Individuals make predictions on the basis of their perceptions and then make decisions on the basis of their predictions.

The sensory and mental functions (identification, prediction, decision) finally culminate in the performance function as the individual *executes* (E) his decisions related to the hazard(s).

An error in any four of the human functions may result in injury or other losses. For example, an individual may identify correctly that a highway is slippery, predict accurately that higher speeds result in a

table 5–12   *Illustrations of the IPDE Model*

Activity	Identify (I) ⟶ Predict (P) ⟶ Decide (D) ⟶ Execute (E)			
Camping	Sleeping over-night in rattle-snake infested area	Stay overnight with the risk of rattlesnake bite and/or sleep loss over worry		
		OR		
		Move to safer area	Move to safer area	Move
Boating	Fishing trip planned in 14 foot motor boat when strong winds (35 mph) are forecast	Risk capsizing from highwaves		
		OR		
		Cancel plans until better weather forecast	Set another calendar date for fishing trip	Schedule another date
Swimming	Friends swim 100 yards to raft in 20 foot deep lake. Farthest you have ever swum is 50 yards.	Risk of drowning from inability to swim 100 yards or from fatigue while attempting to swim 100 yards		
		OR		
		Obtain a rowboat or canoe for transportation to raft	Rent or borrow rowboat or canoe	Obtain rowboat or canoe
		OR		
		Stay on shore and wait for friends' return		
Bicycling	Tree limb blocking bike path	Hitting tree limb could result in tire failure or falling off bike		
		OR		
		Stop and remove tree limb	Remove tree limb for safe passage of self and others	Remove tree limb from bike path

greater likelihood for skidding, and decide that steering the vehicle into the skid direction (turning the steering wheel in same direction that the rear-end of vehicle turns) is the correct action to take. Yet this driver may still have an accident because he applied his foot brake.

Another illustration shows proper identification, prediction, decision, and execution. A ball suddenly rolls into the street ahead of the driver (identification). Prediction of a child chasing the loose ball into the street results in the driver's decision to decelerate and prepare to stop. The driver lifting his foot from the accelerator and over to the foot brake is an example of proper utilization of the IPDE model. The task of all people is to make accurate decisions and execute them at the right time to avoid hazards.

Education and training for improvement of these four human functions is possible and feasible, and in some cases is being accomplished. Yet training based on the IPDE concept still needs to be adapted to many safety education and training programs. Several high school driver education textbooks and other curriculum materials use the IPDE model as a basis for instruction.

IMITATION

There are several ways in which behavior is influenced. Some of the most obvious agents which deliberately attempt to induce specific behavior are television commercials, public schools, and parental discipline.

Behavior is also strongly influenced by what we learn through imitating others. "Do as I say and not as I do" is a saying that reflects the fact that people sometimes learn more from imitation than we would like to admit. A little girl does not dress up in her mother's clothes and high heels because she has been taught to do so; she is doing what she has seen her mother do.

A person's attitudes and behavior are strongly influenced by the people with whom he or she associates. The power of social influence is illustrated by an experimental situation in which 90 students with differing degrees of thirst were faced with a sign over a drinking fountain which read, "Do not use this fountain." The students had been told that the experiment they were to take part in was a study of taste preferences rather than a study of social influence. Differing degrees of thirst were induced by asking the students to eat varying numbers of crackers, some treated with hot sauce. After eating the crackers, the subjects were asked to step into the hall for a few moments on the pretext that the next part of the "taste experiment" was not yet ready to start.

While they were in the hall, the students saw the water fountain and the sign prohibiting its use. One group of students observed someone else who did not conform to the prohibition. The other group of students, a control group, was not exposed to anyone else's reaction to the sign.

The critical question in the experiment was: Could someone else exert any influence on the decisions and actions of the individual? The findings indicated that when students saw someone else violate the prohibition, they were more likely to drink from the fountain themselves than were the students who observed conforming behavior.[13]

Research on imitation tells us that we must behave in the way we want our children and students to behave. It confirms the fact that when your behavior is hypocritical, the teaching is less effective than if you practice what you teach.[14]

The significance of imitation is well documented. With regard to the tendency to imitate and its effects on safety, Michigan State University researchers say that fathers with numerous traffic convictions tend to have sons who have numerous traffic convictions. Fathers with no convictions tend to have sons with no convictions. How a young man drives seems to be influenced more by his family than by driver education or the actions of police and courts.[15]

There are other methods of influencing behavior which vary in effectiveness with the process of imitation. For example, exhortation, often used in encouraging accident prevention, has seldom been very successful in influencing behavior. Most of us would rather learn by example than by being told what to do.

MODIFYING HUMAN BEHAVIOR

There are two general ways by which we can influence the actions of others. One is to concentrate on altering their ideas, feelings, or goals; the other is to change the situation, thereby indirectly affecting their goals, ideas, and feelings. We often combine these approaches.

We strive for prevention of accidents through modification of human behavior by means of one or more of the following *modes of influence:*

1   By conveying new information (education).

2   By advising (effective according to the prestige of the source: his presumed experience, knowledge, and judgment).

3   By giving commands that carry authority.

4   By appealing to values and sentiments (other than those invoked by positions of authority).

5   By giving inducements (offering something valued in return for compliance).

6   By using coercion (threat of harm, the opposite of inducement; it can be a form of inducement: "If you do as I wish, then I won't do what you'd rather I not do").

7   By using force, with or without authority (the threat of force is coercion).

It should be noted that behavior modification usually begins with education and continues down through the influence of each successive mode if the preceding one is not effective.

Dr. William Haddon, Jr., gives some examples of the continuum of behavior modification in accident prevention:

The prevention of accidents through the modification of human behavior is usually approached through (1) education, (2) coercion, and (3) legal sanctions. In general, when educational efforts have failed, coercion has been tried; when this has failed, legal sanctions have been endorsed. However, when neither education nor coercive measures have proved effective, the implementation of the last step has often taken decades. This was seen in the quarter-of-a-century lag between the development of the railroad air brake and automatic coupler and the passage of legislation that forced their general use—a period in which tens of thousands of railroad workers were killed and many more injured. This is also illustrated by the long lag between the required use of safety belts in aircraft and their mandatory installation in new automobiles and by the interval in the United States of some fifty years between the first public recognition that the drinking driver is a highway menace and the enactment of laws permitting his identification through the use of breath and other quantitative chemical tests.[16]

The bases of influence are numerous. We can include among them the most important position in an organization (e.g., a command post in an army), money, social connections, prestige as a result of past performance, knowledge, skill, and physical characteristics (e.g., strength, height, sex appeal).

Major factors that account for the long lag in applying acquired knowledge include the following:

1   New knowledge is emerging in greater profusion with more rapidity than ever before.

2   There are far too few trained personnel, facilities, and resources for us to make use of new knowledge.

3   Various public attitudes toward the accident problem inhibit prevention efforts (as we noted in chapter 1).

4   Measures to reduce accident injury and death demand continuous individual effort.

NOTES

[1]Automotive Safety Foundation, *A Resource Curriculum Guide in Driver and Traffic Safety Education* (Washington, D.C.: Automotive Safety Foundation, 1970), p. 75.

[2]H. W. HEINRICH, *Industrial Accident Prevention* (New York: McGraw-Hill Book Company, 1959), p. 13.

[3]Ibid., pp. 15–16.

[4]DAN PETERSEN, *Techniques of Safety Management* (New York: McGraw-Hill Book Company, 1971), pp. 13–15.

[5]JOHN E. GORDON, "The Epidemiology of Accidents," *American Journal of Public Health,* XXXIX (April 1949), 504–15.

[6]WILLIAM HADDON, JR., "The Prevention of Accidents," in *Preventive Medicine,* ed. Duncan W. Clark and Brian MacMahon (Boston: Little, Brown and Company, 1967), p. 595.

[7]RICHARD E. MARLAND, "Injury Epidemiology," *Journal of Safety Research* (September 1969), p. 102.

[8]U.S. Department of Transportation, *Third Annual Report of the Department of Transportation on Activities Under the National Traffic and Motor Vehicle Safety Act,* October 7, 1970 (Washington, D.C.: Government Printing Office, 1970), pp. 27–31.

[9]The author of the poem is unknown. Quoted from *Farm Safety Review* (May–June 1966), published by the National Safety Council.

[10]WILLIAM FINE, "Mathematical Evaluation for Controlling Hazards," *Journal of Safety Research* (December 1971), pp. 157–66.

[11]Ibid., pp. 158–64.

[12]FREDERICK L. McGUIRE, "A Typology of Accident Proneness," *Behavioral Research in Highway Safety,* I (January 1970), p. 32.

[13]D. L. KIMBRELL AND R. R. BLAKE, "Motivational Factors in the Violation of a Prohibition," *Journal of Abnormal and Social Psychology,* LVI (1958), 132–33.

[14]DAVID ROSENHAN, FRANK FREDERICK, AND ANNE BURROWES, "Preaching and Practicing Effects of Channel Discrepancy on Norm Internalization," *Child Development,* XXXIX (March 1968), 291–301.

[15]WILLIAM L. CARLSON AND DAVID KLEIN, "Familial vs. Institutional Socialization of the Young Traffic Offender," *Journal of Safety Research,* II, no. 1 (March 1970), 13–25.

[16]HADDON, "The Prevention of Accidents," p. 598.

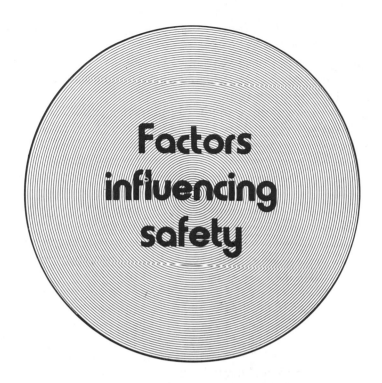

Factors influencing safety

THE SAFETY TREND

6 Probably accidents have always plagued mankind. One of the earliest accounts of safety concern occurs in the eighth verse of the twenty-second chapter of Deuteronomy: "When thou buildest a new house, then thou shalt make a battlement for thy roof, that thou bring not blood upon thine house, if any man fall from thence." From this early admonition until the Industrial Revolution of the 1800s, accidents were the concern of the individual. The Industrial Revolution brought many changes—new hazards and new responsibilities which affected more people.

Factory inspections were introduced in England as early as 1833 and were designed to alleviate some of the worst hazards. But not until the twentieth century was any really effective attack made upon industrial hazards.[1] Governmental regulations and controls were gradually formulated by most states in this country.

The most effective labor legislation was passed between 1910 and 1915 and consisted of workmen's compensation laws. These laws required that the employer contribute to the costs of any work injury, whether or not a worker had been negligent.

Increased interest in safety also resulted in the formation of the National Safety Council in 1912. Initially formed out of concern for industrial safety, this agency was later expanded to include all aspects of safety and accident prevention.

We can see how effective the safety movement has been by examining accident rates for the past several decades. In general, statistics available for work or industrial accidents indicate a definite decrease. However, trends over the years for motor-vehicle accidents have been less encouraging, although mortality rates based on deaths per 10,000 motor vehicles and per 100,000,000 road miles have shown a decrease. Fatal home accidents show an unfavorable trend over the years—there has been little change in yearly totals. Thus death rates for household accidents have dropped because the total population has increased.

The accident problem remains a significant one. There is still much room for improvement.

The National Safety Council reports that from its formation in 1912 to the present, accidental deaths per 100,000 population have decreased 32 percent, and if the rate had not decreased, nearly 1,600,000 more people would have died as a result of accidents.[2] Of course, the success of death prevention is a result of the efforts of many organizations and individuals to alleviate accidental death.

We should be proud of the progress since 1912, but comparisons should be made for the past decade which shows no progress and in fact has worsened. Original concern focused on physical conditions. Since the 1930s, unsafe acts have been emphasized. With no progress shown in the total accident picture, we need to reexamine our techniques for further success. Haddon's concepts may provide hope (see chapter 5).

Organizations and Agencies

Consistent and organized safety efforts have reduced the toll of accidents which otherwise might have reached considerable proportions. Various organizations have emphasized to varying degrees what is known as the "three E" concept of accident prevention: Engineering, Enforcement, and Education. Table 6–1 lists some of the organizations that are concerned with various phases of the "three E" concept. The list is by no means exhaustive or comprehensive in identifying those agencies and organizations with a specific interest in safety.

The safety educator or specialist can keep well informed and abreast of current safety issues by subscribing or referring to the periodicals suggested in Table 6–2.

table 6-1 *Organizations and Agencies*

engineering	enforcement	education
National Commission on Product Safety	National Commission on Product Safety	National Commission on Product Safety
National Highway Traffic Safety Administration	National Highway Traffic Safety Administration	National Highway Traffic Safety Administration
University Safety Centers	University Safety Centers	University Safety Centers
National Safety Council	National Safety Council	National Safety Council
Highway User's Federation for Safety and Mobility	U. S. Coast Guard	American National Red Cross
American Society of Safety Engineers	State and local law enforcement agencies	National Rifle Association
National Board of Fire Underwriters	American Association of Motor Vehicle Administrators	American Driver and Traffic Safety Education Association
Underwriters' Laboratories, Inc.	American Bar Association	American Alliance of Health, Physical Education, and Recreation
National Fire Protection Association	Occupational Safety and Health Administration	American Automobile Association
Insurance Institute for Highway Safety		Bicycle Institute of America
		Motorcycle Safety Foundation
		American Academy of Safety Education
		American Trauma Society

85

table 6–2   *Safety Periodicals*

name of periodical	when published	address
Traffic Safety	Monthly	National Safety Council 425 North Michigan Ave. Chicago, Ill. 60611
Family Safety	Quarterly	National Safety Council 425 North Michigan Ave. Chicago, Ill. 60611
National Safety News	Monthly	National Safety Council 425 North Michigan Ave. Chicago, Ill. 60611
National Safety Congress Transactions	Annually	National Safety Council 425 North Michigan Ave. Chicago, Ill. 60611
Journal of Safety Research	Quarterly	National Safety Council 425 North Michigan Ave. Chicago, Ill. 60611
Professional Safety	Monthly	American Society of Safety Engineers 850 Busse Highway Park Ridge, Ill. 60068
Journal of Traffic Safety Education	Bimonthly except summer months	California Driver Education Association 413 Dahlia Corona del Mar, Calif. 92625
Statistical Bulletin	Monthly	Metropolitan Life Insurance Co. One Madison Avenue New York, N.Y. 10010
Accident Analysis and Prevention	Quarterly	Pergamon Press Maxwell House, Fairview Park Elmsford, N.Y. 10523

Disasters

Chapter 3 deals briefly with the number of deaths resulting from disasters. As you will recall, the number of deaths from disasters is proportionately small when compared with other causes of accidental death; yet events called disasters receive front-page coverage in newspapers and news magazines.

The loss of life from disasters has decidedly influenced attempts to prevent needless death and injury. Table 6–3 presents a list of disasters with their respective death tolls and, more important, includes efforts made for reducing deaths and injuries following these disasters.

The Galveston tidal wave of September 8, 1900, in which approximately 6000 lives were lost, was the most devastating disaster on record in the United States. A cyclone and tidal wave on November 12, 1970, struck East Pakistan, resulting in a disaster of proportions unprecedented in this century (see Figure 6–1). The cost in lives from this natural disaster will never be reckoned accurately — a loss of more than half a million lives has been estimated. Most of you will recognize one or more of the major U.S. disasters listed in Table 6–4.

table 6–3 *Disasters and Their Effects on Safety Measures*

type	location and date	total deaths	results
Fire	City of Chicago, Illinois October 9, 1871	250	Building codes prohibiting wooden structures; water reserve
Flood	Johnstown, Pennsylvania May 31, 1889	2209	Inspections
Tidal wave	Galveston, Texas September 8, 1900	6000	Sea wall built
Fire	Iroquois Theatre, Chicago, Ill. December 30, 1903	575	Stricter theater safety standards
Marine	"General Slocum" burned East River, New York June 15, 1904	1021	Stricter ship inspections; revision of statutes (life preservers, experienced crew, fire extinguishers)
Earthquake and fire	San Francisco, California April 18, 1906	452	Widened streets; limited heights of buildings; steel frame and fire-resistant buildings
Mine	Monongah, West Virginia December 6, 1907	361	Creation of Federal Bureau of Mines; stiffened mine inspections
Fire	North Collinwood School Cleveland, Ohio March 8, 1908	176	Need realized for fire drills and planning of school structures
Fire	Triangle Shirt Waist Co. New York March 25, 1911	145	Strengthening of laws concerning alarm signals, sprinklers, fire escapes, fire drills
Marine	*Titanic* struck iceberg Atlantic Ocean April 15, 1912	1517	Regulation regarding number of lifeboats; all passenger ships equipped for around-the-clock radio watch; International Ice Patrol
Explosion	New London School, Texas March 18, 1937	294	Odorants put in natural gas
Fire	"Cocoanut Grove," Boston, Mass. November 28, 1942	492	Ordinances regulating aisle space, electrical wiring, flameproofing of decorations, overcrowding, signs indicating the maximum number of occupants; administration of blood plasma to prevent shock and the use of penicillin
Plane	Two-plane air collision over Grand Canyon, Arizona June 30, 1956	128	Controlled airspace expanded; use of infrared as a warning indicator

source: Based upon information from *Accident Facts* (1974), p. 21, by permission of the National Safety Council.

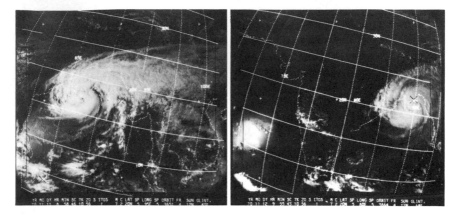

figure 6–1 This cyclone (hurricane) in the Bay of Bengal, 1970, produced the century's worst disaster. This photo was taken from an unmanned weather satellite, ITOS-1. Reproduced courtesy of the National Oceanic and Atmospheric Administration.

The world's worst disaster on record (other than the Biblical account of Noah and the flood) occurred in A.D. 1887; a flood took 900,000 lives along the Hwang Ho River in China's Honan Province.

TECHNOLOGY

We become aware of the impact of technology on safety and accident loss reduction by looking at various innovations (see Figure 6–2 a–d). Whether the innovation be safety lenses (eyeglasses), safety belts (lap

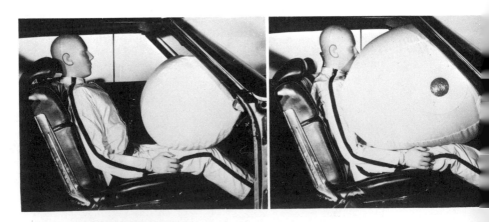

figure 6–2 The automobile protective airbag and safety belts may be the most important safety developments in recent years. Reproduced courtesy of the Na-

and harness types in automobiles), safety hats (steel or other hard material), safety shoes (steel-toed), or safety guards (on electrical saws) — all of which are widely accepted today — we can be sure that formerly they were viewed as quite unacceptable and met with widespread resistance. One prime obstacle to change is *habit*. Only when many people recognize a problem do we consider change and search about for new ways of doing things. Perhaps there are several reasons for the survival of many unsafe practices and technological methods: people are used to these practices and methods, people accept the fact that accidents will happen, and people hesitate to adopt new ways for preventing accidents because it involves effort.

In addition to habit, *traditionalism* often lies behind some resistance to innovation. Not only are people accustomed to present ways of doing things, but they also revere these ways because they link them with the past.

A third factor which leads to resistance to change is *vested interests*. There are always groups of people in advantageous positions who would feel their status threatened by change. Most of the issues in safety presented in chapter 4 represent groups of people with vested interests.

LEGISLATION

Usually laws are enacted as a "last resort" after other attempts to control behavior have failed. Legislation also appears as an aftermath of a disaster. A basic question that merits consideration is: "Can safety be legislated?" There is little doubt that some regulatory legislation, such as

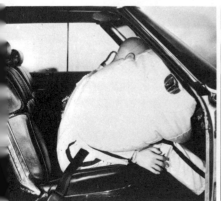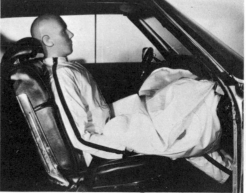

tional Highway Traffic Safety Administration and General Motors Corporation.

table 6–4 *Largest U.S. Disasters by Category*

	type and location	no. of deaths	date of disaster
floods:	Galveston tidal wave	6000	Sept. 8, 1900
	Johnstown, Pa.	2209	May 31, 1889
	Ohio and Indiana	732	Mar. 28, 1913
	St. Francis, Calif. dam burst	450	Mar. 13, 1928
	Ohio and Mississippi River valleys	380	Jan. 22, 1937
hurricanes:	Florida	1833	Sept. 16–17, 1928
	New England	657	Sept. 21, 1938
	Louisiana	500	Sept. 29, 1915
	Florida	409	Sept. 1–2, 1935
	Louisiana and Texas	395	June 27–28, 1957
tornadoes:	Illinois	606	Mar. 18, 1925
	Mississippi, Alabama, Georgia	402	Apr. 2–7, 1936
	Indiana, Ohio, Michigan. Illinois, and Wisconsin	272	Apr. 11, 1965
	Arkansas, Tennessee, Missouri, Mississippi, and Alabama	229	Mar. 21–22, 1952
	Texas and Oklahoma	167	Apr. 9, 1947
earthquakes:	San Francisco earthquake and fire	452	Apr. 18, 1906
	Alaskan earthquake-tsunami hit Hawaii and California	173	Apr. 1, 1946
	Long Beach, California, earthquake	120	Mar. 10, 1933
	Alaskan earthquake and tsunami	117	Mar. 27, 1964
	San Fernando–Los Angeles, Calif., earthquake	65	Feb. 9, 1971
marine:	"Sultana" exploded–Mississippi River	1547	Apr. 27, 1865
	"Titanic" struck iceberg–Atlantic Ocean	1517	Apr. 15, 1912
	"Empress of Ireland" ship collision–St. Lawrence River	1024	May 29, 1914
	"General Slocum" burned–East River	1021	June 15, 1904
	"Eastland" capsized–Chicago River	812	July 24, 1915
aircraft:	Two-plane collision over New York City	134	Dec. 16, 1960
	Two-plane collision over Grand Canyon, Ariz.	128	June 30, 1956
	Jetliner crash into mountainside near Juneau, Alaska	111	Sept. 4, 1971
	Scheduled plane crash near Miami, Fla.	101	Dec. 29, 1972
	Plane explosion–crash, Jamaica Bay, N.Y.	95	Mar. 1, 1962

Today there is so much to learn, and what we don't know can harm us.

What is the point? Simply this — that safety education is vital. If we could learn the things we need to know without safety education, there would be no justification for such a program.

Even today we should and do learn many of the things we need to know through normal life experience. For example, most children learn before going to school that fire is hot. If schools taught only such simple things, they would not be justified.

All items of knowledge are not of equal value. This is why safety educators find themselves battling with those who believe there are more important things in the school day than safety instruction. In safety education the instructor usually decides what is needed and what is to be taught. An agreement on what needs to be learned in this area is of primary importance.

The sooner one learns something he needs to know, the more effective his life will be. Thus, many within the safety education ranks have spoken out in favor of safety instruction starting in pre-kindergarten.

A constant aim of the safety educator should be to find ways to speed up the learning of safety by his students. Common methods in use include the quoting of accident statistics, stressing of safety rules, and application of "scare" techniques. These are among the poorer approaches that could be used. As previously stated, once concepts are clear, behavior can be influenced. Thus, we need to develop safety concepts that allow for productive and effective lives.

The conceptual approach offers much to safety teaching. Not only must a teacher know *how* to teach, he must know what *ends* he hopes to achieve. A differentiation needs to be made between concepts and behavioral objectives since both are end products. Concepts are those ideas which the student is expected to *know,* while behavioral objectives identify what the student will be able to *do* (overt behavior) with what he knows (the concepts). Thus, the student may know the concept "water puts out Class A fires," but actually having him put out a Class A fire is a way the teacher can determine if the student really knows the concept.

Let safety education be identified not as mere topics, admonitions, statistics, or learning activities, but as an accident avoidance approach which has continuity and measurable expectations (with concepts and behavioral objectives), and is not a curriculum "timewaster."

Growth in our knowledge of how to cope with the accident problem has not kept pace with the growth of the problem. Accidents have attracted little interest in the scientific community. America's poor accident record, and its failure to marshal enough scientific and monetary resources to improve the record, concerns those who work in the field of safety education. Safety educators, individually and through such organizations as the National Safety Council, have been outspoken on the need to combat the accident problem.

The task of safety educators is to identify those truths or concepts that will lead toward the goal of accident loss reduction for effective living. As one looks at the world, there are some universal truths discovered, such as the fire triangle, while there are probably innumerable truths yet to be identified (Figure 7–1). Our challenge is to identify these concepts.

INSTRUCTIONAL MODEL

There is no single concept, theory, or method of teaching or instruction, and probably never will be. For example, the Socratic method of teaching stresses inquiry, dialectic (conversation between the teacher and the student), and inductive logic. Those who follow the Jesuit method of education are described as "masters of method"; they emphasize rote learning. Yet both of these approaches and others have been successful to varying degrees.

One of the most recent and useful emphases in education is the so-called systematic approach to instruction. We may compare this "systematic approach" to the vacationing tourist who travels with a predetermined route marked on a road map. Although some good teachers may not adhere to the following ideas, their success was not the result of accidental or "off-the-cuff" inspiration. They succeeded because they were well organized, informed, inventive, and skillful in presenting their concepts to students. This chapter is designed specifically with a framework to help you become a better safety instructor.

Schaplowsky of the U.S. Public Health Service tells us that:

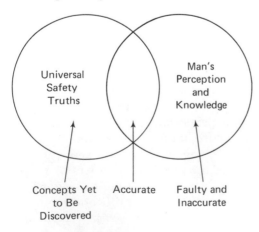

figure 7–1 There are safety concepts yet to be discovered.

[A]ccidents can be prevented by bringing about changes in man's environment and in his behavior. We know that behavior may be changed as a result of an increase in man's knowledge, improvement in his skills or modification of his attitudes.[1]

Schaplowsky continues by citing examples of traffic and scuba-diving accidents, child poisonings, effects of carbon monoxide, and the dangers of ultrathin plastic bags to illustrate the point that many accidents are the consequences of an individual's lack of knowledge. However, successful communication of factual knowledge does not necessarily guarantee successful modification of behavior. This applies to safety, algebra, English, and a myriad of subjects.

The lack of professional qualifications of safety instructors has been implicated in their occasional ineffectiveness in influencing safe behavior. That the safety instructor must be highly qualified is well illustrated by Elkow:

The New York Times editorialized last week on a shocking fact: "[H]alf the operations performed in American hospitals are done by physicians unqualified to perform in accordance with the standards of the American College of Surgeons." Equally shocking is the fact that safety education functions are carried on by persons *who*, at the time of their initial appointment or in some instances individuals currently functioning or about to function, are unqualified to meet the vital functions of preparing youth for safe living in our complex environment.[2]

Courses have been systematically developed for various areas of safety instruction. A project devised for the American Telephone and Telegraph Company by the American Institutes for Research had as its objective "to develop a basic first aid course which would, in seven and one-half hours, produce results at least equivalent to those produced by standard first aid instruction taking ten hours." Another instructional guide based upon behavioral objectives is *A Resource Curriculum in Driver and Traffic Safety Education* of the Highway Users Federation for Safety and Mobility, Washington, D.C.

The instructional model advocated in this chapter features four component parts or four essentially distinct operations. The definitions of the four parts are presented here; later sections of the chapter will be devoted to detailed consideration of each component part. Figure 7–2 depicts a flow chart which illustrates the sequential relationship of the four component parts of the instructional model. *Behavioral objectives* (box A) are the goals the student should attain upon completion of a

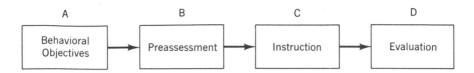

figure 7–2   The instructional model. Adapted from W. James Popham and Eva L. Baker, *Systematic Instruction* (Englewood Cliffs, N.J.: Prentice-Hall, Inc., 1970), p. 13, by permission of the publisher.

segment of instruction. *Preassessment* (box B) is a determination of the student's current status with respect to the behavioral objectives. *Instruction* (box C) describes the activities that should bring about the intended student accomplishment as stated in the behavioral objectives. *Evaluation* (box D) consists of a means of determining how well the student has achieved the behavioral objectives. If the evaluation indicates that the student has fallen short of the standard of achievement (as stated in the behavioral objectives), an adjustment may be required in one of the essential parts of the instructional model, usually in the instructional component.[3]

BEHAVIORAL OBJECTIVES

Most instruction plans lack a clear expression of behavioral objectives. Although most educators believe in objectives, past objectives or goals were based upon what the teacher had to accomplish or ambiguously described what the student was expected to achieve. Behavioral objectives describe explicitly how the student is expected to behave at the conclusion of instruction.

Robert F. Mager recommends that behavioral objectives include the following three parts:

1   Identification of the terminal performance or behavior which the instruction attempts to encourage. The verb in the statement of the objective identifies and names the action expected to be observed in the student.

2   Description of the important conditions under which the behavior is to occur. These conditions might include writing an examination, speaking orally in class, driving on a canyon road, or performing a particular skill on the job.

3   Description of the acceptable level of student performance. Instructors might establish 90 percent correct answers on the examination, pass-or-fail performance of a job with safety checks, or consistently wearing safety goggles while using a grinding machine as standards or expected levels of student performance.[4]

In insisting that the words chosen to state objectives (verbs depicting observable behavior) must not be open to misinterpretation, Mager supplies examples for consideration:[5]

words open to many interpretations:

to know	to appreciate	to enjoy
to understand	to fully appreciate	to believe
to *really* understand	to grasp the significance of	to have faith in

words open to fewer interpretations:

to write	to differentiate	to list
to recite	to solve	to compare
to identify	to construct	to contrast

Examples of a variety of behavioral objectives are presented below. Notice that each states what the student will be doing as he demonstrates that he has achieved the stated objective; each also says something about the level of acceptable performance and under what conditions it should be reached. The form varies but this is not important; what is important is that expected student outcomes are made clear.

Example 1

Using a copy of *Accident Facts,* the student should be able to classify ten home accidents as one of the eight types of home accidents.

Example 2

As part of the final examination, the student should be able to list three disasters which took more than 25 lives in the United States last year.

Example 3

Goal: Be able to point out community safety hazards.
Behavior: Identify dangerous conditions.
Conditions: The student will survey the community determined by the instructor.
Standards: Ten danger conditions.

Example 4

Goal: Be familiar with terms commonly used in safety.
Behavior: Match term with correct definition.
Conditions: Given a list of terms and definitions.
Criterion: 8 correct matches out of 10.

There are different levels of behavior objectives, such as lowest cognitive (rote memory or recall), higher-than-lowest cognitive (application, analysis, synthesis, evaluation, etc.), psychomotor (skills), and affective (attitude) levels. You might refer to the writings of Benjamin S. Bloom, Robert Gagne, and W. James Popham for further information and elaboration concerning different types or levels of behavioral objectives.

PREASSESSMENT

Preassessment is the process used to determine a student's level of attainment in relation to prescribed behavioral objectives. A teacher preassesses a student in two ways: (1) by knowing the student well enough to estimate his knowledge and background for the lesson before the class meets (evaluation at the conclusion of one lesson often aids in effective preassessment for a following lesson), and (2) by determining before or during the class period the student's knowledge of the lesson material and his ability to reach the behavioral objectives through, for example, his response to written diagnostic tests, oral questions, and general discussion. Instructors who preassess their students and instruct accordingly will probably avoid boring students with material already known and frustrating them with advanced material for which students lack the necessary background.

INSTRUCTION

Instruction consists of those activities in which a student engages to help him attain a behavioral objective. Notice that here we place emphasis on those things which a *student* does. Instructors use various methods and techniques which allow the student active participation in reaching the desired behavioral objectives.

There are many instructional methods and techniques. We may differentiate between a method and a technique by suggesting that a technique is a subtype of a method. For example, discussion is a method, whereas the specific types of discussion—question–answer, brainstorming, buzz groups, etc.—are techniques. An accurate guide that tells the instructor the best method or technique is nonexistent. In this section we will present some guidelines for the instructor's use in selecting appropriate instructional activities for his lesson.

Mager suggests that the selection of instructional procedures be based upon:

1   Choosing the technique which has conditions called for by the objective. If the objective calls for the student to analyze accident causes from newspaper accounts, then guided practice with newspaper accounts would be in order.

2   Choosing the technique which causes the student to perform in a manner called for by the objective. If the objective calls for the student to recognize potential community safety hazards, then guided observation through slides, a film, or a field trip to a segment of the community would be appropriate for practice in identifying potential hazards.[6]

Other considerations important to the proper selection of instructional activities are the grouping of students and the use of audio-visual aids. Table 7–1 shows us three kinds of classroom groupings and suggests activities for each. Note that some instructional activities may be utilized in one or more of the groups. In Tables 7–2 and 7–3 William H. Allen presents some factors for our consideration when using educational media or audio-visual aids as part of instructional activities.

In a later section you will find ideas and a suggested sequence for developing and unifying behavioral objectives, content, and instructional activities.

EVALUATION

Evaluation is the process of comparing a student's behavior with the predetermined behavioral objective. Most often evaluation occurs in the final lesson or at the end of a lesson, although we may evaluate through a try-out experience during the lesson or in any applicable

table 7–1   *Grouping for Instruction*

a. teacher alone		b. interaction (between teacher and students or between students)		c. student alone	
1	lecture	1	buzz groups	1	reading
2	films	2	brainstorming	2	research
3	slides	3	question-answer discussion	3	programmed instruction
4	television	4	committee work	4	practice
5	guest speaker	5	debates	5	writing
6	chalkboard	6	role-playing		
7	demonstration				

table 7–2 *Relationship of Instructional Media Stimulus to Learning Objectives*

instructional media type	learning objectives					
	learning factual information	learning visual identifications	learning principles, concepts, and rules	learning procedures	performing skilled perceptual-motor acts	developing desirable attitudes, opinions, and motivations
Still pictures	Medium	High	Medium	Medium	Low	Low
Motion pictures	Medium	High	High	High	Medium	Medium
Television	Medium	Medium	High	Medium	Low	Medium
3-D objects	Low	High	Low	Low	Low	Low
Audio recordings	Medium	Low	Low	Medium	Low	Medium
Programmed instruction	Medium	Medium	Medium	High	Low	Medium
Demonstration	Low	Medium	Low	High	Medium	Medium
Printed textbooks	Medium	Low	Medium	Medium	Low	Medium
Oral presentation	Medium	Low	Medium	Medium	Low	Medium

source: Reprinted from William H. Allen, National Art Education Association government project report, which also appeared in "Media Stimulus and Types of Learning," *Audiovisual Instruction* (January 1967), p. 28, by permission of Association for Educational Communications & Technology.

table 7–3 *Equipment/Media Relationships and Considerations*

instrument	media used	materials production consideration	availability of facilities and equipment	equipment cost
Filmstrip or slide projector	33mm. filmstrips or 2 x 2 slides	Inexpensive. May be done locally in short time.	Usually available. Requires darkened room.	Low
Overhead transparency projector	Still pictures and graphic representations	Very inexpensive. May be done locally in short time.	Available. May be projected in light room.	Low
Wall charts or posters	Still pictures	Very inexpensive. May be done locally in a very short time.	Available. No special equipment needed.	Low

Motion pictures (projection to groups)	16mm. motion picture (sound or silent)	Specially-produced. Sound film is costly and requires 6–12 months time.	Usually available. Requires darkened classroom.	Moderate
Motion picture projection as repetitive loops (8mm. silent) to individuals	8mm. motion picture film (silent)	Special production normally necessary. May be produced as 16mm. film alone or locally at low cost and in very short time.	Not normally available. Will need to be specially procured to meet requirement of instructional program.	Low per unit, but moderate for groups.
Magnetic tape recorder	1/4" magnetic tape	Easy and inexpensive. Usually produced locally.	Available.	Low
Record player	33 1/3, 45, or 78 rpm. disk recordings	Need special recording facilities. Usually commercially made.	Usually available.	Low
Display area	3-D models	May vary in complexity and in difficulty of production. Component parts easy to obtain.	Available.	Varies from low to high.
Television (closed circuit)	Live presentations. Motion picture film. Videotape recordings. Still pictures	Normally requires large and skilled production staff.	Not normally available.	Moderate to high.
Teaching machines and programmed textbooks	Programmed material	Some programs available commercially, but will normally be specially prepared for course.	Not normally available.	Low per unit, but moderate for groups
System combinations	Television. Motion pictures. Still pictures. Audio recordings	Complex. Probably will be done locally to meet specific requirements.	Not normally available	Moderate to high

source: Reprinted from William H. Allen, National Art Education Association government project report, which also appeared in "Media Stimulus and Types of Learning," *Audiovisual Instruction* (January 1967), p. 31, by permission of the Association for Educational Communications & Technology.

way. Evaluation may even take place during out-of-class periods in the form of an assignment.

The development of an evaluation procedure should derive specifically from the condition statement of the behavioral objective. Objectives and evaluation should, in essence, be identical: that is, examination items should be drawn from the behavior specified in the objective to test for it. The following examples indicate objectives and appropriate evaluation:

Example 1

Objective:
   On a written examination, the student will—with 90 percent accuracy—classify fires and indicate which type of fire extinguisher to use for each.
Evaluation:
   A list of fires (wood, gasoline, electrical, etc.) is given to the student. He identifies the fire class (A,B,C) to which each fire belongs and then indicates the best fire extinguisher (carbon dioxide, water, dry chemical, etc.) for each fire listed.

Example 2

Objective:
The student will safely control the steering of an automobile when a tire blows out or the air pressure suddenly diminishes.
Evaluation:
While the student is driving, a flat tire (blowout) simulator will release the air from a normal tire. The student will react effectively to this emergency situation by:

1   Firmly gripping the steering wheel and steering a straight course.
2   Easing up on the accelerator.
3   Braking with a firm and steady pressure (avoid "locking" wheels).
4   Looking for an escape route and driving entirely off the roadway.
5   Securing the car (putting parking brake and selector lever in park).

This prevents the use of tests that are really "guessing games," which often occurs in our schools. If one follows this procedure and students then fail to attain the predescribed goals, the instructor may be responsible; either his plans have been inadequate or he has not carried them out well. However, if the behavioral objectives are achieved, the instructor deserves much credit. When this instructional procedure is followed successfully, norm-referenced or curve grading (which guarantees a definite number of successes and failures) becomes archaic.

LESSON PLANS

The lesson plan is the instructional blueprint that describes those activities which will enable the student or class to reach that lesson's behavioral objectives. Some teachers are criticized for following a lesson plan, but such plans are important. However, there are probably as many different formats for lesson plans as there are instructors: what works well for one instructor may not work so well for another. Most important, the instructor must feel comfortable with his lesson plan.

The lesson plan format in Table 7–4 is a suggested one. The sug-

table 7–4   *Sample Lesson Plan Form*

Title: _____

Objectives:

1

2

Materials needed:

Preassessment:

Ideas To Be Taught	Learning Activities
1	Show:
	Discuss:
	Apply:
2	Show:
	Discuss:
	Apply:

Evaluation:

  In class:

  Following class:

Assignment:

gested plan does not apply to psychomotor (skill) lessons. This plan consists of: behavioral objectives, concepts or ideas to be taught for each behavioral objective, appropriate learning activities, and appropriate evaluation for the behavioral objectives. The ideas to be presented form the content outline.

Table 7–5 depicts a sequence of learning activities entitled *show, discuss,* and *apply* and suggests activities for each. The "cone of experience" shown in Table 7–6 provides additional aid by helping the instructor to determine which experiences or activities will be most effective for *show.* Specific examples of activities for each segment of the "cone of experience" are found in Table 7–7.

Sample completed lesson plans are provided to aid the reader to conceptualize better the ideas of this section (Tables 7–8 and 7–9).

SAFETY INSTRUCTION: SOME PRECAUTIONS

There is a general inclination for safety educators to adopt time-worn instructional methods for accident prevention attempts. Unfortunately, these practices tend only to produce unsatisfactory results. This time-worn method may partially explain why safety and accident prevention education has a less than desirable position in education. Let us examine three common practices: (1) use of statistics, (2) use of scare techniques, and (3) use of rules.

table 7–5 *Learning Activities*

show*	discuss	apply
Show the class what you want them to learn through use of:	Engage the class in discussion to:	Encourage the application of ideas and concepts through:
Objects	Raise questions	Assignments
Pictures	Cite and elicit examples	In-class activities which
Stories	Pose problems	require students to use ideas
Charts	Consider various points	Specific out-of-class projects
Diagrams	of view	which challenge students
Films	Seek reasons	Follow-up measures to ensure
Real experiences		good results
(past and present)		
Recordings		
Role playing		
Textbook content		

*This step should serve as an effective interest arouser and provide a common background experience which can be used later as a reference point for discussion. It is most effective when it is stimulating and eye-catching, although reference to a previous group experience can also be very effective.

source: Adapted from Asahel D. Woodruff, *Basic Concepts of Teaching* (San Francisco: Chandler Publishing Company, 1961), pp. 93ff.

Use of Statistics

The field of safety and accident prevention is replete with figures, statistics, numbers, and rates. There is little literature available on the proper use of accident statistics. Regarding this, William Tarrants, at a

table 7–6 *The Cone of Learning Experiences*

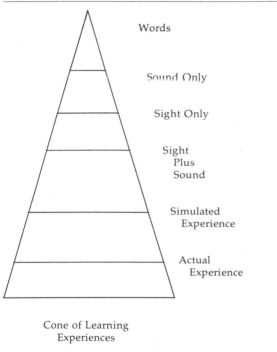

Words

Sound Only

Sight Only

Sight
Plus
Sound

Simulated
Experience

Actual
Experience

Cone of Learning
Experiences

The cone suggests that:

A   Certain experiences are closer to or farther from direct experience.

B   When we use more than one of our senses our learning is more complete. Usually the closer we get to the bottom of the cone the more senses we use.

The cone provides knowledge which enables us to decide the *appropriate* learning experience to use after we consider the following interrelated factors:

A   The readiness of the students in terms of their *experiences* with something.

B   The cost of the experience in terms of money, effort, time or safety.

Often the best instructional decision involves use of learning activities in the lower area of the cone. ⟶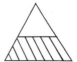

However, the decision to use activities in the upper area of the cone may be appropriate when the two factors above are ⟶ considered.

source: Adapted from Baird et al., *A Behavioral Introduction to Teaching* (Dubuque, Iowa: Kendall & Hunt, 1970), p. 90, by permission of the authors.

table 7–7   *Cone of Experience Worksheet*

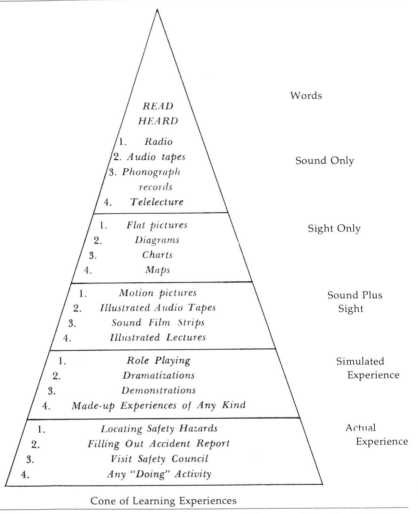

Cone of Learning Experiences

source: Adapted from Edgar Dale, *Audio-Visual Methods in Teaching* (New York: The Dryden Press, 1969).

National Safety Congress, presented information which he felt was pertinent for the safety educator:

We often hear that "off-the-job activities are more dangerous than places of work, since more accidents occur off-the-job" or that "The bedroom is the most hazardous room in the home since more injuries occur in the bedroom than any other room." The originators fail to consider differences in quantity of exposure, type of exposure, age, and other influencing factors.[7]

table 7–8   *Sample Lesson Plan*

Title:
Multiple Cause Concept of Accident Causation
Objective:
After completion of this lesson each class member should be able to define the multiple
cause concept, and identify the implications this concept has for safe behavior.
Materials needed:
1   16 mm. film projector.
2   Film: "The Final Factor" color, 14 minutes, 1968, purchase or lease from AAA Foun-
      dation for Traffic Safety.
3   Copies of a newspaper accident account for each student (double-spaced with wide
      margins).
Preassessment:
Some class members may be well acquainted with the multiple cause concept. Ask which
    are and have them assist you during the lesson by giving illustrations of factors from
    their accident experiences to portray the multiple cause concept.

concept or idea to be taught	learning activities
Accidents generally result from a combination of human-agent-environmental factors acting in a closely interwoven fashion (multiple cause concept).	*Show:* Show the film "The Final Factor." *Discuss:* *Ask:* What is the main concept or idea in the film? *Ask:* What are the implications for safe behavior? *Ask:* Does the multiple cause concept apply to all accidents? *Ask:* Does anyone know of an accident for which several known influential factors existed? *Apply:* Hand out a newspaper account of an accident to each student. Have students circle words, phrases, and/or sentences which might describe factors of accident causation. Write marginal notes if appropriate.

Evaluation:
   In class: The newspaper exercise could be used.
   Following class: During the week read the newspaper. Choose one account of an accident
   and circle the key words, phrases, and/or sentences which might indicate factors affect-
   ing the accident. Write marginal notes if appropriate. Turn the article in next week.
Assignment:
Read sections in the textbook appropriate for the next topic of class consideration.

An early statistician coined a phrase that has since been repeated to
generations: "It's not that the figures lie—it's that liars figure." Although deceptive figures do appear in accident statistics, it is probable
that the largest number of statistical elucidations are compiled by those
desiring to inform rather than misinform.

The practice of citing statistics and then requiring their memo-
rization for an examination is all too common. Typical of the accident

table 7–9   *Sample Lesson Plan*

Title:
Emergency First Aid at an Accident Scene

Objective:
The student should be able to identify recommended first aid procedures for accident cases.

Materials needed:
Situation described below typed and duplicated for each class member.

Preassessment:
Ask for volunteers to demonstrate the systematic examination of a victim for injuries and life-threatening problems.

concept or idea to be taught	learning activities
When accidents occur it is essential that every effort be made to save lives and lessen the severity of injuries. Good first aid training is essential.	*Show:* Hand out copies of the accident situation. Read it to the class or have students read it.

Situation

You are the first to arrive at the scene of a two-car collision. Both cars are upright. A quick survey of the scene reveals the following victims:

Car 1: The driver is unconscious and seated in the front seat fastened by his safety belt. The head of the passenger in the front seat has been thrown through the windshield. He is bleeding profusely about the face, is unconscious, with shallow respiration.

Car 2: The driver is seated in the front seat. He is sweating and appears to be short of breath. He complains of severe pain in his chest and left arm. The passenger has been thrown from the car. He is lying on the road moaning that he cannot move his legs. He appears to feel no sensation in his legs.

Discuss:

1   What is most likely wrong with each victim?
2   Which victim should be treated first and why?
3   What care should be given to each victim?
4   Which victim should be transported first and why?

Evaluation:
   In class: Hand out another typed description of a first aid accident situation to which students may respond individually (similar to an examination).
   Following class: Prepare one accident situation (actual case, if possible) and respond to it by indicating the appropriate first aid measures to be taken.

Assignment:
   Read all assigned material to date in preparation for the final examination.

statistics cited to impress students with the magnitude of the accident problem are the total number of annual accidental deaths, injuries, and property damage costs.

Statistics are not all bad. They can point out and describe problems. It is suggested that the educator use proportional statistics (rates or ratios) rather than quoting numbers and figures, which are usually out of date anyway. For example, rather than saying 115,000 annual accidental deaths occurred, it is recommended that statements similar to the following be used.

1   Accidents are the fourth leading cause of death in the United States.

2   One in four Americans is annually injured enough to require medical attention or activity restriction for at least one day.

3   There is, on the average, one person dying from an accident every five minutes in the United States.

4   Accidents are the leading cause of death among all persons aged 1 to 38 years.

5   Accidents cause more deaths each year than all infectious diseases combined.

Another pitfall is the attention drawn to catastrophes because these events make newspaper headlines. It is significant that a very small percentage of accident catastrophes occur as a result of natural forces such as floods, hurricanes, tornadoes, and earthquakes. The record of national catastrophes reveals that relatively few lives are lost in this way when contrasted with the total number of deaths resulting from other types of unspectacular, unpublished accidents.

Use of Scare Techniques

Ask a former student of a safety class such as driver education what he remembers, and his answer will probably include a description of a film or pictures of bizarre, gory accidents. Their use is common in driver education and industrial safety meetings, and if the safety educator doesn't have access to a "scare" film or accident pictures, then vivid stories or case histories bring images of broken bodies and death.

Experts have come to the following conclusions regarding the use of scare techniques to change or influence behavior:

1   Fear methods tend to be short-term in their effectiveness.

2   Fear techniques can influence behavior by leading to constructive change or by preventing one from doing something dangerous. Strong fear

techniques have been reported to produce no change in behavior, whereas minimal fear techniques have been more successful. Yet it has been reported that those with little experience with the subject matter react favorably after a strong fear appeal. Divergent opinions exist among researchers.

3   Fear techniques can adversely affect some people by causing worry and anxiety.

4   Fear is a learned response.

5   If fear techniques are used too often, a person may become calloused or too accustomed to their use for any desired behavior change to occur.

6   There is need for further research — there is no single answer regarding the effectiveness of scare techniques. Few studies on use of fear techniques exist specifically in safety education. It is advised that until more evidence is shown, the safety educator use fear sparingly.

A fear or scare can shake people out of indifference and apathy toward productive change, and sometimes the use of shock techniques seems justified and necessary. However, in safety education, the use of fear to change attitudes can backfire because fear that generates apprehension can be destructive.

Use of Rules

Typical safety rules are:

1   While hunting see that the safety catch is ON.

2   Wear a life jacket while water skiing.

3   Clear a campfire area at least four feet in diameter.

4   Scuba dive only in parties of two or more.

5   Be sure to sleep with all bedroom doors closed.

6   Store all sharp tools out of the reach of youngsters.

7   Open garage doors when running a vehicle motor inside.

All are admirable. All are in positive terms. Moreover, safety rules such as these usually represent the major causes of accidents: they identify how people are usually injured while in violation of a safety rule. To illustrate, studies of scuba-diving fatalities indicate that most were the result of a safety rule violation. This is probably true in all accident types.

A problem with safety rules is that they are at the lowest cognitive level. There is nothing wrong with the lowest cognitive level or the acquisition of knowledge, but if this is all we are asking of students, we probably should set our sights somewhat higher.

Criteria for determining the appropriateness of using safety rules are:

1   Does the safety rule seem relevant?
2   Is the rule attractive?
3   Can student performance of the safety rule be evaluated satisfactorily?
4   Is the rule accurate in terms of research findings?

The lowest cognitive level of learning, where safety rules lie, may have no bearing upon the affective level of learning. For example, a student may know that a certain specific safe behavior is best and should be followed, but the affective domain will determine whether he follows the safety rule of the lowest cognitive level. The student may know the rule, but if he chooses not to follow the rule, the time and effort expended for safety instruction is wasted.

Another problem with safety rule usage is that if all specific rule listings were compiled they would form several books of encyclopedic size, and even then such listings would probably be incomplete.

Many accidents result because no rule or regulation has ever been stated or taught. Pulling down a garage door with fingers in the gaps between the horizontal boards, rather than using the handle, is an example. The boards close down on the fingertips like the jaws of a vice. There may be rules or a sign someplace warning against such an act, but it's rather doubtful. Rules can't cover all of the numerous human encounters with agents in the environment that are capable of producing physical trauma.

It is becoming increasingly apparent that the way to influence a person's behavior is to help him develop clear concepts of the objects and events which make up his world. There is evidence to support the idea that good thinking and good decisions come from the possession of clear concepts, rather than from specific training in the making of decisions.

The person who can successfully achieve avoidance of accidents must know essential facts about thousands of things in the world. Every blank spot in his safety knowledge is a potential barrier to the attainment of some desire, and every bit of false knowledge he possesses is a potential source of failure and frustration for some objective he may try to accomplish. He is more accident susceptible because of blank spots in safety knowledge and/or the possession of false knowledge.

Woodruff makes note of a series of studies that have led to a recognition of concepts as "the major mediating variable in human decision making and purposive behavior."[8] The actions individuals take are determined largely by their concepts. Therefore, replacing safety rules with conceptual statements is recommended. Listed below are examples of how to change a safety rule into a conceptual statement:

safety rules	to	conceptual statements
1 Clean up litter and junk at home so it won't accidentally catch on fire.		1 Fires start when something that burns (e.g., litter), something hot (e.g., children playing with matches), and air come together.
2 Wear a life jacket while water skiing.		2 Life jackets support a person who may be a poor swimmer or who may be in tiring water situations (e.g., water skiing),

Cognitive Dissonance

Generally, people are consistent in their behavior; however, there is an inconsistency sometimes between what a person knows and the behavior pattern he chooses to follow. We call this *cognitive dissonance*. For example, many people believe that the driver of an automobile should wear a safety belt, but a sizable number of people who believe this do not actually fasten safety belts (70 percent, according to the National Safety Council).[9] Thus, dissonance exists between their beliefs and their behavior.[10]

Values Clarification Techniques[11]

How does an educator teach attitudes? Three techniques are often cited. One is to teach correct concepts and principles and then let the student choose to follow the better ways to behave. Another is to set proper driving models and examples, following the belief that attitudes are caught and not taught. A third technique is to have group discussion with an exploration into feelings, values, and attitudes.

Perhaps there is nothing more frustrating to a teacher than to read in a curriculum guide or a lesson plan—"Discuss: The Effects of Alcohol on Driving" or "Discuss How Emotions Affect Driving." The problem remains—how to discuss.

Overtly, driver education has emphasized cognitive content in the classroom and psychomotor skills in the laboratory phases. Driver educators have attempted a variety of techniques for the affective level. They hold discussions in the hope that values and attitudes will be favorably influenced. They agree with the "good" and question the "bad." They assign a chapter in the textbook and pose "thought" questions. They select and use films and filmstrips.

These teaching techniques have one thing in common. They do have affective input for students. But they have something else in common. None focuses on helping students become aware of their own feelings or attitudes. Without this insight, there can be no improvement in attitudes or values, or reinforcement of good values and attitudes.

Are you looking for a refreshing approach for student involvement and group interaction? Do you want a better way of influencing attitudes? The approach suggested here will give a teacher added tools for what probably is the most important and most difficult area in teaching—value and attitudes.

Value-clarifying strategies described below include:

1   Value Sheets
2   Value Ranking
3   Value Continuum
4   Reaction Statements
5   Agree or Disagree Statements
6   Case Situation

Value Sheets.   A value sheet is a provocative, often controversial, statement designed to stir up strong feelings. Ideas for value sheets often come from essays, quotations, newspaper accounts, poetry, or song lyrics. If the quote or statement does not stimulate the student—positively or negatively—it will make a weak value sheet. The design of this strategy prohibits neutrality.

Each student is given a copy of the provocative statement. After the stimulator, a series of three to six "you-centered" questions are asked: "What is your reaction?" "What are the implications for your own life?" Questions should not be moralizing; they should not have an implied right or wrong answer. The value sheet strategy is usually inappropriate for discussions. The most effective use of value sheets is to have each student respond to the questions in writing, privately and deliberately.

A sample of a value sheet follows:

heart attack victim saves woman from submerged auto as 12 bystanders ignore screams for help

Jim U. has serious heart trouble, but that didn't stop him from saving a trapped woman whose car was overturned in a murky canal—while a dozen bystanders ignored her screams for help.

Mr. U., who can't work because of three recent heart attacks, was going home from a doctor's appointment when he saw a crowd gathering by a canal.

"As I drove by, I looked in the canal and saw a car. At least a dozen people were just standing around," said Mr. U.

"I asked if anyone was still inside. There were four or five guys standing nearby with their hands in their pockets. One said: 'Yeah, there's someone inside the car.' I asked how he knew. He replied: 'Oh, we heard her screaming'."

With no thought of his illness, Mr. U. flung off his shoes and shirt and plunged into the canal. "The windows were rolled up and the doors were jammed by the muddy canal bottom," Mr. U. said. "I heard the woman scream twice, then she stopped."

"Finally I got one of the doors open a little. Water started rushing into the car. It was all black inside and I couldn't see anything." The woman lay helplessly pinned by the steering wheel after her car spun out of control, rolling over the embankment and ending on its roof in the canal.

"I leaned into the car, grabbed her legs and started pulling, but water kept rushing in so fast that we both began drowning," he said. "Finally, I dragged her out feet first. She had lost consciousness and was turning blue. At last, some guys came down and helped me pull her onto the bank. She wasn't breathing, and I gave her mouth-to-mouth resuscitation."

1 Do you think that getting involved pays?

2 Why should people "get involved" when the public has paid and assigned others (e.g., policemen, firemen, etc.) to do so?

3 Would most individuals know how to help—even if they wanted to?

4 Are you willing to help an accident victim? Do you think you are capable of helping? How could you increase your ability to assist others?

5 How would you feel if you didn't assist an accident victim who later died, but could have been saved with your assistance?

Value Ranking.   In exercises based on value ranking, a student is given or prepares a number of items to rate from desirable to undesirable, or from undesirable to desirable.

Ranking of values tends to nudge students; and, of course, students need this nudging. In such rankings there is usually no one "correct" ranking—a factor that should be stressed during the exercise.

When the students have completed a ranking exercise, the teacher can ask them to review their choices and rerank their top choices if they wish to do so. They can then be asked to make a speech or write a composition about what all have in common, or they can make general statements of their positions and what they can or are willing to do about it.

Examples of value ranking follow:

1 Rank according to the driving practice most dangerous.
_____speeding too fast
_____driving left of center
_____failure to yield right of way

_____passing stop sign
_____disregarding signal
_____improper overtaking of another vehicle
_____following too closely

2   Rank according to who are the worst drivers.
_____men
_____women
_____men and women over 65 years of age
_____teenagers

3   Rank according to why people drink and drive.
_____peer pressure
_____show off
_____need to drive to and from drinking place
_____immaturity

4   Rank according to those you would like legal action taken against:
_____social drinking driver
_____problem drinking driver
_____drug abusing driver
_____driver convicted of previous manslaughter
_____underaged driver

5   If you knew that a certain person was a hit-and-run driver, rank according to how you would react:
_____keep the information to yourself
_____notify legal authorities
_____tell your friends
_____tell your parents
_____blackmail him

6   If you were a passenger and the driver was recklessly driving, rank according to what you would do:
_____do nothing
_____ask to get out at the next street corner if he doesn't drive better
_____tell him to drive safer
_____joke about the poor driving
_____offer to drive

7   Rank according to the degree of risk for any individual who engages in them:
_____driving a car
_____drag racing
_____riding a motorcycle
_____playing football
_____use of marijuana
_____sky diving
_____mountain climbing
_____bullfighting
_____smoking cigarettes

Value Continuum.   Controversial issues usually are identified by polarity and either/or type of thinking. To aid students in seeing issues as having varying degrees of alternative choices between two divergent views, value continuums offer an exercise that helps.

Students place a check where they stand on the value continuum line. Afterward, they are asked to defend and express their positions.

Examples of value continuums follow:

mandatory motorcycle helmets _/ _/ _/ _/ _ don't make helmets mandatory

require use of safety belt   _/ _/ _/ _/ _ no requirements on safety belt use

small car safest   _/ _/ _/ _/ _ large car safest

driver license at age 18   _/ _/ _/ _/ _driver license at age 14

Reaction Statements.   In most areas of driver and safety education, one can find statements that are provocative. These statements can be used to end a classroom period, and it will be discovered that students are often still discussing them after the bell rings ending the class period.

These statements can also be used to spark classroom discussions. The teacher can begin a class session by writing two or three of these statements on the chalkboard and asking the class to vote on them. A discussion follows on why they voted as they did.

The following statements represent ideas that could be utilized:

1   The driving age should be 18 years.

2   High school driver education isn't effective.

3   Women are worse drivers than men.

4   Teenagers are the "safest" drivers.

5   Having a driver's license makes you an adult.

6   Showing-off in a car is a way of proving yourself.

7   The name of "motorcycles" should be changed to "murdercycles."

8   A really good driver does not assume risks.

9   Those owners of cars with painted racing stripes will drive as though they are on the race track.

10   Traffic accidents will happen anyway; let's forget education and stress protecting the car occupants more.

Agree-Disagree Statements.   A favorite technique of the author's which has been used for many years is to develop a listing of either belief statements or factual statements. This may resemble the reaction statement technique. The teacher allows time in class for each student to respond by agreeing or disagreeing with each statement. Then the students are formed into small groups of five to six students and instructed that each group is to reach a consensus on the factual information statements. After all the groups have finished, the teacher gives the correct answers to the factual information statements and instructs the students to mark those statements on which they would like more elaboration and clarification.

Examples of factual information statements in driver and safety education are:

1   Smaller vehicles can stop in less time and distance than larger ones.
2   Pumping the brakes helps stop a car more quickly on dry pavement.
3   Studded tires can help stop a vehicle on ice.
4   Bicyclists and equestrians should ride on the left-hand side of the road.
5   Reduce the tire pressure a little before you drive fast on a hot day.
6   Carbon monoxide gas can be seen in the smoke from a car's exhaust.

Examples of belief statements in driver and safety education are:

1   Driver education saves lives.
2   Traffic accidents result mainly from a "loose nut behind the wheel."
3   There is usually just one cause for an accident.
4   There are people who are consistently being injured because they are accident prone.
5   Marijuana is not as bad as alcohol for a driver.
6   Penalties for poor driving (e.g., working at a cemetery or in an emergency room) do not change driving behavior.
7   Scare techniques (e.g., gory movies of accident scenes) cause people to reflect upon their driving and thus become better drivers.
8   People should not be forced to protect themselves (e.g., mandatory safety belts).

Case Situation.   Another activity presents a case situation (usually in one or two paragraphs) followed by forced alternatives for what the student would do if he were in the situation. The procedure is to allow each student to read the case situation individually, then to mark his or her choice(s) among the alternatives. After this, a discussion centers upon which of the choices is best and why. An additional help is for the teacher to be able to document which of the choices may be the best. This is given at the end of the class period.

An example of a case situation follows:

You are the parent of Steve who was apprehended for drunken driving. He was fined and had his license revoked. As Steve's parent, which would you do?

_____ 1   Take away his driving privileges for three months.

_____ 2   Cut off his allowance.

_____ 3   Restrict him to 9:00 p.m. curfew for three months.

_____ 4   Instruct him not to see the friends who were with him again.

_____ 5   Make him pay his own fine by working.

_____ 6   Force him to do extra chores around the house as an additional penalty.

_____ 7   Just discuss the situation with him without punishment.

_____ 8   Tell him it is okay if he drinks as long as he doesn't drink and drive.

_____ 9   Let him know you are disappointed in his behavior.

_____10   Emphasize to him that he has shamed the family name.

_____11   Allow him no more driving privileges with the family car(s) even after his license has been reinstated.

_____12   Others: ....

The preceding represent only a few techniques for values clarification. It is strongly urged that the interested teacher obtain both _Values and Teaching_[12] and _Values Clarification_[13] for more ideas and techniques. These books are hitting education in a manner similar to that of Robert Mager's _Preparing Instructional Objectives_ during the 1960s. Within other disciplines several articles have appeared in their professional literature (e.g., _School Health Review_ and _Journal of School Health_).

Adaptation to safety education and most other subject areas is quite easy. It should be stressed, however, that the total methodology is not as simple as it may appear. Lest anyone think that values clarification is a series of gimmicks and games, be assured that it is a way of teaching, a process that should continually involve students in every class. It is not something to be used when things are dull or as a filler. There is a danger that in the hands of the "busy-minded," directive teacher, it will be a means of forcing the student unyieldingly along another rigid path to nondiscovery.

Values clarification exercises will be effective only to the extent that the teachers share in them and practice the process themselves. Teachers who have experienced values clarification for themselves, and who use it in their teaching, witness their students coming alive as both persons and learners.

Safety Instruction Effectiveness

Evidence to date indicates that safety instruction can be effective. For example, the Utah Fish and Game Department has shown through its mandatory gun-safety training program that firearm accidents can be dramatically reduced. Statistics for 1957, when the program was inaugurated, show that of 165,081 hunters who went afield, 22 were fatally injured. As the program gained momentum, the number of deaths among hunters dropped to twelve in 1959, to seven in 1960, and to five in 1961. Since 1961, the number has fluctuated between four and eight per year. The total number of fatal and nonfatal hunting accidents plummeted from 126 in 1957 to about an annual rate of 20 in recent years. The incidence of juvenile hunting accidents dropped even more spectacularly, plunging from 93 annually to as few as three or four per year. During the same period, the number of licensed adult hunters doubled and the number of juvenile nimrods increased fivefold.

Driver education in American high schools is at present our most popular, most widely applied, and probably most expensive safety instructional program. This course usually consists of both classroom and laboratory phases. In recent years, the majority of United States public high schools provide such a course to students approaching the legal driving age.

One criticism of high school driver education courses is that there is no research evidence in terms of accident and driving violation records to prove the value of the course. Dozens of studies have been made which generally support driver education programs.

A report of the *Secretary's Advisory Committee on Traffic Safety* to the U.S. Department of Health, Education and Welfare (known as the "Moynihan Report") was presented by the press as representing an anti-driver education position. One statement from this report bears repeating and offers a rebuttal to those who oppose driver education:

Now, at the hopeful beginnings of a new era, it becomes necessary to give a new cast to driver education. Although there is no conclusive proof as to the comparative effectiveness of various driver education techniques or, for that matter, the whole of present driver education practice, there is even less proof of the efficacy and value of any alternatives to present practices for communicating to the young person the rudiments of how to handle a car in modern traffic, and the associated social responsibilities. But operational driver education programs must continue. The problem is no different in principle than that for education in general. We have to continue with present systems even while recognized needed improvements are being studied. One would hardly advocate a moratorium on all schooling while looking for proof of better methods.[14]

We now find many who say that the emphasis should be diverted from educational efforts concerned with averting accidents to those efforts which assume accidents will occur and place emphasis on prevention of further loss through the widespread use of passive restraint systems (air bag in automobiles), collapsible steering wheels, and other innovations. Use of these devices will certainly reduce the number of deaths and critical injuries sustained in motor-vehicle crashes.

Walter Kohl offers another very discerning suggestion with regard to the placement of emphasis:

Building more reliable devices, safer cars, better highways, is all to the good, but as one observer said, "it is similar to the attempt of reducing the occurrence of crime by making it harder to steal, or to kill, rather than by improving the social climate." The attitude of people is the basic issue. This attitude cannot be managed, but only improved slowly by the individual's acceptance of a different set of values.[15]

It would seem that through educational efforts we can truly affect attitudes. The critics of safety education programs do not intend to eliminate safety courses but believe these programs should rely on scientific evaluation for their justification rather than on mere "common sense." Any safety educator should want the same.

NOTES

[1]A. F. SCHAPLOWSKY, "What You Don't Know Can Hurt You," *School and College Safety,* National Safety Congress Transactions (Chicago: National Safety Council, 1961), p. 17.

[2]J. DUKE ELKOW, "College and University Advanced Courses in Safety Education," *School and College Safety,* National Safety Congress Transactions (Chicago: National Safety Council, 1961), p. 52.

[3]W. JAMES POPHAM AND EVA L. BAKER, *Systematic Instruction* (Englewood Cliffs, N.J.: Prentice-Hall, Inc., 1970), p. 13.

[4]Adapted from Robert F. Mager, *Preparing Instructional Objectives* (Palo Alto, Calif.: Fearon Publishers, 1962), p. 53, by permission of the publisher.

[5]Ibid., p. 11.

[6]Adapted from Robert F. Mager and Kenneth M. Beach, Jr., *Developing Vocational Instruction* (Palo Alto, Calif: Fearon Publishers, 1967), p. 55, by permission of the publisher.

[7]WILLIAM E. TARRANTS, "Removing the Blind Spot in Safety Education Teacher Preparation," *School and College Safety,* National Safety Congress Transactions (Chicago: National Safety Council, 1965), p. 108.

[8]ASAHEL D. WOODRUFF, "The Use of Concepts in Teaching and Learning," *Journal of Teacher Education* (March 1964), pp. 81–99.

[9]National Safety Council, *Accident Facts* (Chicago: National Safety Council, 1970), p. 53.

[10]See Leon Festinger, *The Theory of Cognitive Dissonance* (Evanston, Ill.: Row and Peterson, 1957), for more information.

[11]Though this section pertains specifically to driver education, it can be adapted to all areas of safety education.

[12]LOUIS E. RATHS, MERRILL HARMIN, AND SIDNEY SIMON, *Values and Teaching* (Columbus: Merrill Publishing Co., 1966).

[13]SIDNEY SIMON, LELAND W. HOWE, AND HOWARD KIRSCHENBAUM, *Values Clarification: A Handbook of Practical Strategies for Teachers and Students* (New York: Hart Publishing Co., Inc., 1972).

[14]U.S. Department of Health, Education and Welfare, *Report to the Secretary's Advisory Committee on Traffic Safety* (Washington, D.C.: U.S. Government Printing Office, 1968), p. 63.

[15]WALTER H. KOHL, "Can Accidents Be Managed?" *Journal of the American Society of Safety Engineers*, XIII, No. 11 (November 1968), p. 12.

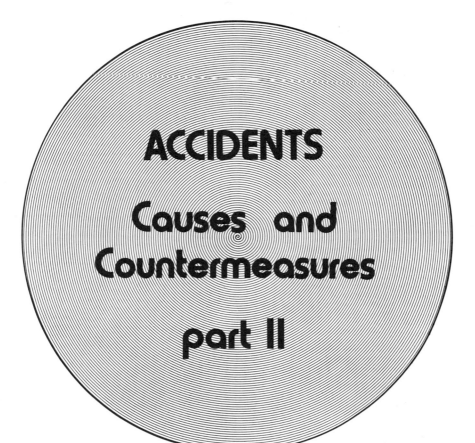

ACCIDENTS

Causes and
Countermeasures

part II

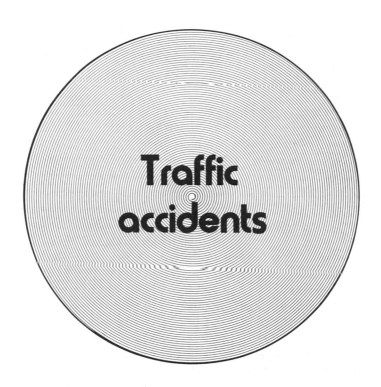

Traffic accidents

Characteristics and Causes

8 Precise pinpointing of reasons for the high rate of traffic deaths and injury losses is not possible. However, some tentative explanations can be offered of those forces that contribute heavily to traffic accident losses.

Role of Alcohol. The drinking driver is the foremost factor in the traffic accident problem. It is well known that excessive drinking and driving are a lethal combination. Just how lethal probably has been underestimated in previous studies and analyses. Reports coming in from accident-investigating teams, medical examiners, and other sources show that though problem drinkers constitute under 10 percent of the driving population, alcohol is involved in more than 50 percent of traffic fatalities, and that the hardcore cases are responsible for at least two-thirds of them.[1]

Surveys carried out in several states indicate that during the evening and late night hours, some 4 percent of drivers have a blood alcohol concentration (BAC) in excess of the established intoxication level of 0.10 percent.[2] This means that one out of every 25 cars on the highway at

127

those times is driven by a drunk—not by a person who has had a drink or two, but a drunk. By any reckoning, this amounts to a version of Russian roulette.

The tragic effects of the involvement of alcohol in driving was extensively documented in a report to Congress by the U.S. Department of Transportation.[3] The use of alcohol by drivers and pedestrians leads to some 25,000 deaths and a total of at least 800,000 crashes in the United States each year. Especially tragic is the fact that much of the loss in life, limb, and property damage involves completely innocent parties.

The problem was first identified in 1904, and was first shown to be serious in 1924. Since then, every competent investigation has demonstrated that the use of alcohol is a very major source of highway crashes, especially of those most violent. In fact, it contributes to about half of all highway deaths and to appreciable percentages of the far more numerous nonfatal crashes.

The role of alcohol is well illustrated by a study made in Vermont.[4] A research team returned to the sites of fatal and serious crashes on the same hour and day of the week when a crash had occurred, and persuaded a random sample of motorists to take a breath test. The investigators found that only 1 in 50 of these drivers could be classified as impaired, in contrast to one of every two drivers responsible for crashes. Thus, half of all drivers at fault in these fatal crashes come from 2 percent of the driving population who had been drinking heavily.

Alcoholics and other problem drinkers, who constitute but a small minority of the general population, account for a very large part of the overall problem.[5] Their involvement in highway crashes and violations after drinking heavily is one of the many tragic derivatives of their deviancy and pathological behavior in society as a whole, and to be dealt with properly must be approached in the larger context.

Fatal and other crashes of teenagers and young adults also frequently involve hazardous amounts of alcohol.[6] Adults who use alcohol, but not identified as problem drinkers by the research to date, are also frequently involved. On the basis of considerable scientific evidence, light drinking, although shown to have adverse effects, is not the source of most of the problem, but its exact role is at present unknown because of insufficient research. It should be clear that the social drinker is not "off the hook" for accident involvement, and it should be remembered that drinking and driving do not mix.

The probability of being involved in a crash can be inferred by comparing the blood alcohol concentration of the population-at-risk (control group of drivers) with the blood alcohol concentration distribution of the drivers actually involved in these crashes for which the control drivers were sampled.

Figure 8–1 shows the relative probability of being responsible for initiating a fatal crash according to the blood alcohol concentration level. With blood alcohol concentrations between 0.05 and 0.10 percent, the probability of fatal crash responsibility begins to increase appreciably, such that at a BAC of 0.10 percent a driver would be seven times more likely to be responsible for a fatal crash than he would with no alcohol. The hazard curve rises very sharply above this lower limit for driving-while-intoxicated (DWI) violation in most states (0.10 percent), such that at a BAC of 0.15 percent a driver would be 25 times more likely to be responsible for a fatal crash, at 0.18 percent he would be 60 times more likely, and at 0.20 percent (namely, at the average BAC found among convicted DWIs and among fatally injured drivers who would have been eligible for a DWI conviction) he would be at least 100 times more likely to be responsible for a fatal crash than if he had not been drinking at all.

The implications of this are very clear: Concentrations of 0.08 percent or higher are incompatible with safe driving, and the higher the concentration, the greater the incompatibility.

Speed.   While the use of alcohol undoubtedly has emerged as a dominant, if not the primary, factor contributing to the causation of crashes, the vehicle is the dominant factor determining the severity of bodily injuries once a crash occurs. Its structural strength, interior padding, seat belts and shoulder harnesses (when worn by the occupants), and the placement of knobs and projections on the instrument panel undoubtedly determine crash survivability. The highest rates of potentially fatal injuries occur to both passengers and drivers when their heads or chests hit the steering assembly, instrument panel, or windshield. Without the protection of proper "packaging," a rider in a crash continues moving at the pre-crash speed of the vehicle and, consequently, hits some part of the vehicle at this speed (called the "second crash").

With the energy crisis came mandatory speed limit reductions and citizen concern over gasoline conservation. With the reduction in the speed limit came a dramatic reduction in traffic fatalities. Speed by itself does not cause more crashes. Excessive speed, improper use of alcohol, vehicle defects, the increase in vehicles and miles traveled, plus many other factors are undoubtedly associated with crash involvement rates. However, a rise does occur in the number of fatalities in crashes

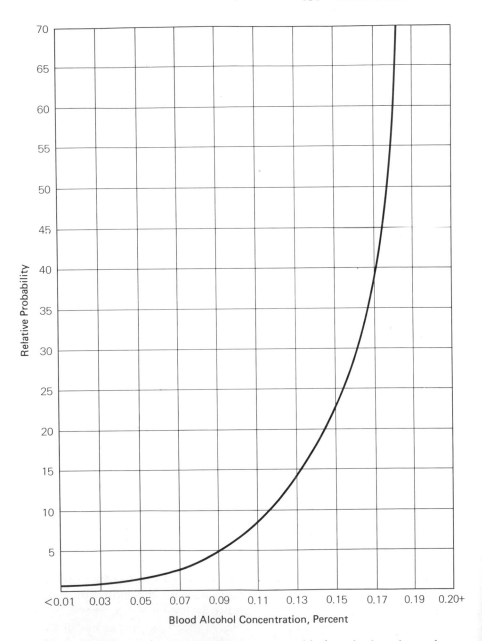

figure 8–1 Relative probability of being responsible for a fatal crash as a function of blood alcohol concentration. Source: M.W. Perrine, J.A. Waller, and L.S. Harris, *Alcohol and Highway Safety: Behavioral and Medical Aspects,* U.S. Department of Transportation, NHTSA Technical Report, DOT HS-800-599, 1971.

with the increase in high speed crashes and their resultant severity. Three out of ten fatalities involve vehicles being driven too fast. Yet studies indicate that more than 50 percent of all accidents happen at speeds under 30 miles per hour.

Vehicle Condition.   Another major factor contributing to traffic death tolls is the state of repair of vehicles in use on the highway. About half of the vehicles in use are estimated to be deficient in one or more aspects of safety performance. These deficiencies are due to normal deterioration with use, improper maintenance, inadequate initial design, or faulty construction.

It is self-evident, for example, that brake failure while a vehicle is in motion almost invariably results in a crash. However, this could be readily overlooked in the subsequent crash investigation. Current routine crash reporting often tends to overlook or understate the role played by vehicle factors in causing crashes and casualties, since most investigations focus on the legal aspects of human fault. In some cases the extent of the damage misleads investigators to think that a defect — if discovered at all — is the result of the crash rather than its cause. It is concluded that much if not most of the crash causation associated with the condition of the vehicle is not being identified and reported.

Medical Conditions.   Research has shown that drivers with epilepsy, cardiovascular disease, or diabetes have substantially higher crash and traffic citation rates than do persons of similar age without these conditions. These facts are mentioned specifically because there is a tendency among some safety practitioners, researchers, and others to treat all deviant driving behavior as if it were subject to change by motivation of one sort or another. These people often completely overlook the fact that some forms of behavior are not subject to modification. The most highly motivated driver with epilepsy or cardiovascular disease will still have trouble on the highway if his physiologic mechanisms are not functioning properly. Furthermore, drivers with chronic medical conditions often appear to have crashes in which the medical impairment, although present, is not clinically obvious. Thus, crashes involving brief episodes of altered consciousness may be attributed to "inattention."

Attitudes.   Regardless of the definition of attitude used, attitudes indicate an individual predisposition to act in a certain manner and are important in determining driver behavior. Actually, little is known about attitudes and driver behavior, and much more work is needed in this area. Research shows that attitude change is possible and that some groups of high-risk drivers can be identified in advance for insurance-rating purposes.

Effects

The automobile, in spite of demonstrable gains in safety, remains a hazardous, expensive, and often tragic (though necessary and convenient) form of transportation.

The traffic accident problem is growing more rapidly than the capability of countermeasures implemented to deal with it. The grim statistics unmistakably highlight the fact that in traffic deaths there is a destructive problem equal in size and complexity to other social ills such as crime, disease, and poverty:

1   Traffic injuries exceed by 10 times all violent criminal acts combined, including homicide, armed robbery, rape, riot, and assault.

2   Traffic crashes rob society of nearly as many productive working years as heart disease and more than are lost to cancer and stroke. Only about one out of five expected man years of life lost to heart disease is in the age interval between 20 and 65; in contrast, seven out of ten man years lost to traffic deaths are in the productive years between 20 and 65.

Danish investigators report a study involving the follow-up of persons who were injured in traffic accidents.[7] They wanted to find out what happens to persons over a number of years after they have been injured. Too often we tend to focus only on the present and immediate effects of traffic accidents rather than the long-range effects. These investigators found that all of the victims in the traffic accidents studied were still alive, although about one-half had been injured about 15 years earlier and the remaining had been hurt about 11 years before the study. Only persons who had been hospitalized for treatment were included in the investigation.

It was found that long periods of disability were more common with pelvic, leg, back, arm, and chest injuries. Disability of longer duration than one year was most frequent in persons with back injuries. A near 75 percent of the injured persons were able to return to the same kind of work they had been doing prior to their accident. In summary, long periods of hospitalization, months or years of disability, and changes in work capacities can be expected for those injured in traffic accidents without fatal consequences.

Vulnerability

The evidence shows that automobiles are especially dangerous for male drivers under age 25. On the basis of public health statistics in the United States, motor-vehicle death rates are at least twice as high for young men aged 20–24 as for older men in their mid-40s. Furthermore, traffic mortality rates since the 1930s have risen faster in the age bracket 15–24 than for any other 10-year age bracket. Pelz and Schuman found that young males aged 18 or 19 had substantially more crashes and received more tickets and warnings than did men either younger or older, and these differences remained after traffic exposure.[8] These researchers found that regardless of whether young men learned to drive early or late, they still showed a clear peak around age 18 or 19.

Kraus et. al. found the following factors more frequent in young drivers with high-accident risk: (1) failed one or more grades in or before grade 8 or had been in a vocational high school course, (2) became a regular cigarette smoker at or before age 16, (3) had first full-time employment exclusive of school vacation time at or before age 17 and before obtaining a driving license, and (4) had been charged with a criminal offense. Furthermore, those who had been in a one-vehicle accident showed still higher frequencies of these factors.[9]

Klein's view is that adolescent drivers are not adults.[10] He believes they can be expected to drive in a deviant fashion, but their deviant driving may conform closely to the norms and values of their own (deviant) group. Thus, according to Klein, efforts to change their driving toward that of the adult population involves persuading them to deviate from their group norms and expectations.

Researchers have found, too, that fathers with numerous traffic convictions tend to have sons who have numerous traffic convictions.[11] How a young man drives seems to be influenced more by his family than by driver education or the actions of police and courts.

Threat

Certain atmospheric or climatic conditions may affect accident frequency by influencing human behavior as well as by creating specific environmental hazards. For example, cold temperatures produce slippery roads and frosted windshields. Cold also results in impaired dexterity and muscular control in persons with cold extremities.

Toxic substances are another factor. For example, carbon monoxide adversely affects people and may go unnoticed by a driver. Carbon monoxide may come from a vehicle's defective exhaust system or through the ventilation system from the exhausts of preceding vehicles.

Low levels of illumination result in traffic accidents. In the United States, over half of the fatalities are at night. Tinted windshields, wet weather (rain, snow, sleet), and sunglasses all affect vision during night-time hours.

Road conditions are an important factor in traffic safety, even though most traffic accidents happen on dry road surfaces. Skidding on wet or icy roads results in vehicle control loss and then injury losses. Highway signs and markers have also adversely affected driving performance. Pictorial signs result in a better understanding of the sign's meaning and warning assuming their proper placement.

An argument often heard is over the issue of small vs. large cars and their relative safety. Research indicates that the likelihood of severe injury or fatality is greater for small car occupants than for large car occupants.[12] However, another study concerning the incidence of accidents (crashes) found no relationship between vehicle size and the frequency of accidents.[13] In other words, small cars are not involved in any more accidents than large cars, but the occupants of small vehicles if involved in an accident are more likely to receive an injury.

It has been said by highway officials that if there is a dangerous obstacle near the roadway, sooner or later it will be struck. The streets and highways are dotted with them — bridge abutments, guard rails designed for strength rather than safety, and sign and light poles embedded in concrete are only a few of the most obvious. To these add the temporary hazards caused by construction work.

About two out of three deaths occur in rural places, but injuries occur more frequently in urban places. Freeways have been shown to be safer than other road types.

Accidents by hour of day vary by day of week. Fatal accidents occur most frequently during the following hours: weekdays, except Friday — evening rush; Friday — late night; Saturday — late afternoon and night; Sunday — early morning. Motor-vehicle death totals vary sharply for different days of the week and different months of the year. Totals run above average from Friday through Sunday, and during the last half of the calendar year. Fatalities are at their lowest levels in January and February. Deaths increase during the summer months and remain at this general level the rest of the year.

The highest death rates are in states of the southeast and Rocky Mountain areas. The leading causes of death are ejection from the vehicle, impacts with the door or side of the car, impacts with the steering assembly, and impacts with the instrument panel. Ejection comes through open doors, open convertible roofs, through windshields, through side windows, and through a roof that may be ripped off. Impact with the side of the car occurs not from striking the doors but from having the side of the car collapse inward on the victim. Steering assemblies pose a danger since the steering shaft points directly at the driver's heart and lungs — it is just like a spear. Fatal injuries sustained in instrument-panel impacts are more often to the head than to any other area of the body. Most injuries resulting in death are to the face and the head.

Countermeasures: Pre-Crash

Alcohol. U.S. Alcohol Countermeasure Program.   In the United States efforts are being made through the National Highway Traffic Safety Administration's Alcohol Countermeasures Program. This program involves a series of community projects, public education, manpower development, and research activity. The Alcohol Safety Action Program is clearly the most extensive and ambitious of any program heretofore. The NHTSA has placed alcohol countermeasures high on its list of priority efforts. Within most states an alcohol safety project has been established and heavily funded (millions of dollars) by the

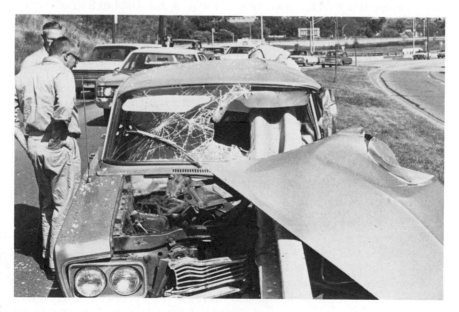

figure 8–2   Guard rail? A common example of highway "safety" design that creates rather than reduces danger, this blunt-end guardrail speared a car through its passenger compartment. Photo from the *Baltimore News-American*, courtesy Insurance Institute for Highway Safety.

NHTSA. Most of these projects run for about three years; after that it is hoped that state and local governments will assume financial responsibility for continued support of the program.

The National Traffic Safety Administration program is based on the concept that alcohol intake by drivers, especially excessive use of alcohol by problem drinkers, is an important key to accident loss reduction. The main efforts are centered around three concepts. The first is identification of the problem drinker through selective enforcement, improved evidence, court records, community agencies, insurance companies, and licensing agencies. The second involves the decision on courses of action by prosecutors, courts, probation departments, licensing agencies, and medical advisors, using such methods as pre-sentence investigation, prelicensing examination, court referral to treatment, license restriction, voluntary treatment, and driver reeducation. The third concept is action to reduce driving after excessive drinking, to reduce drinking to safe levels, and to evaluate the effectiveness of countermeasures taken.

More information is needed on the success of this program. Reports indicate that arrests for alcohol-related offenses are up, and convictions are approaching the 100 percent mark. Also, that traffic fatalities in which alcohol is a factor are down at most of the Alcohol Safety Action Project sites.

It is often suggested that drivers impaired by alcohol should let a passenger drive. Waller found that the passenger is usually equally unfit to drive and is a better driving risk than the driver in only about one out of four cases.[14]

Driessen and Bryk list more than 100 alcohol countermeasures. See Appendix Table 1 for this listing.

Legal Control. Some countries enforce severe penalties for drunken driving. In Finland, for example, one drunken-driving conviction carries a mandatory sentence of three months' labor on a public project. European laws in this area and the enforcement of them tend to be stricter than in the United States. Table 8–1 shows comparative minimum blood alcohol concentrations (BAC) and the penalties for violation.

In the United States at least half of the fatal traffic accidents involve alcohol. Norway reports 15 percent, Sweden reports 10 to 12 percent, and in Denmark the figure is 10 percent. In Czechoslovakia a driver who has consumed any alcohol and drives is subject to arrest. In France, with the highest per capita alcohol consumption in the world, the blood alcohol concentration is 0.08 percent—the same as the lowest BAC in the United States (Utah and Idaho have 0.08 percent BAC). In Finland one drunken-driving conviction carries a mandatory sentence of three months in jail or in a public work project.

The British Road Safety Act of 1967 has drawn worldwide attention. At first it reduced the number of automobile accident casualties, but this effect appears to have been temporary. The act's deterrent power quickly declined because of an unexpectedly small number of arrests. Ross found that the sharp reduction in deaths and injuries which followed enactment of the law was the result of an actual decrease in drunken driving.[15] This decrease was caused by the widespread fear of arrest and conviction under the law, which required a one-year license suspension for drivers found with a blood alcohol concentration over 0.08 percent.

The act authorized police to demand a breath test of any driver involved in an accident and any driver whom they reasonably suspected of having committed a moving violation or of having alcohol in his body. According to Ross, police saw heavy use of the roadside breath test as a threat to good relations with the public. Therefore, they tended to administer the tests only in cases involving erratic driving or when they detected alcohol on a driver's breath after stopping him for another traffic law violation. When the public learned that the breathalyzer tests were being given to far fewer drivers than had been expected, the deterrent effect decreased even though the probability of conviction and license suspension remained high for those who failed the test. Modifications in Great Britain should remedy the problem if the modifications include increased police enforcement.

Reports on states with laws reducing legal minimum drinking age to 18 years show an increased traffic death rate.[16]

table 8–1   *European Control of Drinking and Driving*

country	bac	penalty for violation
Britain	0.08%	Fine of 100 pounds and one year suspension of driver's license or up to four months in jail, or both.
Norway	0.05%	One year suspension of driver's license and three weeks in jail. A second offense leads to license revocation for life!
Denmark	0.05%	One and one-half year suspension of license and 20 days in jail.
Sweden	0.05%	Mandatory two year license revocation; three months' imprisonment; insurance cancellation; DWI in accident bears all associated financial loss.
United States	0.08%–0.15%*	Variable, but generally not as severe as above.

*Most states are currently at 0.10%.

source: Gerald J. Driessen and Joseph A. Bryk, "Alcohol Countermeasures: Solid Rock and Shifting Sands," reprinted with permission from the *Journal of Safety Research,* a National Safety Council publication, Volume 5, Number 3 (September 1973), p. 114.

Apprehending Drinking Drivers. One of the problems in dealing with alcohol-related accidents is the fact that the American public tends to tolerate alcohol use and even drunkenness. Remember the last drunk you saw. A chuckle was probably heard by you or perhaps others heard your chuckle or saw your smile after seeing the staggering drunk meandering down a sidewalk. By the way, who gets the loudest laugh in the movies? Of course—the drunk. Academy Awards have been won by movie stars playing the "funny" role of a drunk.

Traffic Violations. Law enforcement officers apprehend drivers who violate the law by speeding or running red lights. Such offenders can be cited for violating a traffic law, but if evidence is available (e.g., alcohol containers, breath odor, etc.), the driver can be arrested for driving while intoxicated.

Traffic Accidents. There are many reasons for automobile crashes and accidents. Ample research studies have correlated the influence of intoxicating liquor with driving inability. Involvement in a crash certainly can lead to a suspicion of impaired ability because of drinking alcohol.

Physical evidence is sought by a law enforcement officer before an arrest. This evidence may be: (1) liquor containers within the car; (2) witnesses who saw a driver drinking alcohol; (3) breath odor, speech clarity, general attitude, etc.; and (4) testing of a suspect by using such procedures as balancing, walking, touching finger to nose, fetching coins, and turning. Videotapes, sound recordings, photographs, and motion pictures are sometimes used to document behavior.

Spot-Checks. An automobile may be searched for alcohol containers on "probable cause"; that is, on reasonable grounds of belief supported by circumstances which would warrant a man to believe that such items were being unlawfully transported in an automobile. In many states the automobile must be forfeited as penalty if liquor is found. If liquor containers are found, an officer may follow a course of action listed in the previous paragraph in search for evidence.

To summarize, an officer can make an arrest for driving while under the influence of intoxicating liquor from evidence gathered at the scene of an accident, after observing illegal driving behavior and/or during a spot-check.

Implied Consent Law. The alcohol concentration in the blood furnishes an excellent measure of the extent of its influence upon a person, and chemical analysis of the blood itself or of the breath is also an accepted method of ascertaining blood alcohol concentration.

Implied consent laws are now common in most states. This law gives the driver, if arrested, a choice. If the individual refuses to give his consent to a chemical test, thus depriving the law enforcement agency of the opportunity to secure evidence of his blood alcohol concentration, action may nevertheless be taken against the person through legal prosecution or by revoking the driver's license. Such action varies from state to state; the right to a hearing on the question of the legality of the arrest or any justification for refusal to submit to a chemical test is generally preserved. In most states, after a hearing, the person's license is revoked with no driving privilege for one year.

Chemical Tests. A chemical test must be preceded by an arrest based upon reasonable grounds for belief that the person was driving while intoxicated (e.g., breath odor, alcohol container, etc.). The choice of test usually lies with the enforcement agency. The driver has no right to choose his own physician or technician for the administration of the test for the police. The driver may be tested by his own physician, if time permits, in addition to the test administered by the law enforcement agency. In many states a prearrest breath test may be administered to help determine whether or not to arrest an individual.

Blood Alcohol Concentration. With the results of the chemical test, the officer's testimony, and other evidence (e.g., videotapes for replay, liquor container, etc.), prosecution of the arrested driver begins.

An important consideration is the blood alcohol concentration as determined from a chemical test. These tests have been used in the United States since the 1920s. The acceptance of chemical tests has led to laws setting presumptive levels for alcohol intoxication. Presumptive levels are based on alcohol concentration in the blood and do not reflect the amount of liquor consumed. In most states 0.10 percent (Utah and Idaho, 0.08 percent) blood alcohol concentration or higher is presumptive evidence that a person is under the influence of intoxicating liquor. This does not mean that persons having levels below 0.10 percent are not under the influence of alcohol. If other evidence indicates that the person is affected to some degree by the alcohol in his body, he still can be charged with being under the influence.

Adjudication. Several courses of action can follow a conviction of guilty of driving while under the influence of alcohol:

1. Alcoholism Clinic. Persons convicted of drunken driving should be individually assessed to determine if they are problem drinkers. Identification of the problem drinker is the greatest obstacle to this plan of action. Ideally, these treatment programs should provide medical, psychological, and social work resources and should involve the support and participation of the problem drinker's family, employer, and other significant persons.

Much information about the expected values of alcoholism treatment programs is available. However, this approach has not been tried on a widespread organized basis, nor has it been scientifically evaluated.

2. *Driver Improvement Schools.* Enforced attendance at driver improvement schools has been popular. The aims of the improvement schools vary. Some schools act as an alternative to a suspended or revoked license. Others aim at reeducating the driver about his automobile skills. Still others are focused upon changing the drinking patterns of the problem drinker who also drives.

Obviously, there isn't any ready-made, single, easy solution to the problem of driving while drinking. The better improvement schools focus their attention upon abstinence from drinking before driving. Nevertheless, drinking is so widespread and socially acceptable in two-thirds of our adult society that many drivers will not abstain as do the other one-third. So these schools aim at the alternatives which a drinker may follow (e.g., arranging for an unimpaired person to do the driving or using other means of transportation).

It must be pointed out that public education doesn't seem to be very effective with the problem drinker or the alcoholic. It is to be hoped that the future will see an educational program that will prove to be successful.

3. *Jail and/or Fine.* In typical states conviction for driving while under the influence of intoxicating liquor may result in imprisonment for one to six months or a fine of $100 to $299, or both. If another person is injured, punishment cannot be for more than one year in jail nor exceed a fine of $1,000. A drinking driver who causes the death of another person is guilty of a felony and can be convicted and punished for one to five years in the state penitentiary.

A conviction for driving while under the influence of alcohol is followed by an automatic revoking of the driver's license for one year. When the license is revoked, the licensee is required to start over and qualify for a new license after the one-year period. In some states a license may be suspended. There is usually automatic restoration of license privileges at the end of the suspension period.

Regretfully, drivers will tend to ignore driving restrictions dispensed by courts or license administrators if they know they can get away with driving while their license is revoked. A study in California showed that 46 percent of the drivers whose licenses were revoked continued to drive. In most states a person driving while his license is revoked or suspended can be imprisoned in jail for up to six months and/or fined up to $299.

Licensing.   The driver licensing system can be an important way of determining who is permitted access to the highways. A driver's license should be earned, not bought, and renewed on merit alone, not by mailing a check.

Properly administered, the licensing process can help assure that only those who qualify continue to drive. In past years, driver licensing and renewal in many states was considered as little more than a formality. When there were fewer cars, a permissive licensing and renewal policy may have been acceptable. Today, such a policy cannot be afforded or tolerated.

With better vision-screening procedures and improved licensing tests (both pencil-paper and in-car), hopefully, will come more respect for the license (not just as a passport to adulthood, e.g., purchasing of alcohol) and greater discrimination as to driving abilities. The driver license examinations provide the states with their only tool to measure the proficiency of drivers. Therefore, these examinations must yield eventually results which can be correlated with driving proficiency as well as with traffic violations and accident records. The licensing procedure should be constructed as an educational device as well as an instrument of skill measurement. Moreover, it should be diagnostic in nature.

Education. The driver is the least predictable of all the traffic components. To improve the driver's safety skills and habits requires research in some very imprecise fields, such as human behavior modification, motivation, risk taking, and education.

In order to teach the beginning driver, or to upgrade the skills of the veteran driver, it is necessary to know exactly what they are supposed to do and how to do it well. These skills are known in driver education as the driving "task" and "objectives." A study has been completed which defines the knowledge, habits, and attitudes the driver must acquire to operate a vehicle skillfully and safely.[17] (See Appendix Table 2.) Based on the task and objectives, the effectiveness of a variety of training programs can now be judged.

The National Highway Safety Act requires that all states provide for comprehensive driver education programs. Effectiveness of these programs as constituted at present is not quantitatively or even qualitatively known.

The driver education course is typically made available to youth as they approach or reach legal driving age and is provided in the classroom and laboratory. Most beginning driver education courses for youth are found in the secondary schools, while some youth and most adults unable to drive may learn through commercial driving schools. Classroom instruction is similar to classroom sessions in other curricular areas. It precedes or is offered concurrently with laboratory instruction. Laboratory instruction allows a direct application of what is learned in the classroom along with other concepts, values, and skills.

The most widely used form of laboratory instruction is that of a teacher instructing two to four students inside a properly equipped driver education car operating on public streets and highways. One student drives while the others observe and sometimes participate by answering questions, recording observations, or evaluating driver behavior.

The other laboratory alternatives are simulation and multiple-car ranges. The driving simulator method of instruction is defined as "a programmed, group instructional system which employs student interaction with filmed driving environments. The system consists of simulator units, teacher control station, and projection package. Through the interaction of system components, including teacher actions, the students develop proper perceptual, judgmental, and behavioral proficiencies as well as procedural responses and, to a lesser degree, manipulative skills."[18]

A list of simulation's advantages includes:[19]

1   Provides emergency driving situations in the safety of the classroom rather than on the highway and thus reduces the possibility of accidents during the training period.

2   Develops good driving attitudes to a greater degree than the use of the dual-control automobile alone.

3   Standardizes course content without lessening the opportunities for teachers to interject personal teaching techniques and express their individuality.

4   Provides a permanent "driving" record (of skills) for each pupil free from the subjective evaluation by the teacher.

5   The time spent in the simulators decreases the accident frequency rate in the dual-control automobile.

6   Has far-reaching values for the physically handicapped pupils and the negligent operator.

7   Arouses the enthusiastic interest of the pupil in this new type of teaching device.

8   The opportunity of effectively supervising and assisting three to four times more pupils than could normally be handled in the dual-control automobile.

9   Provides an opportunity for more drill time in the development of manipulative skills.

10   Allows flexibility in scheduling.

11   More economical.

The multiple-car range is another innovative laboratory method used in driver education. This method permits several automobiles to be operated simultaneously on a special off-street facility, under direction of one or more teachers positioned outside the vehicles. The teacher typically communicates with students by radio.

The strengths of the multiple-car range method include:[20]

1   Makes for more efficient use of teacher time by enabling one teacher to work with more than one student-operated vehicle.

2   Permits an increased amount of practice on manipulative skills under relatively safe conditions.

3   Allows the instructor to devote extra time to students with special problems while more advanced students continue to practice on their own.

4   Tends to promote an increased sense of responsibility and self-reliance among students by permitting solo operation of practice driving vehicles.

5   Enables the teacher to control the learning environment to meet the needs of learners—in particular, traffic patterns can be varied.

6   Enhances quality while increasing quantity and reducing cost of instruction.

Questions have been raised as to the effectiveness of driver education as an accident countermeasure. For years the public has been led to believe that the nation's driver education programs are effective accident countermeasures. In fact the results of over 50 research studies would indicate that "trained drivers" have better driving records than "untrained drivers." However, the poor quality of research design and other factors tend to render the results of these studies suspect. This has led some to declare that:

... it becomes necessary to give a new cast to driver education. Although there is no conclusive proof as to the comparative effectiveness of various driver education techniques, or, for that matter, the whole of present driver education practice, there is even less proof of the efficacy and value of any alternatives to present practices for communicating to the young person the rudiments of how to handle a car in modern traffic, and the associated social responsibilities. But operational driver education programs must continue. The problem is no different in principle than that for education in general. We have to continue with present systems even while recognized needed improvements are being studied. One would hardly advocate a moratorium on the schooling while looking for proof of better methods.[21]

Most are of the opinion that appropriate education and training programs can affect behavior. Good educational programs can have a significant impact upon accident frequency and severity. Driver education should be an ongoing program throughout the life of an individual and not just a course when he approaches the legal age to obtain a driver's license.

With evidence that the driver causes about 70 percent of the crashes, the question of whether or not driver education programs are good countermeasures is purely academic.

Enforcement.   The role of police traffic supervision for highway safety is the same as in other phases of law enforcement: the protection of life and property and the preservation of order. Traffic police accomplish these goals through:

1   Enforcement of traffic laws — to protect the driver from his own unlawful behavior and that of others.
2   Investigation of traffic accidents.
3   Direction and control of traffic.

It should be recognized that the traffic officer provides a variety of other services designed to facilitate the safe and efficient movement of traffic (e.g., assisting motorists and protecting the highway from damage).

Unfortunately many people think that the traffic court's only function is to punish the violator, but a more important function is to improve drivers by helping them to understand the logic for traffic laws and convincing them to comply as a means of making our roadways safer. Traffic court judges, then, are in a unique position to educate and correct the behavior of motorists.

Traffic codes and laws are ineffective and meaningless without enforcement. The highway system, and the driver in particular, require regulation and supervision and a continuous control. The objective of enforcement with respect to traffic safety is essentially directed toward creating a feeling of surveillance that will induce the vast majority of drivers to follow voluntarily the traffic rules and regulations. There is no question about the importance of enforcement to the success of the entire traffic safety program. The threat of deterrent action, coupled with the ability to apply it, followed by swift, fair, and impartial administrative or judicial adjudication will lead to a more successful traffic safety program. The effect of enforcement procedures as an accident countermeasure suffers from the same problem as most of the other elements of accident prevention — lack of scientific proof of its effectiveness in reducing death and injury on the highways. Research, then, has not provided a basis for concluding that any simple regulatory changes, more stringent enforcement, penalization, and legal factors will have a major effect on traffic safety. This does not mean that enforcement measures should be nullified, especially speed law enforcement. There needs to be scientific research to determine the most effective enforcement techniques. It is believed that the Connecticut traffic safety record (lowest of any state, based on deaths per hundred million miles) is mainly the result of an overall program in which speed enforcement received the most publicity and therefore was held (in the public's view) as the effective countermeasure for reducing traffic fatalities.

Medical.   The Wisconsin State Medical Society has identified the following specific medical conditions that should receive particular attention in respect to the legal operation of a motor vehicle:[22]

1   *Diabetes.* The uncontrolled diabetic should be advised not to drive because of the possible development of disabling complications.

2   *Hyperinsulin States.* Individuals subject to attacks of faintness, giddiness, or unconsciousness should not drive.

3   *Thyroid Disease.* Uncontrolled thyrotoxicosis should be considered a contraindication to driving, also severe myxedema and cretinism.

4   *Muscle Weakness and Hypotonia.* Individuals with these symptoms of various metabolic and/or neurologic conditions may need to be advised to restrict or stop their driving.

5   *Cardiovascular Disease.* Uncontrolled conditions in which sudden death, lapse of consciousness, or pain sufficient to cause loss of control of the vehicle may occur should preclude motor vehicle operation.

6   *Cerebrovascular Disease (includes hypertension and vasomotor instability).* Those with inadequate blood flow to the brain are likely to have attacks of fainting or dizziness (vertigo) and should be advised not to operate a motor vehicle.

7   *Vision.* Optimally corrected vision poorer than 20/40 in the better eye should be considered to be cause for restricted driving privileges. Color blindness is not now considered to be of any great consequence to safe driving.

8   *Hearing.* Hearing loss can be compensated for to enable safe driving. Present state laws usually require outside rear-view mirrors for these drivers.

9   *Skeletal (Orthopedic) Defects.* Acute musculoskeletal injuries frequently produce temporary driver impairment; chronic and permanent effects frequently may be compensated for by special mechanical devices and should be subjected to the test of "demonstrated competence" to drive safely.

10   *Convulsive Disorders.* Most states allow the privilege of the highway to the person whose condition is controlled. Night driving may present particular hazards of "light stimulation of seizures" of which the driver should be advised.

11   *Narcolepsy (uncontrolled sleep).* Persons with this condition should be allowed to drive if it is controlled by medication and medical supervision is maintained.

12 *Mental Deficiency.* Drivers need to have the intellectual capacity, demonstrated by testing, to interpret the basic traffic control signs and to react appropriately. This determination is a function of the licensing authority and borderline applicants should probably have restricted privileges.

13 *Mental and Emotional Disturbances.* There are at present no known testing procedures that can reliably predict a person's ability to drive safely or indicate a significantly hazardous emotional instability such as to warrant consideration for license revocation; certainly many mentally ill persons have periods of functional impairment but these, for the noninstitutionalized person, should be handled as are other temporary impairments. Individuals who have had changes in personality, alertness, ability to make decisions, or actual loss of motor or sensory power, should not be allowed to drive until the condition is stabilized and competence can be demonstrated by appropriate testing.

14 *Alcoholism.* Chronic alcoholics should not drive until such time as there is reasonable medical evidence that the condition is controlled.

Engineering. There are several specific approaches to designing safer roadways. Sometimes the theory of "adequate roads are safe roads" is advanced.

Accidents can result where a driver fails to perceive, or incorrectly perceives, a situation. For example, accidents are more likely to occur where there are a number of things the driver must see and pay attention to at the same time. Such a case is a location with many driveways, intersections, and vehicles on the highway. Or the driver's view may be obstructed, making it impossible to see a potential hazard.

Having perceived a situation, a driver must make a decision. Accidents occur where more than one decision must be made at the same place, or where unusually difficult decisions must be made. Examples of the former are roads with heavy traffic volumes, frequent intersections and driveways, and the like. Examples of the latter are complicated intersections with heavy traffic, or combinations of factors such as curves and traffic signals.

Having perceived the situation and made his decision, the driver must act. Accidents happen where there is insufficient time or space for an action, such as on narrow roadways with narrow shoulders, or where there are obstructions beside the roadway.

Accident rates increase when daily traffic increases. There are also relationships between quality of traffic flow and accidents. Traffic on major roads is not only heavier but it is made up of various types of vehicles and motorists with different purposes, characteristics, and goals. The result is a mix which may have some bearing on the accident rate. For example, studies before and after freeway construction show reductions in rate on both the new and old highway. One result of the changed condition is the unmixing of traffic, that is, long distance traffic operates on one highway, local traffic on another.

Countermeasures: Crash

Millions of traffic crashes occur each year which do not result in death or serious injury. The safety features that will permit motorists to ride out a crash without serious injury consist of: (1) safeguarding occupants in the body of the vehicle, known as "occupant packaging"; (2) improving vehicle design so that the passenger compartment will not be dangerously penetrated or crushed; and (3) removing roadside obstacles or replacing them with "cushioning" devices.

Occupant Packaging.   Occupant protection measures fall into two general categories, active and passive. With the former, individuals must do something for their own protection, such as fastening seat belts. Passive measures protect automatically in an emergency without volition (or action) on the part of the occupant.

Based on scientific research, numerous motor vehicle safety standards have been issued by the federal government which greatly enhance crash survival chances. They specify safety criteria for such potentially dangerous features as steering columns, windshields, instrument panels, seat anchorages, unsafe door locks, and fuel tanks. All of these are passive measures. Lap and shoulder straps are part of the active protection package. Unfortunately, far more people neglect them than wear them.

Experts in traffic safety are in agreement that if universal, or near universal, use of belts were achieved, almost 15,000 lives could be saved in this country each year.[23] Greater use of safety belts is essential since it will be some time before passive restraints are put into mass production, and several more years before they are present in numbers that will noticeably affect statistics. Studies show that at least 30 percent of those who died in highway accidents would have been saved if they had been wearing safety belts. Death in crashes is frequently the result of victims being thrown from the automobile, which the seat belts, or lap and shoulder belts, can prevent. Estimates of the chances of survival and of avoiding injury to ejectees (generally unbelted) have been contrasted with the risks of nonejectees (generally belted). (See Table 8–2.)

In view of the persistently low level of safety belt use in the United States and favorable results in Australia, a mandatory safety belt law is a consideration. Australia and New Zealand are the first nations to have

table 8–2   *Degree of Risk—Unbelted Drivers*

Instant death	30 times as high
At least severe injury	9 times as high
At least nontrivial injury	6 times as high
Any injury	4 times as high

source: U.S. Department of Transportation, *Traffic '72*, A Report on the Activities of the National Highway Traffic Safety Administration and the Federal Highway Administration, 1973.

adopted safety belt laws and enforce them. The immediate effect has been to increase safety belt usage greatly. Moreover, there has been a sharp decrease in traffic deaths and injuries since enactment of the law. However, this is dependent upon enforcement. As mentioned earlier, if the United States, by any combination of laws, standards, projects, or programs could achieve similar goals, almost 15,000 lives could be saved yearly.

The inflatable seat belt is a new concept which combines the conventional lap and shoulder belt with the passive inflatable (air cushion) system. Not only is the wearer protected at all times but, in addition, the system has some of the cushioning and load distribution benefits of the air bag. Like the air bag, the new element is triggered by the crash.

Pregnant women seem to be more reluctant to use safety belts than most other people, and the major reason given is fear of injury to the unborn baby or to self. Dr. Crosby points out that the greatest hazard to the unborn baby is the death of the mother, that safety belts prevent many fatal injuries, and that pregnant women should use safety belts and should use them properly—across the upper thighs rather than over the pregnant uterus.[24] The combination shoulder harness and lap belt should improve the survival chances of both the mother and the unborn child.

Two surgeons at University Hospital in Iowa City report that occasionally an injury due to the wearing of a safety belt is seen.[25] Various types of abdominal injuries have been reported, including rupture of the spleen or liver, lacerations or tears of the pancreas, small intestine, and large bowel, or rupture of the abdominal aorta (large artery descending to the lower part of the body), as well as fractures of the lumbar spine (involving the lower back). The types of injuries reported are typical of those caused by severe accidents when persons are wearing lap belts. One thing should be emphasized about this kind of injury. It is an acceptable medical substitute for what might have occurred if the victim had not been wearing a safety belt. The evidence is clear—regardless of the cases in which a person lived because no belt was used—that safety belts save lives.

Vehicle Design. The second lifesaving aspect of crash survivability lies in designing the vehicle to absorb and deflect collision forces so that the passenger compartment remains a safe haven for occupants. Examples include: front-end, energy-absorbing devices; structural reinforcement; padding; head-rest effectiveness; hood-penetrating windshield deflection.

Roadside Hazards. The third element of crash survivability is devoted to the removal of roadside hazards. It has been said that if there is a dangerous obstacle near the roadway, sooner or later it will be struck. The streets and highways are dotted with them—bridge abutments, guardrails designed for strength rather than safety (see Figure 8–3), and sign and light poles embedded in concrete. Efforts have been made, primarily on high-speed roadways, to remove dangerous objects to provide clear recovery space, install breakaway signs and light supports, flatten slopes, and improve guardrails and median barriers. These improvements have contributed substantially to reductions in traffic accidents, injuries, and fatalities. It has been found that with the breakaway supports and crash cushions, occupants survive collisions with little or

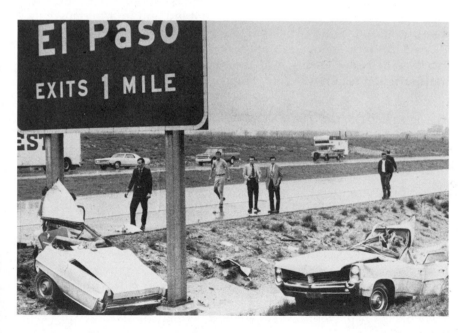

figure 8–3 This car was sliced into two halves by a rigid, unyielding signpost on a so-called "modern" highway—with fatal consequences for the occupants. Photo courtesy Insurance Institute for Highway Safety.

no injury and frequently only minor damage to the vehicle.

Experimental safety vehicles have received a great deal of publicity. The objective of such vehicles is the protection of passengers and drivers from death or serious injury. They will have improved visibility and lighting, better brakes, improved bumper performance, passive restraints, and numerous other features.

Countermeasures: Post-Crash

In the annual total of traffic fatalities, it seems beyond question that some die who would have been saved with prompt and effective medical attention. How many is difficult to determine. Some studies of the problem give some idea of the possibilities that emergency medical services could provide.

It has been estimated by Dr. Mason of the American College of Surgeons that 25 percent of the persons permanently disabled in highway accidents would not have been crippled if proper care and transportation after the accident had been available.[26] Dr. Waller notes that the case/fatality ratio for rural injuries was four times that of urban accidents even though the rural injuries were less severe.[27] He infers that the deaths were related to inadequate first aid and inferior emergency transportation facilities. Dr. Kennedy of the American College of Surgeons Section of Trauma estimates that 20,000 lives may be saved annually with better attention at the scene of the accidents and better transportation facilities.[28] Frey, Huelke, and Gikas note that:

... while the toll of fatalities from motor vehicle accidents continues to mount annually in the United States, there have been few studies performed which would indicate the number of patients that might be salvaged by a more perfect system of care of the injured than now exists.[29]

Medical consultants have observed that, if seriously wounded, their chances of survival would be better in a combat zone (Korea and Vietnam) than on the average city street in the United States. Death rates of battle casualties reaching medical facilities have declined from 8 percent in World War I, to 4.5 percent in World War II, to 2.5 percent in Korea, and to less than 2 percent in Vietnam.[30] Reduction of the time lag from the time of injury to the start of medical care is one of the important elements in the prevention of death and permanent disability in a combat zone.

Because of these observations, an upgrading of emergency medical services is taking place. Noteworthy is the concept of Trauma centers with helicopter Medivac, such as used in Illinois and Maryland and the measures taken to develop or upgrade the skills of ambulance drivers, ambulance attendants, and other rescue workers. The National Highway Traffic Safety Administration initiated the development of an 81-hour basic training course for medical technicians riding ambulances. A 20-hour refresher course has been developed and is available to assure the maintenance of a high level of skill in ambulance attendants. All states have designated someone to coordinate emergency medical service efforts and activities.

Hanns Pacy, a noted Australian authority on traffic accidents, reports that many people die in these accidents because others do not know what to do.[31] The best hospital is of no value if the victim is dead when he arrives. Dr. Pacy says that the proper management of a traffic accident calls for the following procedures:

1 Time of the accident should be recorded at once. It is vital for skilled persons who arrive later to know how long ago an injured person stopped breathing.

2 Rescuers should park properly at the accident scene by slowing down gradually, parking a sufficient distance away so as to leave space for an ambulance or other essential rescue vehicle. Signal lights and/or emergency warning lights should be left on.

3 A primary message should be prepared with an accurate, concise, and complete assessment of the accident situation.

4 Dangers should be controlled through use of flares, flagmen at least 500 yards up and down the highway, turning off of ignitions when engines are still running, control of smoking at the scene, and keeping away from and keeping others from touching any car in contact with a high-tension wire.

5 Removal of injured persons from danger. Generally, injured persons should be removed only by skilled personnel, but sometimes leaking gasoline tanks and smoldering cigarette stubs in the wrecked car may signal a potential explosion, or there may be some other hazard from which the victim should be rescued. The head of an unconscious person must be held up in removals of this nature because kinking of the paralyzed larynx can cause suffocation.

The proper removal of a person injured in a traffic accident should involve a consideration of the victim, the vehicle, and the environment.[32] The vehicle accident that is accompanied by a fire requires an immediate rescue. The technique of "grab and pull" must be accepted. An accident on a high-speed highway, where the hazard of a second collision is imminent, may also justify the "grab and pull" approach, but there may be time for more careful consideration. If a vehicle is submerged beneath water, or is sinking, the "grab and pull" technique is necessary. If a vehicle is teetering on the brink of a cliff, the same technique of rescue may be justified, but the great majority of accidents occur within an environment that permits a calm, deliberate, planned removal of the victim from his car.

Two factors are of significance: the injuries that the victim has sustained, and the position of the injured person. Rapid examination of the victim should be directed toward two life-threatening injuries: respiratory difficulty and severe hemorrhage. Respiratory difficulty demands first attention, but hemorrhage must be controlled to prevent shock.

In answering the question of how a victim can be moved with maximum gentleness and minimum risk of adding to his injuries, three basic principles should be followed: (a) rest is a basic factor in the immediate treatment of many types of injuries; (b) the car should be disentangled from the victim and not the victim from the car; and (c) it is always preferable to put equipment on the victim rather than move the victim onto the equipment. Splints should be applied in the car before removal of the victim.

6   First aid to save lives should be applied. The unconscious person should be kept on his side so that he will not inhale blood or vomitus. Control of bleeding, mouth-to-mouth resuscitation, or other measures, such as cardiac massage, may be necessary.

MOTORCYCLE ACCIDENTS

Characteristics and Causes

The rapid increase in the number of motorcycles registered in the United States over the last decade, coupled with a high fatality rate for motorcyclists compared with drivers of other vehicles, has generated considerable concern among those in highway safety. Much of the hazard associated with motorcycles can be attributed to the nature of the vehicle itself; compared with automobiles, motorcycles are less stable, are less visible to other road users, and offer less protection to the driver in the event of a crash.

Motorcycles are a real part of the traffic. They are here to stay and with the light-weight motorcycles, their mobility, economy of use, and ease of operation, they are becoming even more popular. Once upon a time, the only people who drove motorcycles wore black leather jackets or worked for the police department.

The problem of motorcycle accidents will continue. Besides more and more "bikes" being registered each year, it is now possible to rent one, which exposes people to unknown hazards. Inexperience with a motorcycle greatly increases the hazard of motorcycle riding.[33]

The automobile is the motorcyclist's worst enemy.[34] In these collisions, the motorcyclist is not always to blame. Many people have observed that drivers of larger vehicles do not always realize that motorcycles, and especially motor scooters and motor bicycles, are also motor vehicles and should be treated as such. In many cases, automobile drivers claim they simply did not see a motorcyclist in time to avoid an accident. Speed too fast for conditions is a main contributor to motorcycle accidents.

In terms of miles driven, the motorcycle is the most dangerous type of motor vehicle.

Effects[35]

Fractures are the common injury. The bones most frequently fractured are the leg (tibia and fibula) and hand-wrist area. Common injuries other than fractures are those to the head, resulting in concussion; intrathoracic injuries, in which contusion or crushing injury to the lung or heart are the most frequent types; and intra-abdominal injuries, commonly involving the liver or spleen.

Multiple injuries are common among those seriously injured in motorcycle accidents. The main cause of death is skull and brain injury, usually occurring when the cyclist is thrown against another vehicle or on the roadway.

Vulnerability

Considering that motorcyclists are afforded little or no protection at the time of the impact, it is amazing that they survive as well as they do. Certainly the youthfulness of the motorcycle accident driver must contribute to his survival. All studies show that most victims are young— under 25 years of age.

Female drivers have one-half the risk of serious injury of male drivers, and male cyclists are involved in more accidents than females. Females appear to be susceptible to injury as passengers.[36]

Threat

Most of the research studies on motorcycle accidents have been done on populations and accidents in the "cycle" states; that is, those states where motorcycles are dominant because of favorable weather conditions conducive to year-round riding (e.g., California, Arizona, Florida). The most dangerous hours of the day have been identified as those between 4:00 P.M. and 6:00 P.M. The most dangerous day is Saturday. It has been reported that the rate of serious injury is highest in January, February, and October, and lowest in June. This may not be the case in those states where riding is quite prohibitive during the winter months. It should be expected that summer months in the snowbound states would be the most serious time for motorcycle accidents.

Most victims are within five miles of their residence when involved in an accident, and this is explained by the fact that most riding occurs within five miles of their residence. Most of the accidents occur on dry roads. This is to be expected since motorcycles are not driven much on wet or icy roads.[37]

Countermeasures: Pre-Crash

There exists among traffic safety specialists a controversy as to whether motorcycle safety education programs belong in the school's driver education course. The issue is not whether to have motorcycle safety education, but whether it belongs in the high school curriculum.

The Motorcycle Safety Foundation was established to promote, foster, and encourage motorcycle safety and education. This agency has developed educational materials.[38]

Among other pre-crash countermeasures are:

1   Special motorcycle license recognizing those with skills and knowledge necessary for safe motorcycling.
2   Bright-colored fluorescent vest mandatorily worn to aid motorists in spotting the cyclist.
3   Establish a minimum age of drivers.
4   Control the speed of cycles.

Countermeasures: Crash

Studies suggest that the risk of fatal injury to a motorcyclist in a collision is significantly reduced by the wearing of a helmet. The risk of serious head injury is 50 percent less for those who wear helmets.

The well-designed helmet provides two protective features: it distributes concentrated forces over larger areas of the head, and it reduces force levels transmitted to the head. Individuals and organizations committed to the reduction of motorcycle injury losses must work more actively toward the acceptance and use of this effective and inexpensive method of injury protection for the operator and passenger. Helmets should bear the (ANSI)z90.1 or Snell standards.

Other suggestions for injury loss reduction include: redesigning the motorcycle to make it more crashworthy, restraining the rider from ejection during a crash, and "packaging" the driver/passenger more safely.

PEDESTRIAN ACCIDENTS

Characteristics and Causes

People inside automobiles are relatively protected in a collision. But almost every pedestrian who is struck is hurt. The pedestrian is vulnerable, fragile, and without protection. He does not stand a chance against a vehicle weighing about two tons.

Alcohol is heavily involved in adult pedestrian fatalities.[39] One study showed that more than 50 percent of the fatally injured pedestrians tested had blood alcohol concentrations over 0.10 percent.[40]

Crossing between intersections causes most pedestrian deaths in residential areas. The young and middle-aged pedestrians are most often negligent, while the elderly are the most law-abiding age group, yet the elderly are involved in the highest percentage of fatal accidents. It has also been noted that drivers of motor vehicles with less than 15 years of driving experience are most often involved in pedestrian accidents.

Effects

Pedestrians account for a sizable portion of highway fatalities and injuries. National Safety Council figures indicate that in recent years over 10,000 pedestrians have been killed annually and 120,000 have received disabling injuries.[41] Pedestrian fatalities have increased over the past decade. It has been estimated that 4 percent of all automobiles will strike a pedestrian at some time, and of all those struck, about 6 percent will die.

Because the motor vehicle is the main agent of injury, attention has been directed to its modification to reduce the seriousness of pedestrian accidents. The consequences of a pedestrian accident are dependent upon such factors as vehicle design, vehicle speed, pedestrian height and age, and pedestrian posture at impact.

The injuries to the body are primarily in the form of broken lower limbs and pelvis. Damage to the abdomen and thorax is common and concussions are frequent.[42] Pedestrians are not often "run over" by cars, but rather "run under" or "lifted up and over."[43] A "second crash" effect takes place when the victim rebounds off the vehicle and impacts with the roadway (pavement) or side of the road.

Vulnerability

Pedestrians involved in accidents can be categorized into three age groups: the young who are involved in about half of the pedestrian accidents, with those between four and eight years old being the most vulnerable; the elderly (65 years or older) who are involved in under one-fourth of the cases; and the 15–64 year group accounting for the remainder of accidents, with those between 21 and 50 years old involved in only 20 percent of the accidents. The involvement of males in pedestrian accidents is higher at every age than that of females.

Nine-tenths of the pedestrians fatally injured in a recent year were nondrivers. Their not being familiar with the automobile could explain the large number of accidents involving persons in the young and the elderly age groups. A child's vulnerability to being involved in a pedestrian accident seems to be more acute when the problems of family illness, mother's preoccupation, overcrowding, and absence of playground facilities are present. Knowledge of the area does not seem to be an influencing factor in pedestrian accidents. More residents of areas are injured than nonresidents; however, their exposure rate is higher in the area of their residence. For young children under five years of age, most accidents occur within 100 yards of home; those aged 11 to 15 years are involved in accidents within one-quarter of a mile from home.[44]

It has been thought that the elderly's physical problems, such as slower reaction time, are often responsible for their accident involvement. Though the elderly do suffer from some loss of hearing or poor eyesight, a study in St. Petersburg shows that 95 percent of the elderly population had no limitations on mobility or activities.[45]

Investigators from the University of South Dakota observed that the injury of a child by a motor vehicle is the result of a complex combination of circumstances involving elements of the child's behavior, the behavior of the driver of the vehicle, and a host of environmental factors.[46] In laboratory studies (observational) behavior demonstrated near the curb by kindergarten children was analyzed, and only two types of behavior were selected for detailed analysis: not stopping at the curb prior to entering the street, and not looking for oncoming traffic.

It was found that girls were more likely to run than boys, but more likely to observe for traffic when approaching the street. Only one-third of the children came to a full stop prior to entering the street. Nearly identical numbers of boys and girls stopped. Whether a child stopped at the curb was largely unrelated to whether he had been running or walking during the approach.

Threat

Pedestrian fatalities and injuries are primarily an urban problem. While about 70 percent of motor vehicle fatalities occur in rural areas, the majority of pedestrian deaths (roughly two-thirds) occur in urban areas. Severe injury or death is more likely in rural areas because of the higher impact speed in these areas. Fatality likelihood is greater on roadways of four or more lanes.[47]

Far more pedestrians are injured during the months with more hours of darkness (November through February). A little over half of the pedestrian fatalities occur in darkness. Fridays and Mondays appear to be the worst days for pedestrian accidents.

Countermeasures: Pre-Crash

Lighting.   As previously indicated, a significant portion of the pedestrian accidents occur in the hours from dusk to dawn. A reduction in all nighttime accidents from improvements in lighting can be expected. In addition, crime reduction is a spin-off benefit from such a countermeasure.

Traffic Control.   Identification of the high accident rate areas can determine the placement of vehicular and pedestrian traffic control instrumentation.

Pedestrian/Vehicle Isolation.   Typical of such countermeasures are bridges, underpasses, fences, and sidewalks. Bridges and underpasses are in general quite effective, although they do impose some inconvenience upon the pedestrian. While fencing and bridging all streets and intersections might not prove desirable or feasible, wise use of these techniques in the most troublesome areas could prove effective.

Traffic Flow Planning.   One-way streets eliminate many of the turning type of vehicle/pedestrian encounters. Also, shorter light control cycles are more in keeping with pedestrian tolerance and thus help to avoid crossing violations.

Visibility of the Pedestrian.   Lighting the pedestrian and contrasting him with his background are the two main ways of making the pedestrian more visible.

Education.   There is a real need for better education for both children and adults in traffic safety.[48] An educational program must induce every pedestrian to realize his danger and to accept the responsibility for his own safety. Information about laws and the limitations of traffic control devices and automobiles should be included. Information about problem walkers (children, the elderly, and the intoxicated) should also be presented.

One logical place for information dispersion is the high school driver education course. Though some believe that high school driver education effects may wear off after a period of one to five years, a refresher course such as the National Safety Council's Defensive Driving course could be taken at frequent intervals. This course attempts to develop an efficient use of the visual search process on the part of the driver, thus enabling him to recognize, interpret, and react to driving events more effectively.

In order for traffic safety programs to be effective, the community must be well informed on the extent of the problems facing them. A continuous educational program is very important, for without constant reminders the positive effects will wear off. Many media are available to reach large segments of the population, such as newspapers, radio, television, and magazines. Posters and informative pamphlets can be provided by local and/or national organizations.

One of the most successful concepts in the education of young children is the "safety town," which consists of a model street network with traffic signs, traffic signals, and pavement markings to simulate a real street system.

According to Baker et al., pedestrian injuries will not be effectively reduced by traditional safety campaigns that concentrate on changing pedestrian behavior, because such programs fail to recognize that the pedestrians most likely to be killed are those whose behavior is "hardest to influence." Because of society's "tendency to blame the victim," attention has been focused on pedestrian behavior and diverted from other elements in pedestrian collisions.[49]

Countermeasures: Crash

Vehicle design countermeasures are extremely complex. Suggestions for reducing pedestrian trauma of impact with a vehicle include: reduction in sharp edges and points; attempts to keep the victims with the vehicle rather than being bounced off; allowing damage to the lower extremities rather than to the torso.

BICYCLE ACCIDENTS

Characteristics and Causes

In the past few years, there has been a resurgence of interest in bicycling. Multispeed gearing, improved lightweight construction, stress on physical fitness, and the energy crisis have made the bicycle more appealing to adults. This is evident throughout the country where many dealers are noting that adults of all ages are buying all the five-and tenspeed bikes they can supply.

Unfortunately, the dramatic increase in the number of cyclists has brought an equally dramatic increase in the number of bicycle injuries and fatalities. The Consumer Product Safety Commission estimates that more than 371,000 persons received bicycle-related injuries serious enough to require hospital emergency room treatment (note that most of these do not involve an automobile), and as many as one million injuries required professional medical treatment.

Loss of control is a major problem in bicycle accidents. This may result from some human action such as riding double, stunting, or making an unsafe maneuver. Other important causal factors are mechanical and structural problems and entanglement of body parts in the bicycle.

Bikers are notoriously unresponsive to traffic control measures. This may be explained by the fact that the largest segment of the riding public is composed of children who have not been taught the rules of the road and the hazards inherent in traffic violations. It should be noted, however, that the 15–24 year old group is heavily involved in accidents and that this group usually knows the rules of the road and the inherent hazards.

Effects

Studies indicate that about three-fourths of all injuries to bikers are lacerations, contusions, or abrasions.[50] Fractures and concussions occur in only a small percentage of the injured. The leg or foot is injured most often, but most of the bike deaths are the result of head injuries.

Threat

Injuries and death occur more frequently in urban than in rural areas.[51] As most of the riding is during daylight hours, most of the injuries occur during daylight hours and during clear weather.

One study[52] found that high-rise bikes are not more hazardous than the standard style, while the National Commission on Product Safety reached a contrary conclusion.[53]

Vulnerability

Despite the recent increases in adult bicycle riding, the accident problem predominantly involves children. However, accidents with motor vehicles are in the young adult. It is reported that male riders are nearly twice as likely to be involved in bicycle accidents as females. This probably reflects differences in exposure.[54] One concern is the large number of children who ride their bikes at night, despite the rarity of lights; it is interesting to note, however, that this has resulted in few injuries.[55] Another problem noted is that some children have bikes too large for them to handle properly.[56]

Countermeasures: Pre-Crash

Many believe that major emphasis should be placed on biker education programs. Such programs are designed to teach cyclists of all ages the rules of safe riding and to induce them to observe these rules. Cyclists are shown that they are required to observe the same rules as those that prevail for motorists. It is therefore important to familiarize every cyclist with local traffic regulations.

The basic safety rules:

1   Do not carry passengers.
2   Observe traffic regulations and stop signs.
3   Use hand signals to indicate turning and stopping.
4   Ride single file.
5   Do not ride from between parked cars.
6   Keep to the right side of the road.
7   Keep both hands on the handlebars.
8   Do not speed in busy intersections.
9   Avoid crowds.
10   Give right of way to pedestrians and automobiles.
11   Do not ride when tired or ill.
12   Avoid stunt riding, racing, and zig-zagging in traffic.
13   Do not "hitch" rides.
14   Use caution at all intersections and driveways.

15   Make bicycle repairs off the road.

16   Dismount and walk across heavy traffic.

Unfortunately, educational programs alone are not enough to reduce substantially the frequency of bicycle accidents. Many areas have designed special provisions for bicycles to try to reduce the number of potential conflicts between different kinds of vehicles. For example, construction of bike paths on separate rights of way, and the channeling of bicycle, pedestrian, and automobile traffic on shared facilities.

Grade separations at intersections have been provided in some cities. Channelization will decrease the risk involved in bike riding. This is done through special bicycle lane lines and offset median crossings.

Countermeasures: Crash

There appears to be limited value in concentrating on this phase of reducing death and injuries. Some improvements might be:

1   Encouraging bikers to wear helmets, shoes, and other protective clothing.

2   Insuring that bikes are made with a minimum of protuberances which might injure a falling biker.

3   Providing clear roadsides for bicycle paths.

SNOWMOBILE ACCIDENTS

Causes and Characteristics

For the past several years, increased leisure time has given rise to a corresponding increase in recreational accidents. One of the fastest growing winter sports is snowmobiling. For the hunter and fisherman, the snowmobile is an easy means of transportation to out-of-the-way hunting and fishing areas. Snowmobiles are also used for racing, camping trips, delivering supplies to snowbound places, and just plain "joy riding." As the number of machines increases so have complaints from farmers, other sportsmen, and law enforcement officials about the improper operation of snowmobiles.

The snowmobile is part sled, part motorcycle, part army halftrack type of vehicle, which operates at speeds up to 60 mph over rough snow and ice-covered terrain. Originally designed for rescue work, the snowmobile has been in use by police departments in several northern states and Canada for many years. Snowmobiles have replaced dogsleds for the Canadian Northwest Mounted Police and even for many Eskimos.

The National Safety Council reported 154 deaths from snowmobile accidents in the United States during the 1973–1974 winter season, according to reports from 31 states and a survey of newspaper clippings.[57] For the 1972–1973 season, the Consumer Product Safety Commission estimated that 19,000 snowmobile-related injuries were treated in hospital emergency rooms. The National Safety Council survey showed that collisions with fixed objects, collisions with moving motor vehicles, and drownings were the most common types of fatal accidents. In nonfatal injury accidents, the most frequent types were collisions with fixed objects, collisions with a moving snowmobile or other motor vehicle, and overturns.

The reporting of snowmobile accidents has to date been very haphazard. This is due to the snowmobile's recent emergence as a popular winter recreational activity. Snowmobiles are receiving critical attention from recreational experts, environmentalists, safety councils, and legislators. Noise, property damage, and ecological considerations have been the main concerns. The problem of snowmobile accidents, however, has received little attention, possibly because accidents affect only snowmobile users and their families — not the general public — and because good data on such accidents have been difficult to collect.

Robert Dewar gathered 18 surveys on snowmobile accidents from a variety of sources, including medical journals, conference papers, safety councils, and police and Department of Motor Vehicles reports.[58] He suggests that current reporting was found to be meaningless and that more information is needed. Dewar cautions readers not to draw conclusions from the data in the studies. For example, not all injuries are treated in hospitals or by physicians, which are the sources for most of the studies. In another instance he points out that until it is known what proportion of snowmobile miles are driven over frozen bodies of water, the finding that one-sixth of the fatalities involved drowning is unwarranted.

Effects

Weighing from 400 to 1000 pounds, the easily tipped snowmobile, when overturned, can cause serious arm and leg injuries. Broken bones accompanied by bleeding are not uncommon. Spinal cord injuries have occurred and fatal neck injuries have resulted from encounters with an overhead wire or a fence. Drownings have occurred when snow vehicles have broken through lake ice. Also, cold injury is often associated with a snowmobile breakdown.

Injuries include sprains, strains, fractures, lacerations, contusions, spinal fractures and back strains, concussion, skull fractures, fractures and cuts of the face, hand injuries, rib fractures, dental injuries, frostbite, blindness, and paralysis.

Snowmobiling is often enjoyed at temperatures below 22°F., when the "windchill factor" (wind and cold combined) is at a level where exposed skin begins to freeze. Cold injuries, such as frostbite, can thus be expected. (See Table 8–3.)

For example, if the temperature is minus 30°F. and the wind is calm, a standing man will be very cold. If he starts to move, then wind movement becomes a factor. If he walks at three miles per hour, the exposed parts of his body will be subject to frostbite. If he rides in a snowmobile or in an open truck at 15 mph, frostbite will develop almost immediately.

Frostbite is the freezing of living tissue. The first symptom is a feeling of numbness in the affected part. Degrees of frostbite are:[59]

1st degree: Body part will be red, warm, swollen, and tender; there will be no blisters.

2nd degree: Similar in appearance to first degree, but blisters will form from minutes to hours after the injury and will enlarge over a period of days. In mild forms, the fluid in the blister will be pale, pink, and translucent. In deeper injury, the blisters are sometimes reddish, the fluid is pink, and the surrounding tissue has the appearance of first-degree injury.

3rd degree: Blisters are absent or small and dark colored. The fluid is reddish-purple and the surrounding skin may have a red color and fail to blanch with pressure.

4th degree: There are no blisters and no edema (swelling). The part remains cold and bloodless, varying in color from white to dark purple. There is no feeling and the victim is unable to move injured appendage.

Countermeasures: Pre-Event

Any snowmobile incorporates a certain amount of hazard because these machines do not protect their riders in the event of an accident. Riders are often thrown off. Safety belts for snowmobilers are definitely not recommended.

The individual snowmobiler can develop skills and adopt habits that

table 8–3 *Windchill Factor Chart*

estimated wind speed (in mph)	actual thermometer reading (° F.)											
	50	40	30	20	10	0	-10	-20	-30	-40	-50	-60
	equivalent temperature (° F.)											
calm	50	40	30	20	10	0	-10	-20	-30	-40	-50	-60
5	43	37	27	16	6	-5	-15	-26	-36	-47	-57	-68
10	40	28	16	4	-9	-24	-33	-46	-58	-70	-83	-95
15	36	22	9	-5	-18	-32	-45	-58	-72	-85	-99	-112
20	32	18	4	-10	-25	-39	-53	-67	-82	-96	-110	-124
25	30	16	0	-15	-29	-44	-59	-74	-88	-104	-118	-133
30	28	13	-2	-18	-33	-48	-63	-79	-94	-109	-125	-140
35	27	11	-4	-20	-35	-51	-67	-82	-98	-113	-129	-145
40	26	10	-6	-21	-37	-53	-69	-85	-100	-116	-132	-148

(Wind speeds greater than 40 mph have little additional effect.)

little danger (for properly clothed person). Maximum danger of false sense of security.

increasing danger Danger from freezing of exposed flesh.

great danger

Trenchfoot and immersion foot may occur at any point on this chart

will do much to keep him out of trouble. It is important for the novice to seek instruction in riding and handling a snowmobile. There are a number of snowmobile clubs that encourage their members to take courses in driving and general safety. Some believe that snowmobile training has a place in the schools.[60]

The best places to snowmobile are at resort areas that maintain trails just for that purpose. The terrain is known and there is less risk of getting lost. Help is usually quite near in case of an accident, or in out-of-gas or disabled machine situations. Also, such areas are less likely than other places to involve property owners or conservationists.

Other types of trails — for horseback riding or logging — often make for good snowmobiling. Cross-country riding should be reserved for those who have extensive experience. Any time a new trail is broken, there is always the chance of an unexpected hole or obstruction. Most people who have access to lakes that are used for winter sports can also benefit from local wisdom and experience about weather and ice thickness and safety. Experienced ice sports enthusiasts still go through the ice.

Snowmobiling at night is more hazardous than in the daytime. A snowmobile should have adequate headlights and taillights and a brakelight. Reflecting material should be attached to various parts of the snowmobile so that its general outline will be visible, especially when it is parked and its lights are off.

Studies indicate four main areas of driver imprudence as major causes of snowmobile accidents. The first two are concerned with speed — excessive speed for conditions and excessive speed in unfamiliar areas. The other two are consumption of alcohol and driving in such prohibited areas as a public road or a railroad right of way. Snowmobiles can be so noisy that their drivers may not hear the horn of an approaching automobile or the sound of an oncoming train.

Snowmobiles can be great fun, but they must be used with good sense. The National Safety Council recommends the following ten points for snowmobile safety:[61]

1   Driving instruction is required for the safe operation of a snowmobile.

2   Treat a snowmobile with respect and care due any power-driven vehicle, and recognize the limitations of operating ability.

3   Study carefully the operating manuals supplied by the manufacturer of the snowmobile.

4   Know your legal status regarding licensing, traffic regulations, and responsibilities pertaining to public liability and property damage when operating a snowmobile.

5 Avoid public thoroughfares and when necessary cross at right angles using extreme caution.

6 Do not operate a snowmobile on frozen lakes or rivers without first checking ice thickness and having an intimate knowledge of water currents.

7 Wear protective, warm, windproof clothing; insulated footwear and mitts; shatterproof, tinted goggles; and a safety helmet.

8 For casual snowmobiling, within reach of assistance, carry spare drive belt and spark plugs with tools for installation.

9 For a distant safari, the following pieces of equipment should be carried — snowshoes, emergency fuel, map and compass, ax, knife, water-proofed matches, mess kit, emergency rations, first aid kit, waterproof shelter, survival blanket.

10 Do not attempt distant safaris without an experienced person in charge; use the "buddy system," two or more snowmobiles.

Countermeasures: Crash

Since a snowmobile offers little protection in an accident, it should be mandatory to wear a helmet. It is, in fact, required in some states. Wearing goggles or a face shield to protect the eyes from flying objects and to keep them from tearing in the wind is also strongly recommended.

Frostbite Avoidance[62]

Frostbite is a serious matter. Even "a little nip of Jack Frost" can result in a long period of hospitalization and the loss of fingers or toes (or worse). A person raised in the southern part of the United States is more prone to frostbite than those raised in the North, probably primarily because of his or her lack of knowledge or opportunity to acclimatize to cold.

Depending upon the circumstances, anyone exposed to temperatures below 32°F. is a candidate for frostbite — a partial or total freezing of tissue. Frostbite most commonly occurs in peripheral areas of the body: feet, hands, ears, and nose, in that order. Other cold injuries, such as trenchfoot and chilblains, can occur at higher temperatures depending on such factors as moisture, wind velocity, and length of exposure.

The best way to avoid frostbite is to be prepared for cold — not just cold by the thermometer, but all the conditions that relate to frostbite: cold, wind, and moisture. Wind has a marked effect on heat loss. High wind velocity increases the hazards of cold by increasing loss of heat. If the thermometer reads 20°F. and the wind speed is 20 mph, the exposure is comparable to −10°F.

A rough measure of how hard the wind is blowing is: If you just feel it on your face — wind velocity is about 10 mph; if small branches move, or dust or snow is raised — 20 mph; if large branches are moving — 30 mph; and if a whole tree bends, wind velocity is about 40 mph. Moisture is also a factor in frostbite because moisture conducts heat, and if you are out in the cold and wet, the heat is being conducted away from your body.

Proper clothing is important in preventing frostbite because it insulates the body. Best protection is offered by several layers of light clothing, rather than one bulky or heavy article of clothing. Waffle-weave underclothing is helpful because air is trapped between the skin and the fabric and serves as insulation. If the underclothing is made of cotton or is cotton-lined, it will absorb perspiration and reduce heat loss. For the next layer, nonpermeable, closewoven shirt and slacks are ideal. Over these, a lightweight sweater and down-filled parka provide excellent protection. To protect the ears, wear a parka with a hood with a fur ruff.

Your feet are best protected by light cotton socks next to the skin, and over them woolen or synthetic socks. Boots, high enough to protect the ankles, should be worn. Tight boots constrict circulation and add to frostbite danger. Your hands are best protected by mittens rather than gloves. This allows the fingers to help keep each other warm.

Avoid tight, constricting clothing. Ski parkas with tight wristbands are fine for keeping out snow, but may restrict circulation to the hands. Waterproof clothing is not advised, since it holds moisture in and damp innerwear increases body heat loss.

It's just as important to dress appropriately for the weather when you drive to the ski resort or to a party or when participating in sports. Many people become frostbitten when their cars have mechanical failures. If you don't want to wear your high boots and parka to a party or while you are driving, be sure proper clothing is available in your car. If the weather is subfreezing and your vehicle fails, don't take off your mittens or gloves to make repairs. Do not touch any metal bare handed. Avoid getting gasoline on your hands. It doesn't freeze, but it does take on the temperature of the surrounding area and cools skin by evaporation.

Don't walk through snow in low shoes. If you do not have boots and other proper clothing, stay in the car. As a rule, a rescue team is more likely to find an individual if he remains close to his vehicle, be it car or plane. Certainly, if external heat cannot be provided by a fire or auto heater, but especially if you are outdoors and unable to find shelter (even when you are properly dressed), *keep moving.* Walking or moving your arms and legs will help keep your circulation up and help reduce the chance for frostbite.

Do not take any alcoholic beverages. Alcohol dilates blood vessels.

This is the action that makes your face red and gives you that warm feeling when you drink. But the feeling of warmth is deceptive. Dilated blood vessels near the surface of the skin make your body lose heat more quickly.

Finally, keep your head. Paying a towing fee is cheaper than the frostbite you court if you try to make repairs yourself in subzero cold.

NOTES

[1]JULIAN A. WALLER, "Alcohol and Highway Safety Programs: Comments and Clarification," *Medical Tribune,* December 30, 1971, p. 5.

[2]U.S. Department of Transportation, *The 1968 Alcohol and Highway Safety Report* (Washington, D.C.: U.S. Government Printing Office, 1968).

[3]Ibid.

[4]M. W. PERRINE et al., *Alcohol and Highway Safety: Behavioral and Medical Aspects,* D.O.T. Contract No. FH–11–6608 and FH–11–6899, Report No. HS–800–599, 1971.

[5]U.S. Department of Transportation, *The 1968 Alcohol and Highway Safety Report,* p. 1.

[6]Ibid., p. 2.

[7]M. O. ANDREASSEN et al., "Traffic Casualties-I," *Danish Medical Bulletin,* February 1972, pp. 45–50.

[8]DONALD C. PELZ AND STANLEY H. SCHUMAN, "Are Young Drivers Really More Dangerous After Controlling for Exposure and Experience?" *Journal of Safety Research,* June 1971, pp. 68–79.

[9]A. S. KRAUS et al., "Pre-Driving Identification of Young Drivers With a High Risk of Accidents," *Journal of Safety Research,* June 1970, pp. 55–66.

[10]DAVID KLEIN, "Adolescent Driving as Deviant Behavior," *Journal of Safety Research,* September 1972, pp. 98–105.

[11]WILLIAM L. CARLSON AND DAVID KLEIN, "Familial vs. Institutional Socialization of the Young Traffic Offender," *Journal of Safety Research,* March 1970, pp. 13–25.

[12]JOHN W. GARRET AND ARTHUR STERN, "A Study of Volkswagen Accidents in the United States," *Journal of Safety Research,* September 1969, pp. 115–26.

[13]HARRY W. CASE et al., "Vehicle Size and Accident Involvement: A Preliminary Study," *Journal of Safety Research,* March 1973, pp. 26–35.

[14]JULIAN A. WALLER, "Factors Associated with Alcohol and Responsibility for Fatal Highway Crashes," *Quarterly Journal of Studies of Alcoholism,* 1972, pp. 160–70.

[15]H. Ross, "Law, Science, and Accidents: The British Road Safety Act of 1967," *Journal of Legal Studies,* 1973, pp. 1–78.

[16]Insurance Institute for Highway Safety, *The Legal Minimum Drinking Age and Fatal Motor Vehicle Crashes* (Washington, D.C.: Insurance Institute for Highway Safety, 1974).

[17]A. JAMES MCKNIGHT AND ALAN G. HUNDT, *Driver Education Task Analysis, Volume III: Instructional Objectives* (Washington, D.C.: Report 71–9, March 1971).

[18]Highway Users Federation for Safety and Mobility, *The Driving Simulator Method* (Washington, D.C.: The Federation, 1970), p. 5.

[19]MELVIN T. SCHROEDER, "High School Driver Education—Driving Simulation," *Traffic Safety, National Safety Congress Transactions,* (Chicago: National Safety Council, 1964), p. 50.

[20]RICHARD W. BISHOP, "Multiple Car Driving Range Plan," *Traffic Safety, National Safety Congress Transactions* (Chicago: National Safety Council, 1964), pp. 52–53.

[21]U.S. Department of Health, Education, and Welfare, *Report to the Secretary's Advisory Committee on Traffic Safety* (Washington, D.C.: U.S. Government Printing Office, 1968), p. 63.

[22]State Medical Society of Wisconsin, "Medical Evaluation of Driver Impairment," *Wisconsin Medical Journal,* January 1968, pp. 18–19.

[23]National Safety Council, *Accident Facts* (Chicago: National Safety Council, 1974), p. 53.

[24]WARREN M. CROSBY, "Does It Make Sense for a Pregnant Woman to Wear a Seat Belt?" *Emergency Medicine,* May 1969, pp. 22–23.

[25]SAMUEL D. PORTER AND EDWARD W. GREEN, "Seat Belt Injuries," *Archives of Surgery,* February 1968, pp. 242–46.

[26]Quoted in *Ambulance Services in Michigan Survey Summary* (Lansing, Mich.: Michigan Department of Public Health, 1967), p. 1.

[27]JULIAN A. WALLER, "Control of Accidents in Rural Areas," *Journal of the American Medical Association,* 1967, p. 176.

[28]*Ambulance Services in Michigan Survey Summary.*

[29]C. F. FREY et al., "Resuscitation and Survival in Motor Vehicle Accidents," *Journal of Trauma,* April 1969, p. 223.

[30]L. D. HEATON, "Army Medical Service Activities in Viet Nam," *Military Medicine,* 1966, pp. 646–47.

[31]HANNS PACY, "First Aid for Drivers," *Journal of the American Medical Association,* March 5, 1973, pp. 1151–53.

[32]LOUIS C. KOSSUTH, "The Extrication of Victims from the Accident," *Arizona Medicine,* February 1969, pp. 128–30.

[33]PATRICIA Z. BARRY, "The Role of Inexperience in Motorcycle Crashes," *Journal of Safety Research,* December 1970, pp. 229–39.

[34]National Safety Council, "Motorcycles Data Sheet" (Chicago: the Council, n.d.).

[35]RICHARD S. RIGGINS et al., "Motorcycle Collision Injuries," *Third International Congress on Automotive Safety,* I (n.d.), 4.7–4.9.

[36]National Safety Council, "Motorcycles Data Sheet."

[37]Ibid.

[38]Motorcycle Safety Foundation, *The Beginning Rider Course,* 1974.

[39]WILLIAM HADDON, JR., et al., "A Controlled Investigation of the Characteristics of Adult Pedestrians Fatally Injured by Motor Vehicles on Manhattan," *Journal of Chronic Disease,* December 1961, pp. 655–78.

[40]American Automobile Association, *AAA Special Survey on Alcohol Testing and Pedestrian Accidents, Pedestrian Safety Report,* November 1970.

[41]National Safety Council, *Accident Facts,* 1974, p. 42.

[42]ROBERT B. SLEIGHT, "The Pedestrian," *Human Factors in Highway Traffic Safety Research,* p. 242.

[43]Ibid.

[44]TREVOR O. JONES AND BRIAN S. REPA, "A General Overview of Pedestrian Accidents and Protection Countermeasures," *Proceedings of the Third International Congress on Automotive Safety,* I (1974), 1–6.

[45]SAM YAKSICH, JR., *Pedestrians With Mileage: A Study of Elderly Pedestrian Accidents in St. Petersburg, Florida,* American Automobile Association, March 1964.

[46]NORMAN W. HEIMSTRA et al., "An Experimental Methodology for Analysis of Child Pedestrian Behavior," *Pediatrics,* November 1969, pp. 832–38.

[47]JONES AND REPA, "Pedestrian Accidents and Protection Countermeasures," p. 1–4.

[48]Ibid., pp. 1–8 through 1–16.

[49]SUSAN P. BAKER, LEON S. ROBERTSON, AND BRIAN O'NEILL, "Fatal Pedestrian Collisions," *American Journal of Public Health,* April 1974, p. 318.

[50]PAUL WRIGHT, "An Overview of the Bicycle Accident Problem," *Proceedings of the Third International Congress on Automotive Safety,* 1974, p. 17–13.

[51]Ibid.

[52]JULIAN WALLER, "Bicycle Ownership, Use, and Injury Patterns Among Elementary School Children," *Pediatrics*, June 1971, p. 1048.

[53]*Final Report of the National Commission on Product Safety* (Washington, D.C.: U.S. Government Printing Office), June 1970.

[54]WRIGHT, "The Bicycle Accident Problem," p. 17-4.

[55]WALLER, "Bicycle Ownership," p. 1050.

[56]Ibid., p. 1050.

[57]National Safety Council, *Accident Facts* (Chicago: National Safety Council, 1974), p. 77.

[58]ROBERT E. DEWAR, "Review and Critique of Snowmobile Accident Reports," *Journal of Safety Research*, March 1973, pp. 38-41.

[59]"Frostbite: Emergency Treatment," *Patient Care*, November 15, 1971, p. 76.

[60]ALBERT ABEND, "THE NEED FOR DRIVER EDUCATION FOR SNOWMOBILES," *Concepts*, Fall-Winter 1974, pp. 10-12.

[61]National Safety Council, "Snowmobiles," *National Safety News*, November 1973, pp. 82-83.

[62]Adapted from "Frostbite: New Approaches Plus the Best of the Old," *Patient Care*, November 15, 1971, p. 71.

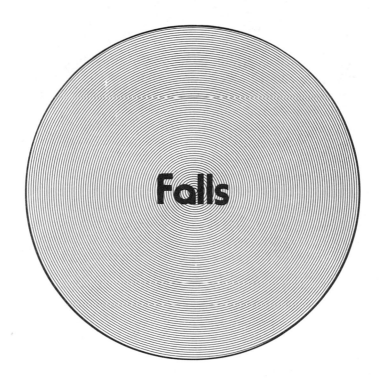

Falls

CAUSES AND CHARACTERISTICS

9 Each year almost 20,000 people in the United States die from injuries sustained in accidental falls.[1] This toll is exceeded only by that taken by motor vehicle accidents.

Injury data on falls are surrounded by many troublesome uncertainties. Statistics on falls are generally underestimated since thousands of falls never get reported. Data for the United States from the National Health Survey show that each year 12 million persons are injured seriously enough in falls to require at least one day of restricted activity or medical attention. No other accident type can match this type for injury involvement.

There is agreement that many personal and environmental factors combine to produce falls, but the manner in which they contribute to any given accident is highly variable. Physical impairment is of obvious significance among elderly people. But many of the conditions which affect us in old age are incipient in subtle forms during younger years, and it is quite possible that physical impairment may contribute to fall accidents at any age. Studies indicate that a range from 3 to 31 percent of home falls are due to physical causes. There are data to indicate that chronic illness plays some role in home accidents.

Often mentioned as contributing factors are "poor judgment," "carelessness," and "in a hurry." None of these has been investigated carefully with respect to falls. It has been reported that some researchers believe that fracture victims, including those injured in falls, have distinctive personality characteristics. This belief should be regarded as unsupported, with no evidence to substantiate it. The physical environment is significant in the precipitation of accidental falls, but few studies are reported in enough detail to show exactly how the environment did contribute.

The term "fall" means the act of dropping or descending in obedience to the law of gravity. The event may be initiated by two different conditions. The first is identified as "loss of balance"; that is, the individual behaves in such a manner as to lose physical control of his own posture. The second condition is identified as "loss of support"; that is, an individual may retain postural control, but lose support from the environment upon which he depends. Sometimes both may be compounded in a single accident. Nevertheless, a distinction between loss-of-support falls and loss-of-balance falls is an important one to recognize from the point of view of injury loss reduction.

J. H. Sheldon, writing in the *British Medical Journal,* contributes to the information about falls in the elderly.[2] One type of cause he describes is the "drop-attack." In the drop-attack the individual suddenly and without warning falls to the ground. There is no time to prevent or to break the fall. There is no loss of consciousness. One explanation is that the movement of the head and neck may affect the blood flow in the vertebral arteries in some individuals.

Tripping is another cause of falls in old age. This comes about because of not lifting the feet, not being able to recover once a fall has started, and a greater likelihood for tripping when tired or in a hurry. Vertigo (dizziness) accounts for some falls in old age, but an attack of dizziness is usually slow enough to allow a person to sit down or hold on to something.

Falls caused by throwing the head back or looking upward are especially dangerous since many times a person will be on a chair or ladder repairing or reaching for an item; the injury is compounded by the fact that the person was higher than the floor and thus has a greater distance to fall. The head tilted backward results in pressure on the vertebral arteries (a kinking effect), which affects the blood supply to the brain.

Standing up rapidly (postural hypotension) accounts for a small number of falls among the elderly. Muscular weakness in one leg, so that it is unable to meet an emergency (e.g., stepping on a loose stone), also accounts for some falls.

EFFECTS

Fall fatalities often evolve from injuries to the head. Fractures of the lower limbs and injuries to the vertebral column are the other leading trauma effects to the body.

The two primary types of brain injury are:[3] (1) bruising when the head forcibly strikes a blunt object (e.g., ground, floor). This contusion causes swelling, which in turn causes pressure on the brain. The pressure disrupts the brain's normal functions. (2) Laceration of the brain tissue from fragments being depressed inward into the skull and brain.

Fractures are classified according to the appearance of the broken bone, as follows:[4]

1   A transverse fracture is a break straight across the bone shaft.

2   An oblique fracture is a break at an oblique angle to the bone shaft.

3   A spiral fracture has the appearance of a spring; the break twists around the bone shaft.

4   A greenstick fracture is a split along the length of the bone. It has the appearance of a green stick that is bent to the breaking point. This type is common to babies and small children, whose bones are soft.

5   A comminuted fracture is a break in which the bone is fragmented rather than being broken into only two pieces.

6   An impacted fracture is one in which the ends of the broken bones are jammed into each other.

About one-fourth of the injuries from falls are sprains or strains, followed closely by lacerations, abrasions, and contusions. Head injuries, including skull fractures, amount to about 8 percent, and fractures 14 percent. Over three-fourths of the deaths from falls result from fractures.

The severity of an ankle injury is determined by three important questions:[5] (1) which way did the ankle turn? (2) at the time of injury, was a snap or pop felt or heard? and (3) has the victim ever had problems with this ankle before? For example, a severe sprain, which often does not swell much, is sometimes less painful than a mild sprain.

THREAT

The National Health Survey reports that about 60 percent of fall injuries occur at home with about 60 percent of these inside the house. This high proportion of falls in the home reflects the great amount of time spent there by young children and by the elderly. Stairs and steps constitute a special hazard for all age groups.

Death rates are highest in the New England and Middle Atlantic states. Falls occur more frequently in urban areas than in rural areas, with farm dwellers having the lowest rates. It has been suggested that poor housing conditions in the core city account for the higher metropolitan rates. Conditions responsible are rickety stair construction, no stairway treads, dim lighting, and clutter.

The months from April through September have the lowest number of fatalities and the winter months (especially December and January) have the highest. Northern sections of the United States with winters of frequent freezes and thaws reflect high rates. Children and youth are most frequently killed during the summer and early autumn, and the elderly have their high rates during the winter months.

About one-fourth of the fatalities occur in falls on the same level (i.e., the floor, ground, sidewalks, or street). Falls on stairs, from ladders, and from one level to another are the leading locations. Most studies show a predominance of falls taking place in the afternoon hours — this parallels the hours of greatest activity in the home, where falls are most prevalent.

VULNERABILITY

The death rate from falls increases markedly with age. Almost three-fourths of all deaths from falls are of persons 65 and older. By age the incidence of injuries resulting from falls contrasts sharply with their deadliness: more than two-fifths of those injured in nonfatal falls are under 15 years of age and only one-tenth are 65 and older. In other words, injuries from falls are a problem of youth. It is clear that while children are more predisposed to falls than the elderly, the fall of an elderly person is far more serious than that of a younger person.

The large number of injuries resulting from falls among children is attributable to their mobility and adventurous activities. Children under five have a much higher death rate than do older children. This may be the result of a predisposition to severe injury-producing incidents and a greater inability to withstand trauma. Falls can be particularly serious when a child is less than one year of age. At this time the brain is growing rapidly and the skull has a thinner wall than at any other time of life. Most injuries are sustained in the head region, perhaps because there is a greater weight in the upper half of the infant's body.[6] The young child is exposed to hazards with which he has had no prior experience. For example, during the crawling stage the child frequently climbs upon and then falls from furniture. Then, while learning to walk, tripping often occurs.

Death rates due to falls are much higher among males than among females in all age groups except ages 75 and older. The "shuffling ten- dency" in old men often results in tripping falls and has been attributed to muscle weakness and the inability to lift the feet. Injuries are greater among females, but this sex difference may be reflecting differences in exposure and activity.

In fractures, medical investigators have speculated that the bone may have snapped before the fall rather than after. Osteoporosis, a bone dis- ease affecting women more than men, in which the bones become in- creasingly porous and brittle, may be the culprit in many fall injuries to elderly people. The area of the hipbone known as the neck of the femur is especially thin and subject to brittleness. Osteoporosis, however, probably accounts for only a small number of total fall injuries.

COUNTERMEASURES: PRE-FALL

There is no single universal safety device on which to base a preventive campaign. As in all accidents, many factors can cause a fall. No two in- cidents are quite the same.

Proper prevention of fall injuries among elderly people can include dietary remedies such as calcium in the diet to ward off osteoporosis.

The fashionable fad of high-heeled, platform-soled shoes has been responsible for ankle injuries (strains, sprains, and fractures). "Falling off the shoe" and landing full force on the lateral side of the ankle is the cause.

Mechanical factors in the design of infant furniture contribute to many falls. A common preventable accident is caused by climbing out of a crib with the side up. Cribs designed with the mattress closer to the floor and the sides raised higher would be one countermeasure. The use of netting might prove helpful, too. A thick rug near the crib to soften any falls is advisable. Dressing tables are the location of many infant falls. Manufacturers should consider adding sides, making a concave surface, and/or lowering the height of such tables.

Some ways of "fall-proofing" a home include:

1   Adding abrasive treads or carpet to stairs to prevent slipping. Tack down any loose carpeting. Never have small rugs at top or bottom of stairs. Stairs will be more visible if you paint a white strip at the step's edge or paint the top and bottom steps white or a light color.
2   Rugs should be made slip-proof by tacking them down, by placing them on a nonslip pad, or by applying a nonslip backing to them.
3   Staircase handrails set out far enough from the wall to allow a good solid grasp are needed on both sides of the stairway. Many modern handrails are too broad or too near a wall for a sudden grasp at the beginning of a fall. There

should be extra support for the handrail at the top and bottom stairs. The rail end should be specially shaped so that you can tell by touch that you have reached the bottom stair.

4   Lighting can end many hazards that cause falls. Provide lights at top and bottom of stairs, in the front of closets and storage areas, as well as night lights in bedrooms and bathrooms. Light hallways well, and keep them free of obstacles.

5   A light for general illumination in each room should be controlled by a switch located directly inside the door so you can light the way ahead of you.

6   Floor wax should be buffed thoroughly to prevent slipperiness.

7   Spilled food or liquid should be wiped up immediately.

8   Use a nonslip rubber mat in the bath. A well-anchored horizontal grab bar, 40 inches above the floor, should be affixed to the wall by the tub. Some new tubs have built-in grab bars.

9   The bathtub should be low, with a flat bottom and a built-in seat at the end of the tub. A standard 14-inch-high tub permits a person to step in for a shower.

10   Shower stalls are safer than bathtubs. One about three feet by four feet is adequate in size. It should have a seat, a nonskid floor, and a well-anchored grab bar about 40 inches above the floor.

11   Install windows that open and close easily. Crank-operated hardware is good. All windows should be cleanable on both sides while you are standing safely inside.

12   All chairs, sofas, and tables should stand firmly on the floor so that they will not slide when someone leans on them.

13   Seats of chairs and sofas should be of proper height and depth for the person using them to sit down or get up easily.

14   Balconies and porches should have strong railings that are inspected often and kept in good repair.

COUNTERMEASURES: FALL

A positive relationship exists between physical fitness and resistance to fall injuries. Recommended practices during an actual fall include: relaxing muscles since injury is more likely with contracted muscles; rolling onto a softer part of the body (e.g., the thighs); and landing on the balls of the feet and letting the bent knees absorb the blow before rolling (this is the secret that allows a parachutist to come down onto hard ground without damage to himself).

In his classic work, published in 1942 and deriving initially from his own crash experience in the Canadian Royal Flying Corps in World War I, Hugh DeHaven showed that death and injury in unintentional decelerations from very high speeds were not necessary.[7] It depended on how the impacting people were decelerated, a point written about and understood by Hippocrates in about 400 B.C.:

Of those who are wounded in the parts about the bone, or in the bone itself, by a fall, he who falls from a very high place upon a very hard and blunt object is in most danger of sustaining a fracture and contusion of the bone, and of having it depressed from its natural position; whereas he that falls upon more level ground, and upon a softer object, is likely to suffer less injury in the bone, or it may not be injured at all . . .[8]

DeHaven provided evidence that the human body is far less fragile than had previously been believed. He also gave support to the idea that the environment is a main cause of damage to people and that the dangerous environment can be eliminated or modified.

It is interesting to note the world record for falling:

The greatest altitude from which anyone has fallen without a parachute and survived is 21,980 feet. This occurred in January 1942, when I. M. Chisov (U.S.S.R.) fell from an airplane which had been severely damaged. He struck the ground a glancing blow on the edge of a snow-covered ravine and slid to the bottom. He suffered a fractured pelvis and severe spinal damage. It is estimated that the human body reaches 99 percent of its low level terminal velocity after falling 1,880 feet. This is 117–125 mph at normal atmospheric pressure in a random posture, but up to 185 mph in a head-down position.

Vesna Vulovic, a 23 year old airline hostess, survived when her DC-9 blew up at 33,330 feet over the Czechoslovak village of Ceska Kamenice on January 26, 1972. She was found inside a section of the tail unit.[9]

NOTES

[1]Metropolitan Insurance Company, *Statistical Bulletin*, October 1968, p. 7.

[2]J. H. SHELDON, "On the Natural History of Falls in Old Age," *British Medical Journal*, December 10, 1960, pp. 1685–90.

[3]HARVEY GRANT AND ROBERT MURRAY, *Emergency Care* (Washington, D.C.: Robert J. Brady Co., 1971) p. 154.

[4]American Academy of Orthopaedic Surgeons, *Emergency Care and Transportation of the Sick and Injured* (Chicago: American Academy of Orthopaedic Surgeons, 1971), p. 89.

[5]ROGER L. BUCK, "It's Only a Sprained Ankle," *American Family Physician*, October 1972, pp. 69–75.

[6]HARVEY KRAVITZ et al., "Accidental Falls from Elevated Surfaces in Infants from Birth to One Year of Age," *Pediatrics*, November 1969, pp. 869–76.

[7]HUGH DEHAVEN, "Mechanical Analysis of Survival in Falls from Heights of Fifty to One Hundred and Fifty Feet," *War Medicine*, July 1942, pp. 586–96.

[8]HIPPOCRATES, "On Injuries of the Head," *The Genuine Works of Hippocrates*, trans. F. Adams (Baltimore: The Williams & Wilkins Co., 1939).

[9]NORRIS MCWHIRTER AND ROSS MCWHIRTER, *Guinness Book of World Records* (New York: Bantam Books, Inc., 1974), pp. 461, 463.

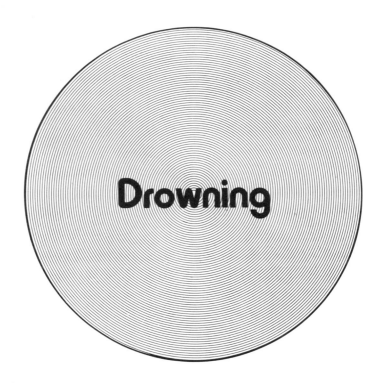

Drowning

CAUSES AND CHARACTERISTICS

10 A person who has been subjected to a severe asphyxial episode resulting from submersion in a fluid medium, with circulatory arrest (heart stopped) and with or without aspiration of fluid, is termed a drowning victim.[1] Near-drowning victims can, of course, undergo post-rescue circulatory collapse or arrest. Thus, the term "drowning" should be used when there is a loss of consciousness and threat to life from submersion in water. When drowning results in death, the term "drowned" should be used. The term "secondary drowning" should be used when the victim has apparently recovered from his drowning but loses his life because of later complications.

Deaths due to accidental drowning fall into two major categories: (1) boating and (2) those associated with swimming, wading, playing in the water, or falling into the water. Preceded in frequency only by motor vehicle accidents and accidental falls, drownings of all types account for about 6 percent of all accidental deaths annually.

Boating

Because of incomplete or inaccurate reporting it is often difficult to pinpoint the specific causes of a boat-related drowning. Sometimes, as in the cases where there are no survivors, the facts are obscure or unknown. Whatever the reported cause, it should be remembered that the so-called cause simply triggers the fatality. For example, capsizing and falling overboard, often referred to as the leading causes of boating fatalities, merely trigger the drowning.

Some indication of the circumstances associated with drowning in boating accidents is available from the United States Coast Guard, which receives and compiles statistics of recreational boating accidents.[2] These reports show that each year more than two-fifths of all drowning victims perish when their boats capsize.

Here is a case with deaths resulting from capsizing:

A West Coast man and his three sons, ranging from 11 to 17 years in age, had made long range plans and preparations for a trip to the off-shore islands in the Pacific waters near their home. The oldest boy and his father even took a course of instruction during the winter to at least obtain some knowledge of the intricacies of piloting and chart work. Their plans included obtaining the equipment necessary to meet the minimum standards provided by federal law. They put aboard extra gasoline, a good quantity of water and food, and all the enthusiasm boys of that age are capable of mustering. The day they selected was chosen because it was a day off for dad. Everything was all set and off to sea they went, in a 17-foot outboard. Late that evening a worried wife and mother called the Coast Guard and an extensive air and sea search was begun. Miles to seaward, an overturned boat was found . . . and that was all.

It was not hard to reconstruct, however, what had most likely happened, for on the day they had put to sea the weather prediction was "northwest winds running as high as 30 knots." Small craft warnings had been displayed.

They had tried to be wise. They had acquired some education in boating matters, but not enough. It takes lots of public information and education to make boating safe for all.[3]

Falls overboard account for more than one-fifth of the drownings. Here is an example of a needless tragedy:

Two families were spending the afternoon on a houseboat on one of our Midwestern lakes. The group included five adults, four children over 10 years of age and two small children, 3 and 5 years old. The older group spent most of the afternoon swimming off the end of the boat, while the little kids played around on deck. The owner was safety conscious. He had rigged railings to protect against accidental falls overboard and had purchased life preservers in sufficient quantity for all hands, including children's sizes for the little ones. Having taken these precautions he was quite at ease and having a good, carefree time himself. After their swim, the older group went into the cabin to dry off and to have a cup of coffee. The mother of the youngest drew her cup of coffee and went on deck to see how the play was going. Her little girl was missing. The tragedy was all too apparent. The little girl had fallen over the side through the opening in the railing left by the swimmers. She was not wearing her life preserver.[4]

The great majority of drownings are attributed to some fault of the operator in his handling of the vessel. Chief among these faults are improper loading or overloading of the boat, disregard of weather conditions, and lack of training and experience on the part of the operator, leading to operation in waters which exceed craft function.

Swimming, Wading, Playing in or Falling in the Water

Drowning can and has occurred in any fluid—paint to milk. Cross found in a study of drownings some unusual circumstances:[5]

Drowned in ten-gallon jar containing rainwater.

Fell head first into pail of milk.

Bathed in Mississippi River while under the influence of canned heat.

Drowned in bathroom stool.

Drowned in washing machine.

Fell into Mississippi River from bridge while working on construction project.

Became wedged head down in basement sump.

Swam across river trying to escape sheriff.

Daniel P. Webster has done several epidemiological studies of drownings in pools[6] and while skin and scuba diving.[7] He found that the most frequent primary cause in swimming pool incidences was unintentional falling or slipping into the water. Next in frequency was the victim's exhaustion, usually related to an overestimation of his ability and to his lack of skill in water survival techniques.

The most frequent contributing cause appeared to be the lack or inadequacy of adult supervision of children and, second, the victim's inability to swim.

The main primary cause for skin and scuba diving drownings is exhaustion which is frequently related to panic. Entrapment or entanglement under ice and underwater ledges, in kelp, and in various lines is another dominant cause. Striking objects in the water and being swept into deep or dangerous water are other primary causes.

In most of the cases of scuba and skin diving drownings, the victim's disregard of one or more of the recognized safety rules or procedures was found to be a contributing cause. Others include overestimation of ability by the divers, solo diving, and swimming or working under water at a distance from the diver's partner.

EFFECTS

With few exceptions, death by drowning is one of three types:[8] (1) dry drowning, when death is due to asphyxia and no water is inhaled, (2) wet drowning, when death results from the immediate effects of the inhalation of water, and (3) delayed effects, when death occurs as a result of the late effects of inhaling water.

Dry Drowning

Autopsies in these cases show that no water has been inhaled, but the findings are those of death due to asphyxia, such as found in strangling. An estimated 20 to 40 percent of all drowning victims do not aspirate water, but rather die from acute asphyxia due to laryngospasm.[9] Whenever a person is drowning there is a period of one to three minutes of breath holding. There is then a violent effort to breathe in air. At this point, spasm of the larynx (upper part of the windpipe) occurs to keep water out of the lungs. This spasm of the larynx may be so severe that all water is blocked from entering the lungs. Under such conditions, neither can air enter the lungs; hence, a person can lose consciousness without water entering the lungs. Dry drownings have the highest recovery rate if the victim can be rescued from the water.

Wet Drowning

The majority of deaths by drowning are due to the inhalation of water. The asphyxia from the spasm of the larynx ultimately causes the laryngospasm to relax and the lungs become partially flooded with water. If, on the other hand, inhalation of water occurs before loss of consciousness, the victim may experience a severe and agonizing pain down the middle of his chest.

The entry of water, fresh or salt, into the lungs, diminishes the oxygen-absorbing area of the lungs and disturbs the degree of electrolyte transfer (exchange of compounds in solution which conduct electricity). In all such cases there is a marked loss of protein from the blood, a factor that is involved in foam production. The characteristic foam that is found in the lungs and respiratory passages occurs because of the disturbance in the normal flow of electrolytes and the loss of blood protein.

The mode of death differs depending on whether the water in the lungs is fresh or salt (see Figure 10–1). Death in fresh water usually follows accidents in rivers, lakes, or reservoirs. In fresh-water drowning, the water in the lungs is absorbed into the bloodstream. The dilution of the blood (hemodilution) results in a lower concentration of sodium in the blood and many of the red blood cells are destroyed (red cells swell slightly and sometimes burst). This disturbance of the chemical balance, when combined with the low levels of oxygen in the body during a drowning episode, causes the heart to go into ventricular fibrillation. Ventricular fibrillation is a rapid, irregular, series of contractions of the ventricular muscles resulting in the loss of the pumping action of the heart. Death in this case is rapid, coming on in about two to three minutes. Swelling of the brain is the most striking characteristic of fresh-water drowning.[10]

When a victim drowns in saltwater, the process is reversed from that of fresh water. In saltwater drownings the principal variation is that fluid is attracted from the bloodstream into the lungs. In effect, the victim drowns in his own fluids as much as in the saltwater itself. Fulmi-

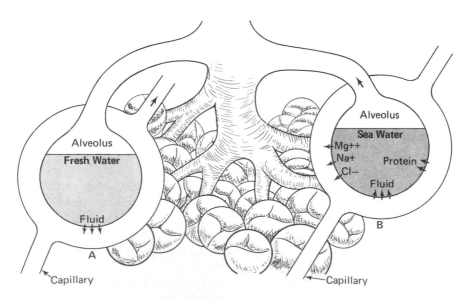

figure 10–1   In fresh-water drowning, water passes into the circulation; in salt-water drowning, fluid passes from the circulation into the lungs. Redrawn after *Patient Care,* June 15, 1972, p. 79.

nating pulmonary edema—a sudden and severe swelling of the alveolar membranes caused by the accumulation of fluid within the lungs— occurs. In pulmonary edema, the increased thickness of the alveolar membrane in the lungs greatly reduces the ability of oxygen to pass across the alveolar membranes.

Chlorinated water, such as occurs in swimming pools where free chlorine is added as a disinfectant, does not pass across the alveolar membranes of the lung and into the bloodstream as fresh water does. Instead, a rapid and severe exudation into the lungs occurs, resulting in pulmonary edema. It is thought that the chemical irritation of chlorine upon the alveolar membranes of the lungs causes this discharge (exudate).

Delayed Effects.   In a few cases people have been rescued from drowning, successful resuscitation has been carried out, and the patient allowed to go home—only to die many hours later from the delayed effects. This results from the irritant action of the inhaled water on the delicate lung tissue. Pulmonary edema sets in and, unless this is promptly treated, it rapidly leads to a fatal result.[11]

THREAT

In the United States the number of persons who die from accidental drowning has increased. Nevertheless, the death rate has remained fairly constant during the past decade.[12] The hazard of drowning varies greatly in different parts of the country, depending on factors such as the proximity and utilization of bodies of water and on the climate. Japan, where much of the population is associated with fishing and aquatic sports, has the highest drowning rate in the world.

Region.   Death rates due to drowning have generally been highest in the Rocky Mountain and Southern states and lowest in the Northeast.[13] In the Northeastern region the percentage of drownings is smaller than the percentage of boats. It is interesting to note that both the Northeast and the Great Lakes regions not only have the better boat-related fatality record, but that the law enforcement programs are the most active in the regulation of boat safety laws.

Location.   The places where the largest numbers of drownings occur are rivers, lakes, ponds, and oceans. This may reflect simply where the largest number of unsupervised exposures occur. Ocean drownings are not as frequent as those in rivers and lakes, perhaps because of the more frequent supervision by lifeguards on ocean beaches.[14]

For infants and children the most frequent place is in the bathtub or in swimming pools. A similar preponderance of drownings in bathtubs is found among the elderly. This may reflect the fact that the very young and the very old are less likely to be engaged in aquatic sports or recreational activities, or it may indicate that infants and children need more supervision in the bathtub and that the elderly are more prone to heart attacks, strokes, or falls (should this occur in a bathtub, drowning could be reported as the cause of death).

Month. More than half of all drownings take place during June, July, and August. Less than 10 percent occur in December through February.[15] It is felt that this reflects the fact that a much larger number of persons are on or in the water during the summer months. In other words, the chance of drowning increases in warm weather because of the increase in aquatic activity and because so many people take their vacations during warm weather and thus have time to indulge in swimming and other aquatic sports.

Day and Hour. About 40 percent of drownings occur on Saturdays and Sundays. About two-thirds occur in the afternoon or early evening hours.[16]

Water Conditions. In about half the cases the water is calm, water temperature is at least 65 degrees, and the weather is clear.[17]

There has been much speculation on the effects of cold water in drowning. Without a doubt, persons submerged in arctic climate water (regardless of how good swimmers they are, or how well equipped with life preservers) can survive only a brief time. It is also known that decreasing the body temperature decreases both the metabolic activity and the demand for oxygen by the brain. This can result in unconsciousness, and then death. Sigal and Mitchell believe that in certain persons cold water triggers the release of a histaminelike substance that causes unconsciousness.[18]

Cold water is more dangerous than cold air because water drains heat away from the body 20 times as fast as air (70 ° air feels warm while 70° water feels cool).

In cold water the skin temperature will drop to within three degrees of the water temperature in two minutes. A heart attack could result in some people. Blood supplies to the arms and legs are reduced making it more difficult to swim. Decreased oxygen in the brain follows, then delirium, unconsciousness, and finally death.

The average person immersed in water at 32°F. will be unconscious in 15 minutes or less. In 40° water he will last 30 minutes; in 50°water he may last 60 minutes; in 60° water he could remain conscious for about two hours.

Keatinge concluded in a study of the survivors of the sinking of the liner Lakonia (loss of 124 lives) that decreased body temperature from submersion in cold water was a significant factor in causing death.[19] He found in laboratory experiments that exercise accelerated and conventional clothing retarded a fall in body temperature while submerged in cold water. He also found that some of the victims of the sinking of the Lakonia were recovered in life jackets that had kept their mouths and noses above water, but were found dead after having spent several hours in the water at a temperature of 64.2°F.

Good swimmers may be more vulnerable to cold water. If Keatinge's theory is true, the good swimmer may stay in cold water longer, swim and exercise more, and therefore, risk hypothermia and unconsciousness to a greater extent. No conclusion can be reached without more specific studies.

VULNERABILITY

Age.   The "teenager" is the age group that is chiefly involved in drownings (nearly one-third of all victims). More than 60 percent of the victims are under 25 years of age.[20] This may reflect a greater degree of exposure to the danger and for longer periods of time than in other age groups.

Sex.   Eighty-five percent of the victims are male.[21] This may reflect the greater exposure of males to aquatic sports and recreational activities, as well as the fact that they are usually more venturesome and risk-taking.

Ability.   About two-thirds of the drowning victims do not know how to swim.[22] Good swimmers do drown and this might be explained by the victims' overconfidence or poor judgment.

Hyperventilation

Craig has obtained valuable information from swimmers who have trodden the fine line between life and death in underwater swimming.[23] Eight such swimmers, all of whom were attempting to swim relatively long distances underwater, were interviewed by Dr. Craig. One of the case studies is cited below:

A good swimmer, age 18, decided to repeat a previous performance he had achieved by swimming under water for three laps of a 75-foot pool (225 feet). He hyperventilated for about one minute, at which time he was dizzy. A significant urge to breathe was not apparent until the beginning of the third lap, when he reminded himself that his goal was 225 feet.

He did not remember swimming most of the third lap. When he reached the end, a fellow student, who was watching the swim specifically, reported that the subject surfaced but that he failed to raise his head. He began to cough and gasp, but regained consciousness in two or three breaths, after his head was held above the surface. The subject did not recall any after effects other than being slightly tired.[24]

All of the survivors studied were considered good swimmers and experienced at underwater swimming. There were other common factors. They all did deep breathing before going under the surface. Seven of the eight had some goal in mind or were in competition with others. The swimmer usually noted the urge to breathe but had little or no warning that he was going to pass out. Some of the swimmers continued to make coordinated movements, and one even executed a turn at the end of the pool beyond the point of remembrance. Observers of these swimmers did not suspect that a problem existed until final collapse occurred.

These events have been investigated by means of experiments to explain why a person might lose consciousness while swimming underwater. It was found that hyperventilation (deep breathing) preceding breathholding and exercise may delay the sensation of the urge to breathe.[25] Before the partial pressure of carbon dioxide increases significantly, the oxygen may decrease to a degree incompatible with high-level cerebral function.

Prevention of this type of accident is the logical answer to the problem, for underwater swimming is quite safe under certain circumstances and may be a useful skill to know. Prolonged or severe hyperventilation should be discouraged before attempting the underwater swim, and the urge to breathe, when felt, should not be ignored for long.

Hundreds, and possibly thousands, of good swimmers have drowned because they have not understood the effects of deep breathing before underwater swimming for distance. When a swimmer breathes deeply repeatedly before he plunges underwater he is lowering the blood content of carbon dioxide. Superficially, this result seems desirable, but what most swimmers do not know is that it is a rising content of carbon dioxide rather than a deficiency of oxygen in the blood that stimulates the brain to a desire to breathe. Thus, the brain is no longer able to recognize the need for oxygen. As the blood content of oxygen falls from the physical effort of underwater swimming, a blackout or loss of consciousness may occur suddenly, as in fainting.

The reduction of carbon dioxide in the blood (which with water provides carbonic acid) also reduces the most important acid part of the body fluid. Respiratory alkalosis is the result of this acid reduction, and this condition in turn interferes with nerve conduction. Another result of carbon dioxide deficit is a constriction of the blood vessels that supply the brain. Many swimmers have survived because friends or lifeguards pulled them out of the water when it was realized they were unconscious. These swimmers have given consistent reports of "going blank," "remembering nothing," and "blacking out," even when they had continued to swim underwater or had surfaced without removing the face from the water.

Four other factors besides the deep breathing itself may increase the hazard of underwater swimming: (1) the swimmer may have a distance goal and be a strongly competitive person, so that he pushes himself, even if he has some warning; (2) some swimmers may be overly sensitive to the effects of deep breathing; (3) strenuous exercise, especially prior to the underwater swimming, can also deplete the blood supply of carbon dioxide; and (4) spectators who could save an underwater swimmer in collapse may not suspect anything because they have seen the swimmer in good health shortly before.[26]

Alcohol

The National Safety Council reports that more than 10 percent of drowning victims were under the influence of alcohol.[27] However, according to Dietz and Baker, the role of alcohol in drowning has been neglected in both the popular press and the public health and medical literature.[28] They cite studies that have implicated alcohol in 7 percent (United Kingdom) to 21 percent (Norway) of all drownings, and in 34 percent of drowned persons aged 15 years and over (Finland). None of these studies was controlled for submersion time or allowed for decomposition of the drowned body. Waller's study in California found 29 percent with positive blood alcohol concentrations and 24 percent with BAC's of 0.10 percent or higher.[29] Dietz and Baker's study of Maryland drownings found 47 percent of the cases with positive blood alcohol concentrations; in fact, all but four were 0.10 percent or higher, the level almost universally recognized as indicating significant intoxication.[30] Because intoxication by alcohol does affect one's judgment, it makes boating, water skiing, swimming, and other aquatic activities more hazardous. The problem of "pseudo-warmth" or the numbing effect of alcohol may cause overexposure to the hypothermic hazards of very cold water. Incidences of intoxicated individuals going swimming at night when a boat was moored in deep water, or jumping off a bridge when intoxicated to win a wager, indicate that alcohol is a significant factor in some drowning cases.

After Eating

Water safety experts have advised swimmers to wait at least an hour after eating before swimming. Most people assume the reason for this traditional safety advice is to avoid "stomach cramps" that may disable a swimmer and cause drowning. Actually, there is no scientific evidence to support this idea. A near-drowned man reported a cramp during his last thirty minutes in the water before rescue but said that it did not prevent him from swimming toward and climbing on the rescue boat.[31] Various studies have led to doubt that vigorous exercise by itself has any significant effect on the process of digestion. For example, some laborers customarily work hard immediately after meals. In a University of Iowa study it was found that a small meal, eaten as late as half an hour before competition, had no adverse effects on swimming performance.[32]

Emotional stress may interfere with digestion. For this reason, the advice not to swim soon after eating is still good advice. It works the heart to provide increased circulation to the digestive organs and oxygen to process food. Exertion is an added burden to the work the heart must do. To avoid compounding the load on the heart, exercise before eating or at least two hours after eating. Never exercise vigorously after a heavy meal. It is suspected that many drownings attributed to "stomach cramps" have actually been cases of heart failure caused by a combination of overexertion and distress from abdominal distention.

COUNTERMEASURES: PRE-IMMERSION

Obviously, to avoid being drowned, either hold your breath until oxygen is again available or never get near water. Neither are realistic countermeasures for preventing drowning. Robert L. Foster of California held his breath for a world's record of 13 minutes and 42 1/2 seconds in a swimming pool.[33] Record breaking of this kind is extremely dangerous. The record of holding one's breath out of water is 5 minutes and 40 seconds and is not recommended because of possible serious ramifications.[34] (See Figure 10–2.)

As mentioned earlier, drowning can occur in any fluid. Avoidance of liquids and especially water is almost impossible. People even drown in their own fluids, as in pneumonia.[35]

SWIMMING

Learning to swim is survival in water with few exceptions. As Lawlor has said, "Most drowning accidents would not have occurred if the victims had been able to swim 50 feet, a distance usually sufficient to survive an emergency."[36] Parents are often unsure as to how old a child must be before he can learn to swim. The Council for National Cooperation in Aquatics (CNCA) has issued a statement that three years of age should be the minimum for organized swimming instruction. The CNCA is a group that includes the American National Red Cross, the National Safety Council, the National Recreation and Park Association, and others.

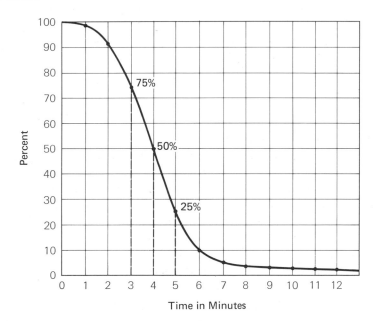

figure 10–2 A graph plotting the chance of a victim's recovery (by percent) against the time elapsed after breathing has stopped. This assumes that competent artificial respiration is administered.

The CNCA statement says that certain considerations affecting a child's learning and safety require a degree of development not attained by most children before they are three years old. By the time a child is three he or she is able to follow instructions on a class basis. A child may develop a lasting fear of water if the lessons prove unpleasant. A child's head is much larger in proportion to the rest of his body, so it is harder for him to hold his head out of the water to breathe.

The CNCA also stresses the importance of parents' realizing that, even though preschoolers can learn to swim, no young child — particularly the preschooler — can ever be considered "water safe" and must be carefully supervised when in or around water. If a child should appear reluctant to participate in the class, encourage him, but never force him to learn to swim.

Parents can encourage younger children to feel comfortable around water, beginning with carefully supervised bathtub play. Wading pools, under the supervision of an adult, and lawn sprinklers also provide excellent opportunities for a young child to accustom himself to water. Most realize that learning to swim is a long, continuing process.

Good swimming ability, although obviously helpful and desirable, by no means completely protects one from the risk of drowning. Indeed, in some instances overconfidence, poor judgment, or excessive risk taking while engaging in aquatic sports that are not adequately protected and safeguarded may trigger drowning among good swimmers. Thus, overestimating one's swimming ability or one's life-saving ability (many succumb trying to save others) can result in a fatality.[37]

SUPERVISION

No single action will prevent all drownings. One measure, however, could prevent a large number — competent adult supervision. Leaving children temporarily unattended is a major cause of drowning according to several studies.[38, 39] Professional lifeguards should be required at all swimming areas other than those at private residences. One report cited two sisters, aged 9 and 11, drowned in Massachusetts while other bathers were nearby in the water and 50 others were at poolside. Having lifeguards is still not the complete answer, however, because of overcrowding or because lifeguards are often assigned other jobs, such as maintaining chair and umbrella rentals, which distract them from their duties.

BARRIERS AGAINST TRESPASS

Fences and walls should not be expected to halt all trespassers. Such barriers can, however, keep out small children and make trespass by older children more difficult.

"DROWNPROOFING"

Fred Lanoue discovered a floating method he called "drownproofing" which has as its objective keeping a person afloat, even though injured or suffering a cramp, not just in a pool but in rough water.[40] One of Lanoue's pupils—severely burned and with one arm broken after his ship had been torpedoed during World War II—stayed afloat for five hours until rescued. Many demonstrations of drownproofing's effectiveness could be cited.

Lanoue's system is based on a simple principle: With a full breath in their lungs, 99 percent of all men are lighter than water. This is also true of about 99.99 percent of all women and children. An average head weighs close to fifteen pounds, so if a man floats vertically (most men float nearer the vertical than the horizontal) about five pounds is in the air, and with women, about eight pounds. (There are factors that may influence this, such as air trapped in clothes, fat volume, etc.) If a man wants to keep his nose and mouth out of water all the time and see where he is going, he must hold up with muscular energy at least five pounds all the time. These weights sound too small to be important, but over a period of time they cause many drownings. The basic procedure is to drop down into the water for a rest of eight to ten seconds between breaths. There is then a positive force always pushing the person up rather than dragging him down. Usually only the back of the head is above water. With little effort, the person comes up for air as needed (see Figure 10–3). Those wishing to learn this method should inquire at a local pool, swim club, or swimming organization.

PREEXISTING ILLNESS

Those who suffer from seizure disorders are especially vulnerable to drowning. Epidemiological studies substantiate this fact.[41] Physician counseling for every patient who experiences periodic lapses of consciousness due to seizure activity (epilepsy), transient ischemic attacks (localized anemia due to blood deficiency), or any other cause should be advised about the special hazards posed by aquatic environments. Such patients should be advised to bathe in the smallest possible amount of water, for it is in the bathtub that exposure is most frequent and the danger least evident.[42]

SWIMMING AIDS

Swim rings, inner tubes, sea horses, and air mattresses are referred to by some as "drowning equipment." Flotation equipment is usually no threat to the capable swimmer who slides off a wet mattress or loses his hold on an inner tube. For the poor swimmer, such equipment allows

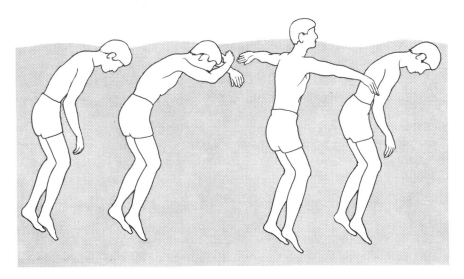

figure 10–3 Drownproofing technique: 1. Rest just below the surface, letting arms and legs hang limp. 2. Slowly raise arms as if to fend off a blow to forehead. 3. Extend arms and float to surface. 4. After rising for breath, rest by hanging limp under water. Redrawn after *Today's Health,* June 1969.

him to have fun but, by giving him a false sense of security, may cause him to go beyond his depth and drown. Foam kickboards, air mattresses, and face masks should never be used where a person would not be safe without them.

SKIN AND SCUBA DIVING

Violations of accepted safety rules contribute to most skin and scuba diving fatalities. Controversy as to the minimum age of a diver indicates that chronological age is a poor guide. However, most authorities agree that participants should be not less than 16 or 17 years of age. Certainly, stamina and swimming ability should rank high as drowning deterrents. Basic abilities for beginning divers are:

1 Tread water (feet only for three minutes).
2 Swim 300 yards without fins.
3 Tow an "unconscious" swimmer 40 yards without fins.
4 Stay afloat 15 minutes without accessories.
5 Swim underwater at least 15 yards with no fins and without a push-off.

A physical examination should be performed by a physician who is acquainted with the special hazards of diving. The Council for National Cooperation in Aquatics has a medical form specific for scuba diving.

BOATING

The causes of boating accidents were cited earlier in this chapter. Here are the major types of accidents and what can be done about them.

Capsizing and Sinking. About half of all small-boat fatalities are accounted here. Improper loading and overloading are probably the chief factors in capsizing. The records are full of cases in which too many people set out in a boat built for fewer persons; one person moves, and the boat turns over. According to the Coast Guard, you can roughly estimate the number of people that can be safely taken aboard a small boat by multiplying its length by its width and dividing that figure by 15. Federal law now requires that each new boat carry a capacity plate stating its maximum safe weight load. The number of seats in a boat is not a reliable indicator of how many people it can safely carry. Additionally, the operator's view may be obstructed and the boat improperly handled.

Collision. The most frequent kind of boating injury results from one craft striking another, or a floating object, or a person. Some operators of boats don't look where they are going, while others don't know the "rules of the road" — on which side to pass another boat, who has the right of way, how to signal intentions.

Falling Overboard. Slipping while refueling or pulling up an anchor, while pulling in fish or firing guns, or simply standing up are the main causes. Fishermen and hunters with heavy clothing and boots are especially susceptible to drowning if they fall overboard. Heavily implicated is the use of alcohol. Most accidents of this type could be prevented by adhering to this rule: Never stand up in a small boat. Also, don't ride the gunwales and don't jump in to rescue someone unless all other approaches have failed.

Unsafe Boats. Boats wear out and break down just like automobiles, and many accidents can be attributed to such malfunctions as broken steering cables, fuel-line problems, and stalled engines.

No Lifesaving Devices. Requirements for lifesaving equipment on recreational boats have been established by the U.S. Coast Guard. Previous Coast Guard requirements for recreational boats applied only to motorboats, but now sailboats, canoes, and rowboats come under Coast Guard jurisdiction. The authority for boating requirements comes under the Federal Boat Safety Act. The most significant part of this act is the establishment and enforcement of minimum safety standards. For example, load capacity, safe powering, flotation in a swamped or damaged condition (see Figure 10–4), a "good Samaritan" clause (provides protection to someone giving assistance to a boat in trouble), safety education, and enforcement are provisions found in the Federal Boat Safety Act.

Ignorance.   This is probably involved in accidents of all types and not just boating accidents. Novices frequently start their boats in gear, causing them to lurch forward; they anchor from the stern, instead of the bow, a maneuver which can drag the boat under. The Coast Guard has a home-study course available along with lecture slide shows for the beginning boater. Extensive courses are available from them and the Red Cross.

COUNTERMEASURES: IMMERSION

Life Jackets.   There is confusion in the nomenclature of lifesaving gear. In official U.S. Coast Guard language, there is no such thing as a "life jacket"; instead there are Personal Flotation Devices or PFDs.

The distinction is an important one for boatowners expecting to abide by U.S. laws governing inland and coastal waterways. The Coast Guard approves four types of PFDs. Recreational boats of 16 feet or longer (excluding canoes and kayaks) must carry for each person on board one Coast Guard approved wearable flotation device—either Type I, Type II, or Type III (see Figure 10–5). Those larger boats must

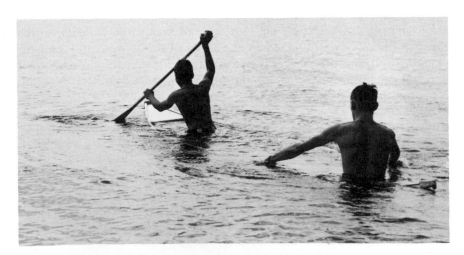

figure 10–4   Stay with the boat—it floats! Photo courtesy of the National Safety Council.

Type I: Life Preservers *Must be labeled: "Designed to turn unconscious wearer face up in water." Must be colored orange or red.*

160.002[1]
Kapok (Jacket Type)
Minimum buoyancy:[2]
Adult—25 lb.
Child—16½ lb.

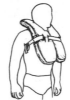

160.055
Plastic Foam (Bib Type)
Minimum buoyancy:[2]
Adult—22 lb.
Child—11 lb.

Type II: Buoyant Vests *Must be labeled: "Designed to turn unconscious wearer face up in water."*

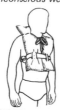

160.047
Kapok or Fibrous Glass (Bib Type)
Minimum buoyancy:[3]
Adult—16 lb.
Medium child—11 lb.
Small child—7¼ lb.

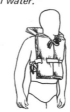

160.052
Plastic Foam (Bib Type)
Minimum buoyancy:[3]
Adult—15½ lb.
Medium child—11 lb.
Small child—7 lb.

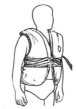

160.064
Foam-filled Vests
Minimum buoyancy:[3]
Adult—15½ lb.
Medium child—11 lb.
Small child—7 lb.

Type III: Special Purpose Water Safety Buoyant Devices *Must be labeled: "Designed to keep a conscious person in a vertical or slightly backward position in the water."*

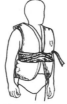

160.064
Foam-Filled Vests
Minimum buoyancy:[3]
Adult—15½ lb.
Medium child—11 lb.
Small child—7 lb.

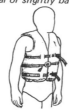

160.064
Ski Vests
Minimum buoyancy:[3]
Adult—15½ lb.
Medium child—11 lb.
Small child—7 lb.

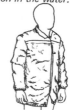

160.064
Sleeved Jackets
Minimum buoyancy:[3]
Adult—15½ lb.
Medium child—11 lb.
Small child—7 lb.

[1] *Coast Guard approval number: 160 indicates life-saving equipment, second three numbers specify the kind of equipment. Manufacturer's numerals follow.*
[2] *Child: under 90 lb.*
[3] *Medium child: 50-90 lb.; small child: under 50 lb.*

figure 10–5　Personal flotation devices—summary of U.S. Coast Guard designations. Redrawn after *Consumer Reports,* August 1974, p. 613.

also have aboard at least one throwable device, such as a ring buoy or buoyant cushion. Boats less than 16 feet long and canoes and kayaks of any length need merely carry a buoy or cushion for every occupant.

What sets Type I preservers apart from the other devices is their high buoyancy (the weight they can support). They must also be "designed to turn unconscious wearer face up." The right type of life jacket for your needs may well exceed the legal minimum requirements. No matter what the size of your boat, if you often venture well out to sea or on very large lakes, Type I devices are the only prudent choice. For most kinds of recreational boating, however, Type II devices should do. They can keep even unconscious wearers afloat and alive; they are reasonably comfortable, and they are inexpensive. Type III vests have the advantage of being far more comfortable out of the water. That is about their only advantage. For water skiing, only a well-securing ski vest should be worn to cope with high-impact forces during a fall. A skier wearing a bib device is courting a broken neck.

It may be overly cautious to insist that everybody wear PFDs on board boats at all times. Recreational boating is supposed to be fun, and being saddled with an effective life jacket subtracts from the fun. PFDs should, of course, be worn in boats at all times by infirm persons, small children, and nonswimmers. They should always be kept close at hand for others.

Coast Guard data indicate that the use of life preservers and other flotation devices can and does save lives. It is interesting to note, however, that about 10 percent of those drowned in boating accidents used a flotation device. The Coast Guard lists the reasons for such drownings:[43]

1 Injury before drowning (explosion, fire, fall, or electric shock).

2 Physical ailment (heart disease, diabetes, etc.).

3 Exposure (too long a time in very cold water).

4 Water conditions (strong current or high waves).

5 Improper use (failing to fasten ties on jacket or vest, or attaching buoyant seat cushion to one's back—which floats victim face down in water).

6 Inadequate device (nonapproved by Coast Guard, old or defective; or adult using a child's device and vice versa).

7 Miscellaneous (trapped in sinking vessel, weighed down by excessively heavy clothing, under influence of alcohol, drugs, or panic).

While holding onto a capsized boat, victims have been known to lose their hold, become separated from the boat, and drown. The idea of having handles or grips on the bottom of all boats to facilitate using the

overturned boat itself as a life preserver is a possibility. Current regulations require flotation ability of canoes, rowboats, sailboats, and
power motorboats even when tipped over or full of water.

COUNTERMEASURES: POST-IMMERSION

Rescue.   The adage of "reach, throw, row, then go" offers the best sequence for attempting to rescue a person from water. Frequently a
single drowning accident is turned into a double or triple one by the
unskilled or inadequate efforts of incompletely trained individuals to
save drowning persons. When anyone is floundering in the water, it is
prudent not to grapple with him because in his desperation he will
have epinephrine (adrenalin) to augment his strength. It is always best
to give him a pole or rope.

Whether or not the rescuer is a good swimmer, there is a concept of
improvising flotation aids which can be applied to most rescue attempts. When no standard rescue equipment is available, the rescuer
can usually find something that floats to hold up an exhausted swimmer
or floundering victim of a water mishap until he is rescued or has recovered enough strength to kick or paddle his way to safety. There are lots
of things that float — gallon vacuum jug, ice chest with clamp-on lid, ca-
noe paddle, fallen tree branch, spare tire in a car's trunk are examples.[44]
An interesting disclosure is that victims seldom cry out or thrash about
in the water; this may be a factor in drownings when lifeguards are
present.[45]

Swimwear.   Dietz and Baker observed that persons in a drowning
situation disappeared and that the difficulty of locating a body underwater may be a contributing factor to drowning.[46] They suggest that
clothing manufacturers construct clearly visible swimwear. Perhaps a
luminescent material or coloring the swimwear yellow or orange would
aid detection of the submerged.

Submerged Automobile.[47]   Each year people are rescued from cars
that have plunged into water. Each year many passengers in cars that
plummet into water do not survive. The annual number of car sub-
mersions is not great. Probably only 200 to 300 of the thousands of traffic fatalities will be drownings. Because of the drama involved with
each case, each is attended by much publicity. Some uninformed drivers resist wearing safety belts because they feel that their exiting from
their submerged vehicle may be hampered. Actually, being securely
belted is likely to prevent the driver and other occupants from being

seriously injured or knocked unconscious. The chances of getting out of a submerged car are many times better for the uninjured.

When a car is driven into deep water it will float like a boat for a short time. Then, of course, it will sink, and the heavy end will go first. If one or more windows are open at the time of the submersion, and the car is not collision damaged, the occupants merely have to open the door and swim to the surface. Rescue of the injured, nonswimmers, children, and any panic-stricken passengers may be necessary.

Cars with all the windows closed are different. In deep water, there will be great pressure on the doors and windows, making it almost impossible to push the doors open. A large air bubble will be maintained for many minutes within the car. Rolling down a window will relieve the pressure on the door, but exiting must be done quickly. Electric windows pose a problem and usually necessitate breaking the glass to get equal pressure before a door can be opened.

Lighting. Underwater lighting in a swimming pool aids location of an immersed body. Spotlights on boats could avert collisions and could also be of assistance in locating floating persons who would otherwise drown.

NOTES

[1] "Saving Near-Drowning Victims," *Patient Care*, June 15, 1972, p. 78.

[2] U.S. Coast Guard, *Boating Statistics*, published annually.

[3] D. W. SINCLAIR, "Who Gets Killed Boating—Where, How, and Why?", *National Safety Congress Transactions, Public Safety*, 1964, p. 28.

[4] Ibid., pp. 28–29.

[5] WAYNE D. CROSS, "Accidental Drownings in Iowa," *Annual Safety Education Review*, 1965.

[6] DANIEL P. WEBSTER, "Pool Drownings and Their Prevention," *Public Health Reports*, July 1967.

[7] DANIEL P. WEBSTER, "Skin and Scuba Diving Fatalities in the United States," *Public Health Reports*, August 1966.

[8] FRANCISCO M. WONG AND WILLIAM J. GRACE, "Sudden Death After Near Drowning," *Journal of the American Medical Association*, November 16, 1963, pp. 202–3.

[9] STANLEY MILES, "Drowning," *British Medical Journal*, September 7, 1968, pp. 597–600.

[10] A. A. MINTZ et al., "Pediatric Grand Rounds: Freshwater Drowning," *Texas Medicine*, August 1973, pp. 83–87.

[11] JOSEPH S. REDDING et al., "Resuscitation from Drowning," *Journal of the American Medical Association*, December 23, 1961, p. 75.

[12] "Accidental Drowning," *Statistical Bulletin*, June 1972, p. 6.

[13] Ibid.

[14] PARK E. DIETZ AND SUSAN P. BAKER, "Drowning Epidemiology and Prevention," *American Journal of Public Health*, April 1974, p. 304.

[15] "Accidental Drowning," p. 6.

[16]National Safety Council, *Accident Facts*, 1972, p. 77.

[17]Ibid.

[18]C. SIGAL AND J. C. MITCHELL, "Essential Cold Urticaria: A Potential Cause of Death While Swimming," *Canadian Medical Association Journal*, September 12, 1964, p. 609.

[19]W. R. KEATINGE, "Death After Shipwreck," *British Medical Journal*, December 25, 1965, pp. 1537–41.

[20]National Safety Council, *Accident Facts*, p. 77.

[21]Ibid.

[22]Ibid.

[23]ALBERT B. CRAIG, "Underwater Swimming and Loss of Consciousness," *Journal of the American Medical Association*, April 29, 1961, p. 255.

[24]Ibid., p. 256.

[25]"Hyperventilation: Peril for Underwater Swimmers," *Patient Care*, June 1, 1974, p. 69.

[26]W. D. SNIVELY AND JAN THUERBACK, "Voluntary Hyperventilation as a Cause of Needless Drowning," *Journal of the South Carolina Medical Association*, June 1972, pp. 253–58.

[27]National Safety Council, *Accident Facts*, p. 77.

[28]DIETZ AND BAKER, "Drowning Epidemiology and Prevention," p. 309.

[29]J. A. WALLER, "Nonhighway Injury Fatalities: The Role of Alcohol and Problem Drinking, Drugs and Medical Impairment," *Journal of Chronic Diseases*, 1972, p. 33.

[30]DIETZ AND BAKER, "Drowning Epidemiology and Prevention," p. 306.

[31]KEATINGE, "Death After Shipwreck," p. 1539.

[32]"Athletics' Speed is Optimal Despite Pre-Event Feeding," *Medical Tribune*, May 1966.

[33]NORRIS MCWHIRTER AND ROSS MCWHIRTER, *Guinness Book of World Records* (New York: Bantam Books, Inc., 1974), p. 45.

[34]Ibid.

[35]"Drowned and Almost Drowned Again," *Emergency Medicine*, June 1974, p. 222.

[36]JOHN LAWLOR, "Safety Education in Our Future," *Parent's Magazine*, August 1969, p. 28.

[37]EDWARD PRESS, JAMES WALKER, AND ISABELLE CRAWFORD, "An Interstate Drowning Study," *American Journal of Public Health*, December 1968, p. 2285.

[38]Ibid.

[39]ANTHONY I. ADAMS, "The Descriptive Epidemiology of Drowning Accidents," *Medical Journal of Australia*, December 31, 1966, p. 1258.

[40]FRED LANOUE, *Drownproofing* (Englewood Cliffs, N.J.: Prentice-Hall, Inc., 1963).

[41]ADAMS, "Epidemiology of Drowning Accidents," p. 1259.

[42]DIETZ AND BAKER, "Drowning Epidemiology and Prevention," p. 309.

[43]U.S. Coast Guard, *Boating Statistics*, issued annually.

[44]"Find a Float," *Family Safety*, Summer 1971, p. 30.

[45]WEBSTER, "Pool Drownings and Their Prevention."

[46]DIETZ AND BAKER, "Drowning Epidemiology and Prevention," p. 310.

[47]"If You Go In, You Can Get Out," *Family Safety*, Summer 1969, pp. 20–21.

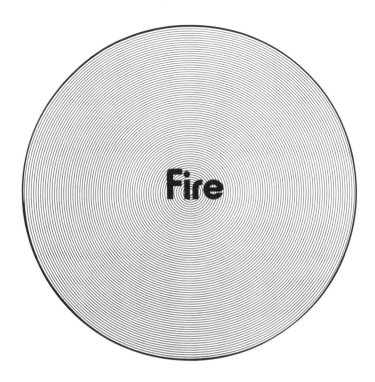

CHARACTERISTICS

11 Fire is a burning that destroys or changes what is burned and usually produces heat, flame, light, and sometimes smoke. All fires require the same three basic ingredients and burn according to the same principle (see Figure 11–1). Fires behave in different ways, however, depending on the nature of the ingredients involved.

The three ingredients necessary for every fire are:

1 *Fuel.* Fuel can be organic, such as wood, or inorganic, such as metal. It can be in the vapor or solid state, although many times only the vapor state is involved in the combustion process. For example, gasoline, a liquid, is commonly thought of as a fuel; but it is only the vapors that are involved in the burning process. Combustion of finely divided metals is a process that does not involve the vapor state. Steel wool, for example, will burn or oxidize rapidly in the presence of heat and oxygen.

2 *Heat.* Heat is necessary to initiate oxidation. The heat can be applied by various means such as direct conduction, thermal convection, or radiation. No matter where the heat originates, the combustion process cannot proceed without it.

3 *Oxygen.* Oxygen is almost always obtained from the surrounding atmosphere which contains about 21 percent oxygen.

The process of burning can be described as follows: When a fuel becomes hot enough, its vapors mix with oxygen in the air, causing a chemical reaction that releases heat, flame, and smoke. The fuel itself does not burn. The vapor it gives off is what burns. A fire spreads because the heat feeds into new fuel and raises it to the ignition point. To extinguish a fire one removes one of the ingredients—by cooling the hot fuel or by separating the fuel and the oxygen.

Each fuel has its own "ignition temperature." The ignition temperature is the temperature to which a fuel must be heated in order for its vapors to combine with the oxygen and start to burn. The ignition temperature may also be called the "kindling point."

Solid fuels (ordinary combustibles) do not produce vapors until they are heated to their ignition temperature. At this temperature, the vapors given off combine immediately with oxygen and burning begins. Some

Chemistry of Fire

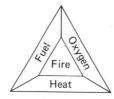 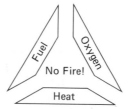

Oxygen — The air we breathe. It is also self contained in some plastics and gun powder.

+

Fuel — May exist in anyone of three forms, such as: a solid (wood, paper), a liquid (gasoline, alcohol), or a gas (acetylene, hydrogen). Since oxygen is a gas the fuel must also be in a gaseous state for chemical combination; or simply, for combustion to occur.

+

Heat — Is made up of both temperature and quantity. There must be a sufficiently high temperature, but there must also be a sufficient quantity of heat. Heat converts the fuel into a gaseous state to combine with the oxygen. One match will not ignite a log but a thousand matches burning together would probably provide enough heat (quantity) to ignite the log. The temperature of a thousand matches is the same as for one but the quantity is greater.

=

Fire — The result of combining oxygen, fuel and heat, the three sides of the triangle.

Remove any one of the three sides of the triangle and the fire ceases to exist.

figure 11–1 Chemistry of fire. Redrawn after *Safety Journal,* American Telephone and Telegraph Co.

examples of solids are: cotton sheets—464°F., paper—about 450°F., wood—about 500°F. As a comparison of temperatures, a match flame has a temperature of about 2000°F.

Flammable liquids are, by far, one of the most hazardous materials found. These include any number of solvents, ethers, alcohols, fuels, and cleaning solutions. It is important to minimize the use of, or preferably completely eliminate, flammable liquids wherever possible. For example, nonflammable liquids can be substituted in many cases for flammable cleaning solutions and solvents.

Flammable liquids give off vapors at temperatures lower than their ignition temperatures. For example, gasoline begins to give off vapors at about −45°F., but its ignition temperature is about 536°F. Kerosene gives off vapors at about 100°F., but its ignition temperature is 444°F. Although the vapors will not combine with oxygen and start burning on their own at these lower temperatures, they are capable of starting to burn when a flame or spark quickly heats them to their ignition temperature. Often the vapors, though invisible, are present and can easily be ignited. The vapors usually travel near the floor.

Most common heat sources usually produce temperatures higher than the ignition temperatures of most common fuels. Thus they can easily raise the fuel to its ignition temperature. For example, the heat produced by a match flame or an electric arc is about 2000°F., and the heat produced by a lighted cigaret ranges from about 550°F. to 1350°F. They are well above the ignition temperatures of paper, wood, cotton, gasoline—the common fuels.

Plastics are becoming more common. They exhibit a wide range of reactions when exposed to fire. Plastics may be grouped into classifications of thermoplastic and thermosetting. Thermoplastics become soft and pliable when exposed to heat, whereas thermosetting plastics generally cannot be resoftened once set. Almost all plastics are somewhat flammable.

Thermoplastics, such as polyethylene, cellulose acetate, and a few others, melt and drip flaming globules when exposed to fire. This tends to increase their fire hazard since the globules can drip on other combustible materials and ignite them, or they may become embedded if in contact with human skin. Polyvinyl chloride will not drip while burning but will form hydrochloric acid vapors if burned in the presence of moisture. This is a severe toxicologic problem. Foamed plastics and foamed rubber products both are highly flammable and emit large quantities of black smoke while burning.

Burning starts in different ways, depending upon the ingredients involved. Ordinary burning begins when heat—usually from friction, a flame, a spark, or a heated surface—is high enough to ignite the vapors of a fuel. Electrical current or spark is another way. Spontaneous heating occurs when a fuel increases its own temperature without drawing heat from its surroundings. In other words, it "heats by itself." This usually happens through fermentation or chemical action. Spontaneous heating of a material to its ignition temperature results in spontaneous ignition. The fire starts "by itself." Fuels that have a high spontaneous ignition are oily clothing or rags, silk and other fabrics, and damp hay. Explosion and fire occur when something is ignited in a confined space such as a container, room, or building, causing quick chemical changes that make the fuel gases expand rapidly with great force. Some examples are firecrackers, rockets, and blasting caps. Aerosol cans may also explode if heated.

Flammability (how easily and how fast something burns) depends on the ingredients involved. The kind of fuel affects flammability. Some fuels have lower ignition temperatures than other fuels and, therefore, burn more easily. For example, paper is easier to burn than metal. Some fuels burn very slowly (asbestos and cement), sometimes only smoldering and never really flaming, while others burn very quickly (soft wood and paper). The shape and form of the fuel also affects flammability. Usually a light, airy form burns more easily than a heavier, more solid form. For example, a crumpled-up newspaper sheet burns more easily than the folded sheet of newspaper. The rate and period of heating is another influence. Long exposure time to heat increases the possibility of burning. For example, a log surrounded by heat from paper and kindling is much more likely to ignite than a log that has a match held against it for a few seconds.

In general, fires spread very quickly. As a fire burns, it gives off heat. This heat warms other fuels in the area to their ignition temperatures and they begin to burn. As a fire grows, it can produce so much heat that it even heats fuels that are a distance from the fire.

CAUSES

It appears that considerably more than half the nation's fires are caused by the careless actions of man. The rest have environmental causes, such as hazardous products, defects in the home, and lightning. A more detailed analysis of the causes of building fires is provided annually by the National Fire Protection Association (see Table 11–1). These are approximations only. Heading the list of causes are heating and cooking, and electrical. These two causes account for the greatest number of fires and the largest amount of fire loss.

Ignorance and indifference contribute substantially to the extraordinary magnitude of the fire problem in the United States. The problem

table 11–1   *Estimated U.S. Building Fire Causes**

	percent of fires	percent of dollar losses
Heating and cooking	16	8
Smoking and matches	12	4
Electrical	16	12
Rubbish, ignition source unknown	3	1
Flammable liquid fires and explosion	7	3
Open flames and sparks	7	4
Lightning	2	2
Children and matches	7	3
Exposures	2	2
Incendiary, suspicious	7	10
Spontaneous ignition	2	1
Miscellaneous known causes	2	6
Unknown	17	44
total	100	100

*NFPA estimates.

has not reached the American consciousness with the same force as, for example, the far less lethal problem of air pollution. In contrast, poliomyelitis, which in the peak year of 1952 killed about a third as many people as died by fire in that year, has been virtually eradicated because of the public attention it received. Americans supported research and control programs to attack the polio problem. Little concern has come forth regarding the grave losses by fire. There are even those in the fire services who pay lip service to fire prevention and then do little to promote it. The public has an image of firefighters as people rescuers and fire suppressers, not as a professional corps of fire preventers. Building designers give minimal attention to fire safety in the buildings they design and are content to meet only the minimal safety standards of the local building code.

Fire, it seems, just isn't a personal threat. There is an old saying in the fire protection field to the effect that fires have three causes: men, women, and children. It takes the careless or unwise action of a human being, in most cases, to begin a destructive fire. Few private homes have fire extinguishers, much less fire detection systems; and often when fire strikes, ignorance of what to do leads to panic behavior and aggravation of the hazards rather than to successful escape.

EFFECTS: PEOPLE

Fire is a major national problem.[1] During one hour there is a statistical likelihood that more than 300 destructive fires will rage somewhere in this nation. When they are extinguished, more than $300,000 worth of property will have been ruined. At least one person will have died. Thirty-four will be injured, some of them crippled or disfigured for life.

Annually fire claims nearly 12,000 lives in the United States. Among causes of accidental death, only motor vehicle accidents, falls and drownings rank higher. Most of fire's victims die by inhaling smoke or toxic gases well before the flames have reached them. (See Figure 11–2.)

The scars and terrifying memories live on with the 300,000 Americans who are injured by fire every year. Of these, nearly 50,000 lie in hospitals for a period ranging from six weeks to two years. Many of them must return, over and over again, for plastic and reconstructive surgery. Many never resume normal lives.

The price of destructive fire in the United States amounts, by conservative estimate, to at least $11.4 billion a year. Beyond calculation are the losses from businesses that must close and from jobs that are interrupted or destroyed. Fire is one of the greatest wasters of our natural resources (refer to chapter 17, Forest and Grass Fires).

Appallingly, the richest and most technologically advanced nation in the world leads all the major industrialized countries in per capita deaths and property loss from fire.[2] (See Figure 11–3.) While differing reporting procedures make international comparisons unreliable, the fact that the United States reports a death-per-million-population rate

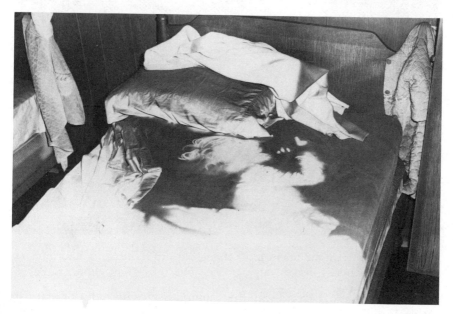

figure 11–2   Most of fire's victims never see the flames. Photo by O.H. Willoughby, courtesy of the National Fire Protection Association.

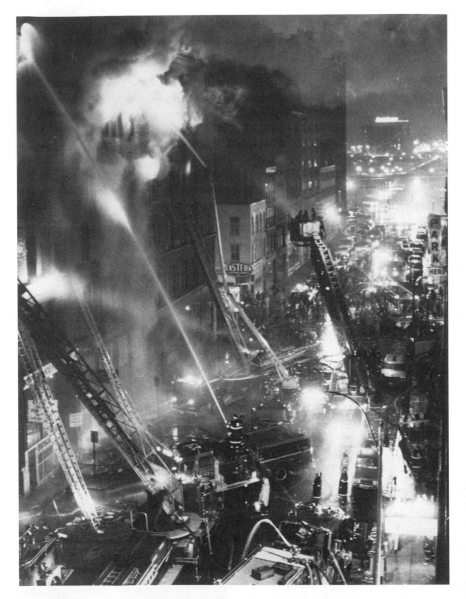

figure 11–3 The United States leads the world in fire losses. Photo from *The Boston Globe*, courtesy of the National Fire Protection Association.

nearly twice that of second-ranking Canada leaves little doubt that this nation leads the other industrialized nations in fire deaths per capita.

There are many effects of fire injury, but they can generally be categorized into primary or secondary effects.[3]

Primary Effects of Fire Injury

The two main primary effects of fire are tissue loss and inhalation of hot combustion products and toxic gases. The most familiar aspect of fire damage to a human is burn damage.

Burn damage to human skin is described by increasing severity with the terms *first, second,* and *third degree.*[4] Categorizing a burn into any one of these three groups depends upon the amount of heat to which a particular type of skin is exposed and the length of exposure time. First- and second-degree burns can be classified as partial-thickness burns (both the epidermal and the dermal layers are involved). Each type of burn has an effect on the body which is distinctive enough to require different first aid or more complex types of treatment.

The redness of the skin caused by exposure to a low heat source is an inflammatory response designated as *first degree.* If the burn is extensive enough, pain and swelling occur. Sometimes the red area feels hot, indicating the tiny blood vessels are swollen because more blood is being pumped to the area. This is one of the body's physiological reactions to the trauma of heat.

Second-degree burns result when the outer (epidermal) cells have been destroyed by heat, and when there is partial destruction of skin appendages. These burns are characterized by a very red, moist surface that is sensitive to light touch. As this is a partial-thickness wound, blisters usually result. Indicators such as these explain the skin's reaction to the heat trauma. Healing depends upon how many of the damaged cells are able to survive and multiply to the extent of resuming their normal functions.

Third-degree burns are marked not only by excessive heat destruction of cells in the dermal layer, but can also be characterized by destruction of muscle, fat, and even bone tissue. In addition to the pain and shock from such a trauma, the extensive injury of a third-degree burn literally bares the internal tissues to infection. The dry, white center portion of a third-degree burn may misrepresent the infectious activity underneath this insensitive covering. A purplish area surrounds the center, indicating sluggish circulation that can result in death of the tissue. Beyond this area is a moist, bright red area that is sensitive to a pinprick.

These descriptions of the three types of burns are classic examples; each type is not always readily visible. Most burns are a combination of degrees, with untreated second degree sometimes changing into third degree. Often one or more of the severity indicators described is very difficult to detect.

Once the skin ceases as a protective barrier and the blood vessels can no longer supply oxygen to the tissue in the burn area, the metabolic system is disrupted to the extent that major body functions can become impaired. The more skin that is damaged, the more severe the injury. Accordingly, extent of burn is measured by the percentage of body surface involved. This can be determined in several ways.[5] In adults (16 years of age and over), the "Rule of Nines" applies; for infants and children, the percentages by age as tabulated on the Lund and Browder chart are more accurate (see Figure 11–4). The fact that the area of one surface of the *patient's hand* is about one percent of the total body surface is very useful in estimating the size of small or oddly shaped burns.

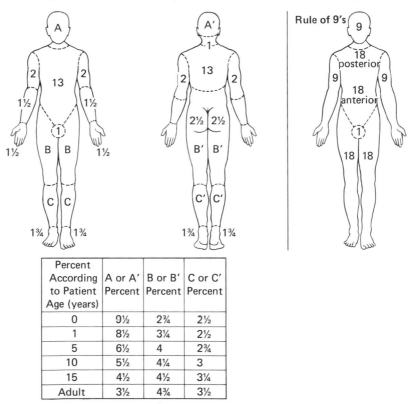

Percent According to Patient Age (years)	A or A' Percent	B or B' Percent	C or C' Percent
0	9½	2¾	2½
1	8½	3¼	2½
5	6½	4	2¾
10	5½	4¼	3
15	4½	4½	3¼
Adult	3½	4¾	3½

figure 11–4 Determining the extent of burn injury. On the left is the burned victim and Lund and Browder's figures for percentage burn according to age. On the right is the "Rule of Nines" diagram appropriately marked with the indicated percentage burn. The "Rule of Nines" is the most commonly used method for determining the extent of burn injury, but it is more accurate to use the Lunn and Browder method of determining the relative percentage that selected areas of the body contribute at various ages. Redrawn after Carl Jelenko, III, "Emergency Treatment of Small Burns," *Hospital Medicine,* January 1975, p. 94.

Burns may be classified as minor, moderate, or critical (see Table 11–2).

Inhalation is the second general category of primary fire effects. As previously stated, most of fire's victims die by inhaling smoke or toxic gases well before the flames have reached them. A person caught in a burning building may have from a few seconds to an hour to escape, to reach an area of refuge, or to be rescued. Ninety seconds frequently is the maximum time that passengers would have to escape from a burning aircraft.[6]

Table 11–3 shows the difference between long- and short-term exposures to products of combustion. In Table 11–4 is a list of the most significant items and the levels at which they may be fatal or cause irreversible damage in seconds.[7]

Heat.   Table 11–5 shows the temperature in buildings during fire tests after certain lapses of burning time. Extremely high temperatures as a result of exposure to fire conditions can cause an immediate reaction in humans. (Temperatures above 300°F. can cause death in minutes.) Death can occur when the mucous membranes lining the respiratory system secrete fluids and thereby fill the lungs with liquid. A victim of fire's heat can drown in his own liquid. In addition, hot smoke with a high moisture content is a special danger since it destroys tissues deep in the lungs by burning.

Carbon Monoxide.   Often called the silent killer, carbon monoxide is one of the most common and dangerous poisons. It is dangerous because it is a gas that is practically colorless and odorless; and it can kill

---

table 11–2   *Classification of Burns**

minor burns
Second-degree burns of less than 15 percent of body surface area (less than 10 percent in children).
Third-degree burns of less than 2 percent of body surface area.
moderate burns
Second-degree burns of 15 to 30 percent of body surface area (10 to 30 percent in children).
critical burns
Second-degree burns of greater than 30 percent of body surface area.
Third-degree burns that involve the face, hands, feet or over 10 percent of body surface area.
electrical burns
Burns complicated by respiratory tract injury (smoke inhalation), extensive soft-tissue injury or fractures.

---

*Bruce E. Zawacki and Basil A. Pruitt, Jr., "Emergency Treatment of Burns," *American Family Physician*, July 1970, p. 63. *Adapted from Artz, C.P. and Reiss, E.:* THE TREATMENT OF BURNS. *Philadelphia: W.B. Saunders Company, 1957.*

table 11–3 *Tolerance to Selected Combustion Products*

combustion products	minutes	hazardous levels for times indicated		
		½ hour	1–2 hours	8 hours
Heat (°F.)	284	212	150	120
Oxygen (%)	6	11	14	15
Carbon Dioxide (ppm)	50,000	40,000	35,000	32,000
Carbon Monoxide (ppm)	3,000	1,600	800	100
Sulphur Dioxide (ppm)	400	150	50	8
Nitrogen Dioxide (ppm)	240	100	50	30
Hydrogen Chloride (ppm)	1,000	1,000	40	7
Hydrogen Cyanide (ppm)	200	100	50	2

note: There is considerable variation among investigators as to what level of a particular gas constitutes a life hazard.

source: Calvin H. Yuill, "Physiological Effects of Products of Combustion," *American Society of Safety Engineers Journal,* February 1974.

table 11–4 *Lethal Levels for Momentary Exposure*

Heat	300°F.
Oxygen	6.0
Carbon Monoxide	1.28%
Carbon Dioxide	12.0 %

source: Calvin H. Yuill, "Physiological Effects of Products of Combustion," *American Society of Safety Engineers Journal,* February 1974, p. 37.

table 11–5 *Standard Time/Temperature Curve*

time (hr: min.)	temperature (°F.)
0:05	1000
0:10	1300
0:15	1399
0:20	1462
0:30	1550
0:45	1638
1:00	1700
2:00	1850
3:00	1925
4:00	2000

source: Calvin H. Yuill, "Physiological Effects of Products of Combustion," *American Society of Safety Engineers Journal,* February 1974, p. 38.

within minutes, depending upon the concentration in the air. Carbon monoxide enters the bloodstream rapidly, since the blood has a 250-times-stronger affinity for it than for oxygen.[8] As CO replaces oxygen in the blood, life can be stopped. Carbon monoxide is liberated when a carbon fuel is burned and its concentration is dependent upon incomplete combustion (e.g., smoldering fire). Generally then, a hot, fast fire, with plenty of oxygen, will produce a minimum of CO; while a slow, cool fire, with a limited amount of available oxygen, will produce more.[9]

Carbon Dioxide.   This gas is also colorless and odorless and is a product of fire. The hazards of carbon dioxide are (1) it can replace oxygen in the blood and (2) it increases the respiratory rate so that other gases present (e.g., CO) will be inhaled more rapidly.[10]

Oxygen Deficiency (Hypoxia).   The depletion of the oxygen supply can be extremely dangerous (see Figure 11–3). Normally there is 21 percent by volume of oxygen in the air we breathe. If that figure drops to 15 percent breathing becomes labored and is accompanied by dizziness and headache. Nausea and even paralysis may occur at 10 percent, and at 6 percent unconsciousness occurs. Below 6 percent death occurs in minutes. Brain damage can occur at 12 to 15 percent.

Smoke.[11]   Obscured and irritated vision result from smoke. If a path of escape cannot be seen through the smoke, the person becomes disoriented and remains in the fire area long enough for other injuries — burns, heat, and toxic gas inhalation — to occur. Probably most of the deaths listed as "smoke inhalation" on the death certificate were really caused by hypoxia or inhalation of toxic gases. Hot smoke sears the mucous membranes and death occurs. If smoke is cool, it may cause swelling (edema) of lung tissue or chemical pneumonia. Smoke particles may have injurious interactions with body tissues over an extended time period.

Other Gases.[12]   Without elaboration, other gases resulting from combustion include: sulphur dioxide, nitrogen dioxide, hydrogen chloride, hydrogen cyanide, phosgene, hydrocarbons, and aldehydes. There is evidence that the hazard of two or more toxic gases is greater than the sum of the hazards of each. There is not enough known about toxicity.

Panic.   Though not a physical product of fire, panic often occurs when fire breaks out and has been the cause of injuries and deaths due to trampling or jumping from windows too high off the ground.

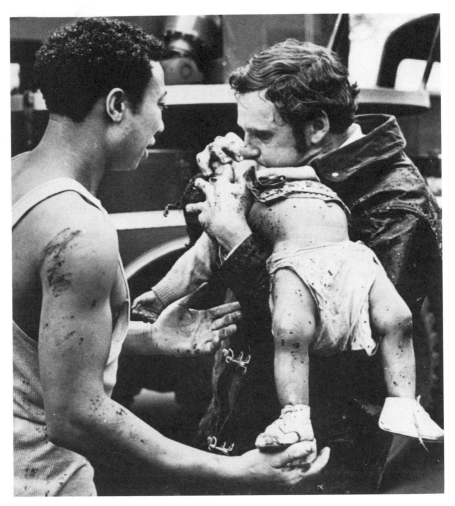

figure 11–5   Artificial respiration giving the "breath of life." ©1970 *Buffalo Courier-Express;* photo by Ron Moscati.

Secondary Effects of Fire Injury

Consequences accompanying the loss of blood and fluid are shock (or low blood pressure) and infection (results in most burn deaths).[13] Bacteria and fungi can enter through areas of skin loss. Much of the burn therapy in hospitals is concerned with the prevention and early detection of infection. The inability to eat (from damage to the gastrointestinal tract) results in lost energy needed by the body to repair itself.

Fire kills. But fire has its living victims, too—those who grieve the loss of loved ones—those who manage to get out alive (while others close to them may not have)—those who are left homeless or jobless or impoverished. The victims most poignant to consider are those maimed and disfigured by burn injuries. About half of these victims are children. Their scars, psychological as well as physical, often last a lifetime.

The victim is not the only one to endure psychological wounds. If the victim is a child, parents are likely to feel guilty for what has happened. Some parents find it impossible to accept and love a disfigured child. Nurses, who must inflict considerable pain on the patient over long periods of treatment, are subject to stress. In many burn care facilities there is a 100 percent turnover in nursing staff every six months.

The average hospital stay for a burn victim is over three times that of medical and surgical patients. An individual's hospital stay and later treatment can add up to $60,000 or more. (Reducing fire accidents, therefore, should be among the top priorities in the national effort to control health care costs.)

If the severely burned victim is fortunate, he or she will be treated in one of a dozen "burn centers" in the United States. In these special facilities, patients receive expert medical and surgical care from the outset, and physical and emotional rehabilitation through the long weeks of recovery. The process can be best described through an actual case history:

It is the fall of 1970. Eight-year-old Susan and her older brother are playing in their garage. An unsealed can of gasoline tips over and, an instant later, the pilot light of the nearby water heater ignites the vapor. In the flash fire and explosion, Susan's face and arms are badly burned, her dress set afire. She is rushed to a local emergency room, where she is treated for shock. Because the burns are extensive and predominantly third degree (the most severe kind), the doctors arrange for her admission to a burn center, 100 miles away.

There, intensive care begins. The wounds are cleaned and treated with antibacterial agents; intravenous lines are inserted; and a catheter is placed into the bladder to collect urine, which serves as a guide to the fluid needs of the body. Nurses in the intensive care unit keep a close watch, lest she go into shock or turn blue from smoke inhalation injury. Later she is anesthetized and wheeled into surgery, where a doctor begins debridement, the cutting away of burned tissue. The wounds are covered with antibiotic dressing, and Susan is given penicillin to ward off infection.

More debridement operations follow. Doctors and nurses continue to monitor closely Susan's fluid management and the functioning of her vital organs. On the third day, having survived the acute phase in which fluid imbalances can be fatal, Susan is taking food by mouth, and the intravenous lines are removed. For the first time, she complains of pain from her wounds.

On the seventh day there is a marked change in Susan. She refuses food, she is unruly. But the staff members have seen this kind of behavior often, for it signals the onset of guilt or fear of parental reaction about the accident. After conferring with staff, Susan's parents discuss the accident, assuring her they were concerned but not angry. Her mood soon brightens. But there will be other periods of irritability. Having less than the normal amount of skin is a depressing condition, and it is common for patients to be difficult, irascible, or complaining until the wounds heal or are successfully skin-grafted.

During the second and third weeks, operations are performed to remove further dead skin. As so often happens, the wounds become infected and for a time her life is in jeopardy. In the fourth week grafting operations begin — four in all, staged at 10-day intervals. Between operations, Susan undergoes intensive physical therapy, since grafted skin tends to contract and hamper the body's movements. Despite all precautions, contractures of her neck, right wrist, and right hand begin to develop, drawing her chin toward her chest, her wrist backward, and her fingers out of joint. Though Susan is discharged after 80 hospital days, the deformities already developing grow worse, despite frequent physical therapy and splinting. She is readmitted twice during the ensuing 4 months for reconstructive surgery.

More plastic surgery awaits her. It will never totally erase the scars. And despite the efforts of the psychiatrist on the burn center staff, Susan still carries psychological scars. She is introspective, self-conscious, and overly dependent on her father.[14]

EFFECTS: PROPERTY

Available statistics give some idea of where the hazards lie in our man-made environment. The vast majority — close to 95 percent — of America's fire losses, both life and property, result from fires in the built environment. Fires in buildings account for most of these losses. Of the nearly $2.7 billion in property losses sustained yearly, about 85 cents out of every dollar lost is attributable to a building fire. What types of buildings are involved offers a key to where the emphasis should lie in the effort to reduce the nation's fire losses.

Residences.   About seven out of ten fires occurring annually are in residential occupancies. The chances are that the average family will experience one fire every generation serious enough to have the fire department respond.

Commercial and Industrial Fires.   While commercial occupancies make up about 14 percent of all building fires, they result in 25 percent of the property loss in building fires. Likewise, industrial fires are only about 16 percent of all building fires but account for 36 percent of the building property loss.

Major Fires.   Those fires producing major property losses are a tiny fraction of total fires. In most cases the building was not sprinklered in the area where the fire originated. The National Fire Protection Association defines as a major fire one in which three or more die, or one in which property losses are $250,000 or greater (or both).

Property is damaged or destroyed by:

1   The actual burning and charring that turns materials to ashes.

2   Smoke, which leave things blackened and often leaves a strong odor that is hard to eliminate.

3   Water and other results of firefighting (walls and doors that have been torn down, broken windows, etc.).

THREAT

The mortality due to fires and conflagrations begins to rise with the onset of cold weather and the increased use of heating equipment.[15] Peak mortality usually occurs in January, when the death toll is more than three times that in July or August. Geographically, the highest death rates from fires are reported from the South and Southwest. Residents of Utah have one of the nation's lowest fire death rates; those who live in neighboring Nevada have one of the highest. The same relationship applies to the neighboring states, Ohio and Kentucky. Even within a single state, the relationship between human and environmental factors can differ.[16]

The rapid expansion of the mobile home industry has added a new dimension to the home fire problem. Mobile homes are now the most commonly built type of single-family dwelling unit. Unfortunately, safety research and consumer education about mobile homes have not paralleled their production gains. The home fire potential in many mobile dwelling units is great.

More than 80 percent of the fatalities occur in the home. On an annual basis, roughly one percent of homes are damaged or destroyed by fire. Nonmetropolitan areas have higher death rates than metropolitan areas, possibly reflecting a lack of fire departments, local rather than central heating, and a shortage of emergency medical services in these areas.

VULNERABILITY

Fires are the leading cause of death from nontransportation accidents among children 1–4 years of age and the second leading cause among youngsters 5–14 and persons 45 and over.[17] The death rate from fire among children under 5 and the elderly over 65 is three times that of the rest of the population. Though together these young and old make up only 20 percent of the American population, they account for 45 percent of the fire deaths. (See Figure 11–6.)

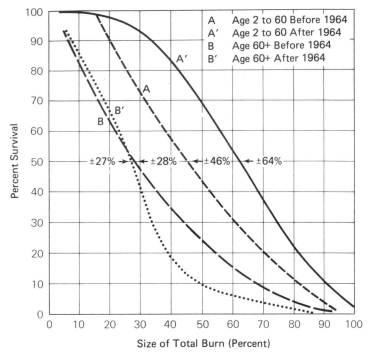

figure 11–6   Survival versus total burn by age groups. Redrawn after Carl Je-lenko, III, "Emergency Treatment of Small Deep Burns," *Hospital Medicine,* January 1975, p. 92.

The decreased agility of older people makes them particularly vulnerable to the hazard of having their clothing ignited by fire. In addition, because of their infirmities, the elderly often find it very difficult to escape from a burning building. The danger to very small children lies in their being left at home alone or with inadequate supervision.

Death rates are higher among males than females. Male mortality from fire is about one and a half times the female mortality at all ages combined.[18, 19]

COUNTERMEASURES: PRE-FIRE

Education

Among the many measures that can be taken to reduce fire losses, perhaps none is more important than educating people about fire. Americans must be made aware of the magnitude of fire's toll and its threat to them personally. They must know how to minimize the risk of fire in their daily surroundings. They must know how to cope with fire, quickly and effectively, once it has started.

Most fire service professionals agree that public education about fire has the greatest potential for reducing losses, and that there is a need for greater education of the public in fire safety. Most of these professionals believe that most fires occur because of public apathy toward good fire prevention practices.

The special target of educational efforts designed to prevent fire loss should be those fires caused by human action. It is estimated that over 70 percent of the building fires can be attributed to the careless acts of people.

The prevention of fires due to human carelessness is not all that fire safety education can hope to accomplish. Many fires caused by faulty equipment rather than carelessness could be prevented if people were trained to recognize hazards; and many injuries and deaths could be prevented if people knew how to react to a fire, whatever its cause. As one writer has summed up the problem:

A significant factor contributing to the cause and spread of fire is human failure — failure to recognize hazards and take adequate preventive measures, failure to act intelligently at the outbreak of the fire, failure to take action which would limit damage.[20]

These failures cannot be legislated out of existence; they must be dealt with through education.

Day in and day out, firefighters see the evidence of human failure. They see pennies in fuse boxes and 30-ampere fuses where 15-ampere fuses ought to be. They see the tragic consequences of trash or flammable liquids stored near furnaces, overloaded electrical circuits, gas heaters improperly vented. They find the victims of fire who have died in their sleep because they failed to take the routine precaution of always sleeping with bedroom doors closed. They find the charred bodies of those who took a fatal gamble with fire: who opened a hot door, who dashed through smoke instead of crawling along the floor, who might have survived the gauntlet if they had held a wet cloth over nose and mouth. Organizations like the National Fire Protection Association and the National Safety Council have based their fire safety messages on these common failings. Firefighters and others have brought these messages into the homes and classrooms of America. And still, thousands of Americans die needlessly every year.

A cynic might remark that this widespread ignorance shows that Fire Prevention Week, school programs in fire safety, and all the posters and pamphlets on fire prevention are wasted efforts. Yet, we do not know how much worse the annual fire record would be if there were no educational efforts. Moreover, we do know that public education programs can dramatically reduce fire losses. Studies provide evidence of this. Though small in scope, the studies are among the few in which results of fire prevention efforts have been measured.

An intensive fire safety education program was directed at an area of southeast Missouri where the fire death rate was far higher than the national average.[21] The first step was to study the pattern of fires and burn injuries and their causes. Then a field staff was trained to administer the program. Civic groups, fire departments, local officials, and the mass media cooperated with the program. The public got fire safety messages every way they turned — from audiovisual demonstrations, educational programs, and media broadcasts. The result: the fire death rate dropped 43 percent in three years — from 12.9 to 7.4 per 100,000 population. For each dollar invested in the program, $20 was saved in anticipated property losses, medical expenses, and earnings losses. Two years after the pilot program was terminated, the death rate was still falling — five times faster than that of the rest of the state.

Incidents have demonstrated that when people have fire safety on their minds, fires decrease in number. In these cases, people were fire-conscious because they knew normal fire protection was not available to them. When snowstorms immobilized all traffic, and when fire trucks were tied up in riot-torn areas, the number of fires dwindled to a fraction of the normal.

A long-term success in fire safety education is the Smokey Bear campaign. Billions of dollars have been saved through this campaign. See the chapter on Forest and Grass Fires for more information about the Smokey Bear program and its effectiveness.

Public Education.   A number of efforts — by professional societies, the insurance industry, fire departments and other governmental agencies — are reaching *some* portions of the American people effectively.

Private Organizations. Through posters and pamphlets, the National Fire Protection Association brings a fire safety message to millions of Americans every year. The National Fire Protection Association is instrumental in promoting the annual Fire Prevention Week campaign, the Sparky the Fire Dog campaign in schools, and seasonal fire prevention campaigns in the spring and at Christmas.

The American Insurance Association annually distributes pamphlets to schools, hospitals, and other organizations. Its films reach an audience of more than two million people each year. Through the special training it provides to thousands of fire inspectors working for insurance companies, the American Insurance Association has an indirect but considerable effect on public education.

The Federal Government. With the very contrasting exception of the Forest Service's Smokey Bear program, the federal government is involved in only a limited way in fire safety education — except in government installations. Each federal agency has responsibility for internal fire prevention. There is no program in the federal government directed toward the public at large to prevent fire losses.

Fire Departments. Local fire departments make significant contributions to public education — through inspections of dwellings and commercial establishments, through distribution of reading material on fire safety, and through cooperation with schools.

In sum, a variety of ways is being tried to heighten public consciousness of fire safety. The very fact that the educational efforts come from a multiplicity of sources in a variety of ways probably serves to heighten public awareness of fire safety. Yet, it is safe to assume, given the sheer number of efforts, that some programs are far less effective than others. What is needed is a mechanism for evaluating these programs so that weak efforts can be replaced by coordinated support of efforts of proven effectiveness.

School Fire Safety Education.   Habits of fire safety are best instilled during the years of childhood, especially since youngsters are particularly prone to fire accidents. That fire safety education in schools can be effective is illustrated by a pilot study supported by the Bureau of Community Environmental Management of the Department of Health, Education, and Welfare.

In 1971 a demonstration project was begun in Memphis, Tennessee, to determine the effectiveness of teaching safety concepts to young school children. Forty-three elementary school teachers attended a 22-hour series of workshops on an injury control curriculum. Emphasis was placed on teaching burn prevention concepts. The teachers returned to their classes and taught what they had learned to 1016 children, ranging from kindergarten to the third grade. In the study area, burn injuries have decreased by 17 percent, while in a control area with similar population, burn injuries have increased by 100 percent. Because of the success of the pilot project, safety education is now being taught to all elementary school children in the Memphis school system.

Among the states requiring fire safety education, Iowa, Minnesota, and New York appear to have the most complete curricula in the field. New York law calls for 15 minutes of fire education a week in all grades, kindergarten through ninth grade (over and above time spent on fire drills), while Minnesota requires 60 minutes a week of health and fire education. While some states do have legal requirements and well-developed curricula, conversations with state officials reveal that implementation of these programs is not well enforced or programs are non-existent in many schools. One state teaches the dangers of ammunition, homemade bombs, and fireworks in the second grade but does not get around to the subject of matches until the third grade.

It is pointed out that the absence of a statewide fire education program does not necessarily mean that there is no fire education in the state. Local school boards, fire departments, or other groups may be filling the void — at least in part. Some communities have exemplary programs. In Santa Ana, California, a city of 165,000 people, an imaginative program in the classrooms is supplemented by demonstrations by the fire department, a parade at the end of Fire Prevention Week, a poster contest, and a carnival for school children in May. Civic groups are as deeply involved in the program as the schools and the fire department.

But the Santa Anas are the exception, not the rule. The nation's widespread ignorance about fire safety and the failure of many states to provide even minimal education in the subject underscore the need for federal intervention. The National Commission on Fire Prevention and Control recommends that the Department of Health, Education, and Welfare include in accreditation standards fire safety education in the schools throughout the school year.

Because fire safety has been ignored in the education of teachers, there are few educators with the knowledge or qualifications to teach it. The Commission recommends fire safety education courses for educators to provide a teaching cadre for fire safety education. The Commission recommends to the states the inclusion of fire safety education in programs educating future teachers and the requirement of knowledge of fire safety as a prerequisite for teaching certification.

Further, the Commission recommends an all-media campaign of public service advertising designed to promote public awareness of fire safety. Major emphasis should be placed on fire prevention in the home. This campaign should include national and regional efforts by all communications media directed toward specific fire-prone groups, such as the young and the elderly. The campaign should cover seasonal fire hazards, and should be geared through language, background, and program timing to the important recipients. Mass media education should not only create an awareness of fire hazards and fire safety, but should provide specific instruction on what to do and what not to do and motivate changes in attitudes and behavior.

Evaluation is an especially important phase of the recommended programs. Effectiveness of fire safety messages is best not left to guesswork. The best techniques of persuasion (admittedly, a field underdeveloped as a science) must go into the message; the most exacting standards of testing must go into the evaluation of results. The latter is true whether results are being measured in terms of attitude changes, elimination of hazards, or decline in fire accidents. In all such testing, results should be compared with a control group, consisting of a similar population, that has not received the fire safety message.

Special Opportunities. While it is premature to say what techniques work best, a project sponsored by the Department of Health, Education, and Welfare suggests approaches that could be adopted on a much wider scale. It was tried in Norfolk, Virginia, in 1969. Specially trained paraprofessionals, called Injury Control Technicians, went from house to house in the target area in the company of housing-hygiene inspectors. The technicians acted as home environment counselors to help residents of the area identify injury hazards and, where possible, eliminate them. (All kinds of hazards were pertinent, but fire hazards were a major consideration.) The advice of the technicians was welcomed by the residents and, as a result, an average of five important hazards per household was eliminated. In a second project, 500 specially trained paraprofessionals, called Health Educator Aides, are now working in 36 cities.

There are a number of Americans in occupations where, if they had special training in fire safety, they could favorably influence the safety of others:

Attendants in nursing homes, hospitals, and institutions for the handicapped should have special training to handle their difficult responsibilities during fire emergencies. Evacuation is usually a slow process and, with certain patients, sometimes impossible; and emergencies can be compounded by irrational behavior of patients.

Employees of restaurants, hotels, and places of public assembly should be trained to lead patrons to exits, to extinguish small fires, and to render first aid.

Physicians are valued counselors on a host of subjects ranging from nutrition to behavioral problems. Their advice on fire safety could be especially important to families with young children or elderly relatives in their care.

Millions of preschool children spend part of their time under the care of teachers and workers in nursery schools, day care centers, and Head

Start programs. In these contacts lie valuable opportunities for lessons in fire safety appropriate to the preschool age group.

There are approximately 20,000 resident managers of major (150-330) units) federally assisted housing facilities for low-income families. Currently these managers are being offered training opportunities in such subjects as administration, management of physical facilities, and human and family relations by the federally funded National Center for Housing Management. If these resident managers had special training in fire safety, they could affect the well-being of ten million Americans who live in these federally assisted housing projects.

These special situations merit special attention.

The need for thorough inspection programs by fire departments still exists. Trained firefighters can bring to residential inspections an expertise exceeding that of paraprofessionals for whom fire safety is a part-time concern.

A National Program for Fire Safety Education.   The National Commission on Fire Prevention and Control believes that an overall reduction of at least 2 percent per year in life loss, property loss, and injuries is a realistic and conservative goal for a national fire safety education program.

Multimedia Public Service Education. This nationwide program should be directed to the public at large through all forms possible, with an approach similar to the Smokey Bear campaign.

Intensive Local Education. This part of the program should be aimed at that 5 percent of the nation's population in areas suffering the highest loss of life from fire: Alaska, several southern states, and the poor sections of large cities. Various pilot projects have achieved significant reductions of fire incidence and burn injuries and deaths within one to two years. The project in Missouri resulted in a 14 percent reduction per year in fire deaths. The volunteer fire department of East Aurora, New York, reported a 28 percent reduction in the number of fires and a 52 percent reduction in dollar losses, achieved through a public education campaign. In Rochester, New York, spot announcements on television during station breaks contributed to a 15 percent annual reduction in smoking-related fires and an 18 percent annual reduction in fires caused by children and matches.

Cost-effectiveness as high as 20 to 1 — that is, $20 saved in losses prevented for every dollar spent on education — has been reported. Where volunteers are used or the media donate space or time, cost-benefit ratios can be even higher.

Education of Children in Schools. Continuous education of children of elementary school age can result in an annual 10 percent reduction in deaths and injuries within that group and an equal reduction in child-caused fires, especially those involving children and matches.

Inspection.   Many have found a checklist to be effective in inspecting a home for fire hazards. The list below is just an example of what can be done; it is by no means comprehensive.

1   Is smoking in bed strictly forbidden?

2   Are matches and lighters kept out of reach of children?

3   Do you make sure all electrical appliances purchased have the Underwriters' Laboratories tag attached?

4   Do you use the correct size fuse (15 amp for lighting) in each circuit of the fuse box?

5   Are all the extension cords exposed and not run under rugs and furniture?

6   Do you have heating equipment checked by a competent service man regularly?

7   Do you keep rubbish cleaned out of the attic, basement, closets, garage, and yard?

8   Is paint kept in tightly closed metal containers?

9   Are gasoline and other flammable liquids stored in safety cans and kept out of reach of children?

10   Do you prohibit the use of gasoline, kerosene, or similar materials for cleaning purposes?

11   Do all family members know how to report a fire?

12   Is there a prearranged escape route from the home in case of fire?

13   Are there sufficient outlets for all appliances to prevent overloading the electrical wires?

14   Are curtains that are located near a stove made of nonflammable material? If not, are they securely fastened to prevent them from blowing over the flame?

15   Is the gas stove equipped with a gas pilot in good working order?

16   Is there a recently inspected fire extinguisher in the home?

17   Are flammable materials, such as oily rags, kept in a closed metal container?

18   Are furnace, chimney, and flues cleaned regularly?

19   Are solid doors on bedroom doors and at tops of stairways?

20   Are fires rekindled with gasoline or kerosene?

21   Are flammable liquids labeled as such?

22   Are curtains, drapes, upholstery, and carpets selected with flammability in mind?

23   Is portable heating equipment used with special caution?

24 Are extension cords used in lieu of permanent wiring?

25 Are home furnishings and bedding selected on the basis of ignition possibilities?

Building Design and Codes

High-rise buildings are prevalent. Their contributions to the hazards of fire include: air conditioning system spreading smoke throughout the building; elevators malfunctioning; sealed windows that cause heat to build up; utility channels and other gaps in walls and floors that spread smoke and gases; overcrowded exitways; upper floors beyond the reach of ladders.[22]

High-rise buildings are not the only modern creation in which design impairs fire safety. In many homes stairwells help to carry fire and the products of combustion upward to sleeping areas. Slim horizontal windows under the eaves of single-story dwellings hamper rescue efforts.

Fire safety lags behind the other considerations in the design of buildings. Some of the reasons for this are: there is little incentive to invest in fire safety; building codes have characteristics that encourage the opinion that they are nuisances; tested uses and actual uses of materials can be two different things; and the knowledge on which fire safety standards are based is deficient.

The two most important codes from the standpoint of fire safety are the building code and the fire prevention code. Typically, two-thirds to three-fourths of the provisions of a building code apply to fire safety, as do all the provisions of a fire prevention code. There are ample examples of tragic fires in buildings that met all local building code requirements. Another problem with the codes is the diversity among cities. What goes in one town won't go in another—and many times for no good reason at all.

A law is effective only to the extent that it is enforced, and so it is with a fire prevention or building code. Many serious building fires have been the result not of code deficiencies, but of lax enforcement (sometimes because of corruption). A fire-resistant floor, for example, is an insufficient barrier to smoke and fire if the architect allows gaps in the floor or a workman punches a big hole in the floor to allow a pipe to pass through.

Vigilance is needed in the review of plans and in inspection during construction. Once construction is finished, compromises in fire safety may be hidden from view. The training of inspectors is, in many places, inadequate.

Codes could be strengthened by requiring that homes be equipped with early-warning fire detectors and alarms, and that automatic sprinkler systems be installed in buildings where many people congregate. These measures would probably not only pay for themselves in damages prevented, but also permit savings by relaxing requirements for other fire safety features. These two requirements might be the most important in providing fire safety within our building environment.

Product Design

It is not just the large structures of the built environment that need improved design if fire losses are to be reduced. Many products need design improvement. Heating and cooking equipment, faulty wiring, and electrical appliances are major fire causes.

The National Commission on Product Safety has identified color television sets, floor furnaces, hot-water vaporizers, and unvented gas heaters as specific fire or burn hazards. Under "unfinished business" — possibly hazardous products the Commission did not study — were listed electric blankets, dryers, hotplates, extension cords, and space heaters.

It is a complicated matter to make consumer products safe from fire and burn hazards. When kitchen range controls were at the front of the stove, children could reach them and cause burner accidents; now that they are at the back, they can be hazardous to the clothing and skin of people reaching for them over hot burners. No doubt today's appliances could be made completely safe, but food wouldn't get cooked, toast wouldn't get toasted, and clothes wouldn't get ironed. Advances are possible. Within the grasp of technology are burners that can be activated only by the weight of specially designed, snugly fitting pans.

Matches pose a special problem. An issue arises as to whether a foolproof match is possible. It remains to be seen if it is. It would appear that such could be developed, but it is costly. When you are talking about costs, the human versus the economic costs, somehow safety always seems to come second to money. Each time the government sets a standard on a product, the cost of that product goes up, but each time the government does not set a standard, we pay the human cost.

When clothing catches fire, the extent and depth of burns are more severe than skin burns on uncovered areas; from the standpoint of fire safety, the human species would be better off naked. One study found that clothing burn victims were four times more likely to die than burn victims spared clothing fire. Their burns covered nearly twice as much body surface.

Various studies indicate that 40 to 66 percent of all burn cases involve the ignition of clothing. One investigator assigned an "avoidability rating" for various types of burns. The preventability of clothing and flame burns ranked highest. In fact, the severity of clothing burns was nearly double that of the next type of burn, involving hot substances.

In rating fabrics as safe or unsafe, many factors must be considered. Cotton and rayon generally burn the fastest. Synthetic fibers possess a somewhat lower potential for injury. Fabrics made of animal hair, pure silk, and wool are the least hazardous. Napped surfaces usually burn quickly. In general, the heavier the fabric the higher its flame resistance. Long, loose-fitting garments are more dangerous than closer-fitting clothes.

The power to set flammability standards for fabrics now resides with the Consumer Product Safety Commission. Only a few standards have been promulgated: those for children's sleepwear, rugs, small carpets, and mattresses.

In 1938, the National Fire Protection Association published its "Model State Fireworks Law" which, where enacted, prohibits the use of all fireworks except those in supervised public displays. Fireworks continue to cause unnecessary losses even in states that wish to eliminate them, because federal, state, and local laws regulating transportation, sale, and use are a confused and futile patchwork.

Downey and Einhorn have made specific suggestions for fire prevention aimed at hospitals.[23] Many of the suggestions are also applicable to schools and homes:

1   Tight-weave carpets are better than high-pile ones. The greater the surface the more it burns.

2   Don't use paper draperies or paper clothes.

3   Avoid the use of carpets in hallways and access routes.

4   Don't use flexible urethane foam in furniture.

5   Don't use indoor/outdoor carpeting, some of which is highly flammable.

6   Don't use polypropylene wastebaskets. Such baskets result in molten pools of liquid that burn for 45 minutes to two hours.

7   Avoid electric overloads. Especially in rural areas, there is a tendency to overload electric systems.

8   Unplug television sets that have quick warm-up equipment. Some models maintain a low level of current in the tubes at all times and have been involved in an unusually high number of fires.

9   Consider having a ground exit from each room.

10   Make frequent inspections of detection and alarm systems and wiring.

11   Make sure circuit breakers work.

12 Be extremely cautious with cork bulletin boards. When hanging vertically, tests have shown they may burn to ashes within 60 seconds.

13 Restrict smoking to special rooms with minimal-combustion products.

14 Comply with the Life Safety Code of the National Fire Protection Association. This might be the simplest way to be better protected from fire.

Fire's Do's and Don'ts

Educational materials distributed by the National Fire Protection Association, the National Safety Council, the American Insurance Association, and others emphasize the major gaps in everyday knowledge and practice.

before a fire starts

1 Remove trash and stored items of outlived usefulness, particularly from the vicinity of furnaces and heaters and from hallways and exit areas.

2 Exercise care in the use of electricity. Do not overload electrical outlets with many appliances, use only appropriate fuses, and do not hang electrical cords over nails or run under carpets. Have cords replaced when they begin to fray or crack, and have electrical work done by competent electricians.

3 Do not store gasoline or flammable cleaners in glass containers, which can break, and avoid storing them inside the home. Do not keep more flammable liquids on hand than you really need.

4 To avoid the danger of spontaneous ignition, dispose of rags wet with oil, polishes, or other flammable liquids in outdoor garbage cans.

5 Inspect your home and workplace often for these and other hazards.

6 Plan for escape from every area of the home, discuss escape routes with your family, and actually rehearse escape. Look for exits upon entering restaurants, theaters, and other public buildings. You might have to find your way out in thick smoke or darkness.

7 Sleep with bedroom doors closed. In the event of a fire, you will gain precious minutes to escape.

8 Learn how to extinguish common fires in early stages the best way. Roll a person whose clothing is on fire; use a proper portable extinguisher or even a handful of baking soda to extinguish a fire on your stove.

9 Clothing afire is a prelude to tragedy. Buy garments, such as children's sleepwear, that meet federal flammability standards as they become available. Do not wear (or permit children to wear) loose, frilly garments if there is any chance at all of accidental contact with a stove burner or other source of fire.

10 Exercise extreme care with smoking materials and matches, major causes of destructive fire. Do not leave these where children can reach them.

11 Invest in fire extinguishers, escape ladders, and—most important—early-warning (smoke or products-of-combustion) fire detector and alarm devices.

COUNTERMEASURES: FIRE

Home Fire Detection[24]

Most who die in home fires die during the nighttime hours. Usually it is smoke, toxic gases, or lack of oxygen — not fire itself — that kills them.[25] Lives could have been saved if the victims had been awakened to the presence of a fire in its early stages. There are on the market approved devices designed to detect smoke or other products of combustion — not heat alone, which can be detected only in a fire's advanced stage — and sound an alarm.

Many devices have been available for years. But they were expensive and required connection to the electrical system because batteries were not considered fail-safe. Units powered by batteries are now permitted if the unit has a built-in method of alerting the occupants when the batteries grow weak or if something is not working properly.

The detector should be placed between the bedroom sleeping area and the rest of the house. The purpose, obviously, is to provide a defense against fire in another portion of the house while occupants are asleep in the bedrooms. Additional smoke detectors can be placed in other areas of the house for even earlier warning. In homes with two or more bedroom areas, a basic detector should be located outside each bedroom area. A detector in the bedroom itself would be a wise investment if there is a special need, such as a young child, an invalid, or a bedtime smoker. Although your nose is a more sensitive smoke detection instrument than any mechanical gadget, when you are asleep the smoke detector on the ceiling will sense the fire long before your nose on the mattress will.

Some believe a system of heat detectors is an adequate substitute, but only if there are many more of them located throughout the house. Only devices approved by nationally recognized testing laboratories, such as Underwriters' Laboratories or Factory Mutual Research Corporation, should be used.

Fire detection systems have become legal requirements for residences in some places. Since 1958, Quincy, Massachusetts, has required fire detection and alarm devices in all new single-family dwellings. The Village of Bayside, Wisconsin, has a similar ordinance, and also requires that occupants perform maintenance checks on the detection systems and report on a standard form to the chief of public safety annually or face a $200 fine. In Ohio the state fire code now requires a single-station fire detector in all new one-, two-, and three-family dwellings.

Certainly the technology of early-warning detectors can be improved and, with a substantial market assured, the costs of these devices can be brought within the reach of low-income families.

Evacuation

In spite of all precautions and prevention activities, fires will still start and lives will be threatened. No house can be made completely fire-proof. Not everyone instinctively flees from a burning home; children often panic and hide in closets or under beds. Being prepared and knowing what to do in case a fire breaks out can mean the difference between life and death. All families should have some sort of family fire escape plan, which should include the following procedures:

1   Everyone should sleep with his bedroom door closed at night. A closed door can delay the spread of fire and keep out deadly gases and smoke for the few extra minutes needed for escape. Sleep with a window partially open so that a fire cannot pull all the oxygen from the room.

2   Draw a floor plan of your home and mark an escape route and alternate route from each room in the house. Explain how to exit through windows, breaking the glass with a heavy object. Exits from second-story windows may require a rope or folding ladder. Never go out a window head first; back out of the window and hang from the sill with your hands before dropping to the ground. Dropping from a window should be a last resort.

3   Give special consideration to very young children and elderly persons when mapping escape routes.

4   Agree on a way in which any family member can sound an alarm — pounding on walls, yelling, whistling, etc.

5   Instruct family members not to waste time getting dressed or collecting prized possessions.

6   Make sure that every family member knows how to test a door. If panels or knobs are warm, keep door closed and use alternate escape route. If not, brace foot and hip against door and open cautiously to prevent superheated air from blowing it open.

7   If you are forced to remain in a room, stay near a slightly opened window. Place towels (wet, if possible) or cloths in the door cracks. To reach the other side of a smoke-filled room, crawl with your head about 18 inches above the floor. Cover the nose and mouth with a pillow or wet cloth, or hold your breath. (There is mounting evidence that the danger of respiratory damage can be diminished by use of a wet cloth.)

8   Decide on a meeting place outside the house where everyone will assemble as soon as they are outside.

9   Call the fire department as soon as everyone is out of the house. Use a neighbor's phone or a call alarm box. Speak clearly and plainly, making sure you give your full name and address.

10   Hold a practice drill once you have set up escape routes; then repeat drills periodically (every six months).

The National Fire Protection Association and the Fire Marshals Association of North America have devised a program called Operation EDITH (Exit Drills In The Home).[26] In a community that adopts Operation EDITH, well-publicized efforts are made to encourage families to devise—and rehearse—plans for getting the family out of the house in the event of a fire.

Decals have been designed which can be easily attached to the windows of rooms frequented by children (e.g., bedrooms and playrooms). Firemen can spot the decal from the outside and clear that particular room first.

Home Fire Extinguishment

Although prevention is best by far, home provision for extinguishing fires is also worthwhile. Such provision, however, should not lead to delay in summoning the fire department at once when fire strikes.

Fire control measures are based on the fact that flammable material burns only if the temperature is above its kindling point and a sufficient supply of oxygen is present. Accordingly, extinguishing measures are: (1) cool the burning material or (2) exclude oxygen, or both.

Fire extinguishers for the home have certain advantages, but cheap, easily contrived devices—for example, buckets of water and sand— serve well for many situations. Most homedwellers are aware about the extinguishment qualities of baking soda. Fire extinguishers are so constructed that their contents can be directed on a fire fairly accurately. Most of them operate by spraying water, inert gas, or inert gas chemical that forms a blanket over the flame to exclude air.

A universally available agent for cooling is water. It serves well against all burning material except grease, oil (causes this fire type to spread), and electricity. Provision for quick use of water may include the placing of pails or basins in strategic spots on shelves or brackets, such as in the basement and attic, or garden hose near selected outdoor and indoor faucets, installation of water reservoirs in or about farm buildings and remote dwellings, and the acquisition of portable hand pumps with water tanks of at least two gallons capacity, such as are used to spray insecticides. Water should not be used on electrical fires since water is a conductor of electricity.

Excluding oxygen is accomplished by such means as throwing sand or a wool blanket, wet towel, or wool rug over a flame, or placing a lid on a dish of burning material, or wrapping heavy material around a person whose clothes are afire. Woolens do not ignite nearly as readily as cotton and synthetic materials. If the door to a closet or any small compartment where burning occurs is closed, the flames may subside because of lack of oxygen. It is not essential to exclude oxygen completely. The burning process consumes oxygen from the air; when the proportion of oxygen in the air falls from a normal 21 percent to less than 15 percent, the burning subsides. However, if the material remains hot the fire may resume when air is again admitted.

Although portable extinguishers are a well-recognized item for use in an emergency, their limitations should not be overlooked. Such equipment is intended for use only on small fires, or in the interim between discovery of a fire and the arrival of professional firefighters. In addition, the effectiveness of any extinguisher is governed by its size, and the capabilities of the individual operating it.

To be effective, portable extinguishers must be:[27]

1   The right type for each class of fire that may occur. Fires are classified according to the following categories:[28] Class A—fires in ordinary combustible materials, such as wood, cloth, paper, and rubber; Class B—fires in flammable liquids, gases, and greases; Class C—fires that involve energized electrical equipment where the electrical nonconductivity of the extinguishing media is of importance (when electrical equipment is deenergized, extinguishers for Class A or Class B fires may be used safely; Class D—fires in combustible metals, such as magnesium, titanium, zirconium, sodium, and potassium.

2   In sufficient quantity to protect.

3   Located where they are ready for immediate use. Distribution should be decided according to the area and arrangement of the building, severity of the hazard, anticipated classes of fires, and the distances to be traveled to reach the extinguishers.

4   Maintained in perfect operating condition, inspected frequently, checked against tampering, and recharged as required. They should be inspected monthly and recharged yearly. A tag showing maintenance and recharge data should be found on each extinguisher.

5   Operable by people who can locate them promptly and use them effectively. Unless a person has had actual experience in the firing of a portable fire extinguisher, he is in for a big surprise if ever called upon to use one in an emergency. The feel, the weight, the experience of firing, and the length of time a unit will operate are all important aspects in the effective use of a portable fire extinguisher.

The pump-tank extinguisher or stored-pressure type using water is recommended as first choice for homes. Most home fires are Class A. This extinguisher is portable and the water container can be replenished quickly. If desired, an antifreeze charge can be added. Models that throw water 45 feet can be obtained. The 2½-gallon size probably suffices; larger sizes are available. The soda-acid extinguisher, so often seen in commercial buildings, cannot be replenished so readily and must be recharged annually. It, too, finds its use against Class A fires, permits quick action, and can be hung on a wall.

As added protection in addition to the pump-tank type, the carbon-dioxide extinguisher may be purchased; it is useful against Class B and C fires. The dry-chemical type is effective against all fires, especially B and C. Although the other kinds of extinguishers have their advantages under certain circumstances, they are not so generally recommended for the home. The foam type leaves a messy deposit on home furnishings. The vaporizing liquid type sometimes uses carbon tetrachloride, a toxic chemical especially dangerous when used in confined spaces. The carbon dioxide and dry chemical types are effective against Class B and C fires and have some value against Class A, and the carbon tetrachloride is effective against electrical fires, Class C. Thus, like the carbon-dioxide extinguisher, they are useful against automobile fires. The water-delivering type may conduct electricity.

Considering the great loss of life and property caused by fires, it is highly advisable to make provision for quickly controlling small fires. Fire extinguishers, or the home-devised improvisations, cost little by comparison.

NOTES

[1] *America Burning,* The Report of the National Commission on Fire Prevention and Control, 1973.

[2] HOWARD W: EMMONS, "Fire and Fire Protection," *Scientific American,* July 1974, p. 21.

[3] WILLIAM BERMAN, "Medical Aspects of Burns," *Journal of Environmental Health,* November 1973, p. 217.

[4] American Academy of Orthopaedic Surgeons, *Emergency Care and Transportation of the Sick and Injured,* 1971, p. 138.

[5] BRUCE E. ZAWACKI AND BASIL A. PRUITT, "Emergency Treatment of Burns," *American Family Physician,* July 1970, p. 61.

[6] CALVIN H. YUILL, "Physiological Effects of Products of Combustion," *ASSE Journal,* February 1974, p. 36.

[7] Ibid.

[8] SIDNEY KAYE, *Handbook of Emergency Toxicology* (Philadelphia: W. B. Saunders Co., 1961), p. 6.

[9] National Safety Council, "Carbon Monoxide—The Silent Killer," *National Safety News,* December 1973, p. 80.

[10]YUILL, "Products of Combustion," p. 38.

[11]BERNARD W. MAYER et al., "Acute Smoke Inhalation in Children," *American Family Physician,* April 1973, p. 80.

[12]YUILL, "Products of Combustion," p. 39.

[13]BERMAN, "Medical Aspects of Burns," p. 218.

[14]*America Burning,* pp. 11–12.

[15]"Mortality from Fires and Conflagrations," *Statistical Bulletin,* December 1973, p. 6.

[16]RICHARD E. GALLAGHER, "The Interaction of Man and Environment in Accidental Fire and Burns," *Journal of Environmental Health,* November 1973, p. 221.

[17]"Mortality from Fires and Conflagrations," p. 6.

[18]Ibid., p. 7.

[19]ALBERT P. ISKRANT, "Statistics and Epidemiology of Burns," *Bulletin of the New York Academy of Medicine,* August 1967, p. 636.

[20]DEUEL RICHARDSON, "The Public and Fire Protection," *NFPA Quarterly,* July 1962, p. 4.

[21]U.S. Department of Health, Education, and Welfare, Public Health Service, *A Community Action Approach for Prevention of Burn Injuries,* Burn Injury Prevention Pilot-Demonstration Project.

[22]"The Low-Down on High-Rise Fires," *Family Safety,* Winter 1972, pp. 18–21.

[23]GREGG W. DOWNEY AND IRVING N. EINHORN, "Need More Research to Improve Fire Prevention," *Modern Hospital,* April 1972, pp. 87–89.

[24]REXFORD WILSON, "The Home Fire Management Program," *National Safety Congress Transactions,* Home Safety, 1973, p. 11.

[25]REXFORD WILSON, "Night Killer," *Family Safety,* Spring 1973, p. 10.

[26]WILSON, "The Home Fire Management Program," p. 11.

[27]"Portable Fire Extinguisher Guidelines," *National Safety News,* June 1974, p. 57.

[28]OSHA Act Regulations for Portable Fire Extinguishers," *National Safety News,* June 1974, p. 69.

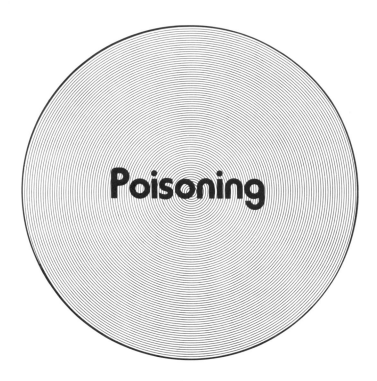

Poisoning

Characteristics and Causes

12 Poisoning by ingestion occurs when any solid or liquid that tends to impair health or cause death is introduced into the body. One man's medicine could be another's poison.

Since the earliest times, man has sought to protect himself against the danger of disease. In the past our defenses were limited to disease control, but more recently we have turned toward preventive measures. This approach has paid rich dividends in the eradication of smallpox, diphtheria, tetanus, and poliomyelitis, and during the last decade, in the prevention of measles, mumps, and rubella.

Another great scourge confronts us—poisoning by solids and liquids, most of which are advantageous to our daily living and are commonly found in every household. With about 90 percent of the accidental ingestions occurring in children under five years of age, the burden of protecting them rests on the adults.[1]

There has been an increased awareness in recent years of the importance of accidental poisoning by solids and liquids. Probably more children under five years of age die of accidental poisoning in any American city than from the classic and feared infectious childhood diseases. Poisoning in children is the result of lack of supervision, even though an adult may be in the house, negligence in storage or disposal of poisonous substances, and curiosity combined with children's inability to read.[2]

This chapter is concerned with accidental poisoning. It would be almost impossible to list all poisons, because a great many substances are harmless if used in the proper way but are poisonous if used in the wrong way or in the wrong amount. For example, nearly all drugs and medicines are potentially both beneficial and poisonous; the effect is determined by the method of use and by the amount taken into the body. The effect of a poison depends on several factors: amount of intake, toxicity of substances, age and body weight of the victim, and individual tolerance.[3]

Effects

The ways in which poisons act are extremely varied and complicated.[4]

Primary Effects.   The first primary effect, which is often cited, is the caustic effect: certain poisons (e.g., strong acids and alkalis) bring about a chemical destruction of the tissues by mere contact. The expression "burning" is appropriate here, since these substances actually cause lesions in the upper digestive tract. If the victim survives, he will have permanent scars.

A second primary effect of poisons is cytotoxicity: disturbance of the normal function of the cells of certain body tissues. This disturbance may result in the death of the cell. Although a disturbance of cellular metabolism of this kind can bring about a necrosis of the tissues similar to that produced by caustic substances, it can also be a temporary disturbance that may be reversible and cure itself when the poison is eliminated.

A third primary effect concerns certain products to which some individuals are exceptionally sensitive. This sensitivity may be acquired or inherited.

Threat

It has been estimated that in the United States as many as a million persons accidentally ingest toxic substances each year, with about 3500 deaths resulting.[5] In general, medicines are accidently ingested most frequently in cold months, with petroleum products, paint solvents, and pesticides more often in warmer months.[6] It is believed that poisonous liquids may be ingested most often in the warm months by infants and young children because of thirst. Research to determine the influence, if any, of hunger and thirst on the frequency of poisoning accidents and the types of poisons would be valuable.

Pica (an abnormal craving for nonfood or unnatural food substances) is not fully understood. Nutritional deficiencies were formerly thought to be responsible for the habit, but this theory has been challenged. Pica is most likely to occur in a child who has a high level of oral activity associated with anxiety and a cultural background that reinforces the habit of eating unnatural foods.[7]

It can be concluded in cases of accidental poisoning that the substances ingested were not only easily accessible but were also not in their proper locations (left on furniture tops and on the floor). The kitchen exceeds all other areas in the home as the place for accessible poisonous liquids and solids, with the bedroom and bathroom following in prevalence.

Lack of awareness of the potential hazard of poisonous substances is common, plus the fact that those getting poisoned are nonreaders. The words "caution" or "warning" or "poison" do not mean a thing to the preschool child. It is thought that the traditional skull and crossbones may even attract children with its pirate connotation.

The threat of poisoning comes from many substances in everyday use (e.g., medicines, cosmetics, cleaning agents). Equally shocking is the fact that 95 percent of poisonings in children under five occur while they are under the supervision of parents or other responsible adults.[8]

There is a general understanding that careless storage is a major cause of accidental poisoning, yet there is no clear-cut evidence that this is true. In a study reported by Sobel, of 400 families no significance was found (1) in the degree of hazard in poisoned vs. nonpoisoned homes, (2) in storage habits between poisoned and nonpoisoned groups, or (3) in storage habits one year later even though there may have been a poisoning in the interim.[9]

One would think that pediatricians would be quite sensitive to safe storage practices. However, a surprise survey of medications in the homes of 12 pediatricians with young children disclosed that only one pediatrician had all of his medications securely locked up.[10] A second pediatrician had 23 of his medications locked in a steel file box; however, he had 12 other medications in three other accessible sites in the home. There was a common disregard in the homes of these pediatricians of a basic principle of poison prevention which they probably tell their patients: "Keep all medications out of reach of children."

In a similar study of 52 poisoned and 52 control families, it was found that there was no significant difference in the poisoned and the control groups in storage habits or in the mother's knowledge regarding toxicity of substances.[11] This study suggests that storage patterns of poisonous agents and parent's knowledge of poison potentials are not the important variables in determining which child is accidentally poisoned.

Most poisonings in the United States are from the ingestion in the home of toxic substances stored in accessible places in the original container with the top closed. The most common substances reported in accidental poisonings are medications. In one survey, the average home contained 30 containers of medication.[12] Each year an estimated 400 containers of toxic or potentially toxic substances (e.g., medicines, petroleum products, cosmetics) enter the homes of families in the United States.

Vulnerability

In the preschool ages poisoning by solid and liquid substances has decreased markedly in recent years, but the danger of this type of poisoning continues greater among very young children than at any other period of life. Mortality from accidental poisonings remains higher among males than among females at all ages.[13]

During the 1960s and 1970s an increase in deaths due to accidental poisoning by solid and liquid substances has occurred primarily at the adolescent and adult levels. This is especially true for women. There may be a correlation with the popularity of drug abuse; many of the poisonings were accidental overdoses of drugs by young people aged 15 through 24. Poisoning by barbiturates and other hypnotic drugs is common among adults who attempt suicide. Since this text is concerned with unintentional injury and trauma, suicides will not be discussed.

A profile of poisoned children shows that they are more likely to be impulsive and overactive, and are discipline problems for their parents. Children are prone to accidental poisoning when usual family patterns are interrupted (e.g., moving, pregnancy, illness, death, or marital problems).[14]

The possibility of poisoning is related to the developmental patterns of the child. The six-month-old will put anything in his or her mouth. A one- to two-year-old child will empty cupboards and experimentally taste most things. By age two and one-half or three years, the child is adventurous and has access to any unlocked drawer or cupboard in the home. The four-year-old tends to be more selective in what he ingests, preferring things that taste good (e.g., flavored children's aspirin, vitamins).

Countermeasures: Pre-Ingestion

Poison Prevention Packaging.   The United States through the Consumer Product Safety Commission administers a federal law entitled the Poison Prevention Packaging Act. This law seeks to protect small children from swallowing poisonous chemicals and harmful drugs by requiring "child-resistant" packaging on products considered dangerous.

To administer this law, a testing method for determining the effectiveness of a safety closure is used. It calls for the testing of 200 children between 42 and 51 months of age, evenly distributed as to age and sex. The tests specify a resistant effectiveness of not less than 85 percent without a demonstration and no less than 80 percent after a demonstration of the proper way to open the package. Adults must also be tested, with the requirement that not less than 90 percent of them are able to open the container after instruction.

Some of the products required to be packaged in child-resistant containers are: aspirin, furniture oil polishes (containing 10 percent or more petroleum distillates), methyl salicylate (oil of wintergreen), household liquid drain cleaners, and thousands of products in the future. The closures cannot be made completely child-proof. A balance has been struck that will protect most children without making the packaging so cumbersome that adults will refuse to use it and thus nullify the entire program.

Studies have demonstrated that widespread community use of child-resistant containers for prescription medications can significantly reduce childhood poisoning (see Figure 12–1).[15] As safety closures become available, they should help alleviate the accidental poisoning problem — but they cannot eliminate it. They will not work at all unless parents buy potentially poisonous products in safety packaging, keep the products in them, and properly close the containers after use. And even if the safety closures are used exactly as intended, they cannot prevent all poisonings. According to the testing protocol, two out of ten children may be able to open them. The same precautions that have always been necessary will still be necessary.

Education.   In the past, most poison prevention programs have been directed toward using the mass media for public education programs. National Poison Prevention Week is conducted in March of each year.

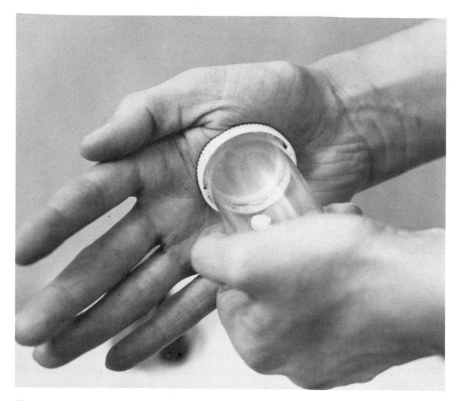

figure 12–1   Child-proof safety caps. Photo courtesy of the National Safety Council.

The purpose of the observance is to alert the American people to the dangers of poisoning. Research is needed on the effectiveness of the efforts made.

With most of the poisonings occurring in young children, the education programs are aimed at the parents, even though it is difficult to prove how effective they are. Many organizations, such as the National Safety Council, National Clearinghouse for Poison Control Centers, National Planning Council for Poison Prevention Week, and the American Medical Association, have abundant amounts of prepared material that can be useful for parent education.

By the time a child reaches school, he has passed the most dangerous poisoning time. Television would do well to stress poison prevention concepts on children's programs and advertising spot announcements.

Poison Control Centers.   The Bureau of Product Safety operates the National Clearinghouse for about 600 autonomous Poison Control Centers throughout the United States. The Clearinghouse supplies the centers with emergency information for common household products and drugs that may be accidentally ingested. In return, the Poison Control Centers voluntarily submit poisoning reports to the National Clearinghouse.

There are differing philosophies about the use of poison control centers, both among the centers themselves and the physicians who utilize them. Some centers discourage calls directly from the public — preferring to deal with or through physicians — and will either call the private doctor or have the victim do so. Other centers will handle lay calls without hesitation and without involving the physician.

The first Poison Control Center in the United States was set up in Chicago in 1953.[16] Most of these centers are manned 24 hours every day of the year to provide emergency service, improve first aid for poisoning, and provide information to physicians concerning poisonous substances. With few exceptions, the centers have not been engaged in prevention programs as they should be.

Specific Poisoning Problems.   *Lead.* Lead poisoning results from ingestion of lead-containing paint in old, dilapidated houses. Prevention of lead poisoning consists of preventing children from eating the paint. This can be accomplished by: (1) removing leaded paint or covering it; (2) warning occupants about the danger; and (3) keeping a child suspected of eating lead from further exposure.

It is estimated that about 200 children die annually and 200,000 have sustained brain damage.[17] It has now become a rare experience to see a child in the hospital in a coma because of lead poisoning, although this was not an unusual experience even within the present decade. Large numbers of children have been discovered with abnormal blood levels by means of routine screening tests. In two large cities where nearly 400,000 children were tested high blood levels of lead have been detected in apparently normal or well children, and it is not known for certain if they are in danger of damage to the nervous system and brain from that quantity of lead. There may be the possibility of subtle damage to the nervous system. A blood level of lead of 40 micrograms per 100 milliliters of blood is considered abnormal by U.S. Public Health Service standards. Twenty percent or more of large groups of children are being found with these blood levels.[18]

Surveys in some large cities have shown that from 40 to 80 percent of the houses in slum areas still contain hazardous quantities of flaking lead paint that was applied many years ago.[19] However, one source reports that lead responsible for poisoning is not always from chipped paint in old houses.[20]

Plants.[21] The vast majority of plants are not poisonous. There is no rule of thumb by which to ascertain which plant is poisonous and which is not. The only reliable rule is: Don't eat anything unless you are absolutely sure it is safe. A realistic estimate of the number of plant poisonings yearly would be around 15,000 cases with more than 100 deaths.

Aspirin.[22] A surprising number of people do not regard aspirin as a medicine. Children's aspirin accounts for much of the accidental poisoning ingestion (one-fourth of childhood poisoning cases). From 60 to 90 tablets of five-grain aspirin constitute a fatal adult dose; if the victim is allergic to aspirin, smaller amounts can be fatal. It is important to determine whether baby aspirin (1/4 to 1/2 gr.), children's aspirin (1 1/4 gr.), or adult aspirin (5 gr.) was ingested. A toxic dose for a child is more than 0.15 gm. per kg. of body weight. The law limiting the number of 1¼ gr. children's aspirin to 36 per bottle is only a beginning in the prevention of aspirin poisoning. Child-proof containers, better labeling indicating its dangers and signs of poisoning, and restriction of advertisements making exaggerated claims about aspirin is recommended.

The American public annually buys 12,000 tons of aspirin. These sales amount to almost 300 aspirin tablets per person each year. Most investigators believe that aspirin does not achieve its pain-relieving capacity by acting on the brain unless an overdosage is consumed. Large amounts of aspirin will act on the brain to increase the rate and depth of breathing. Large doses of aspirin may also cause hemorrhage in the stomach. It tends to prevent the clustering of blood platelets and may thus hamper the clotting of blood.[23]

Rules to help make a home "poison-proof":[24]

1   Keep household products and medicines out of reach and out of sight of children, preferably in a locked cabinet or closet—even a fishing tackle box or suitcase can be used. If you must leave the room for even an instant, remove the container to a safe spot or take the child and/or container(s) with you.

2   Store medicines separately from other household products and keep these items in their original containers—never in cups or soft-drink bottles.

3   Be sure that all products are properly labeled, and read the label before administering. In a dark room, turn the light on to do so.

4   Since children tend to imitate adults, avoid taking medications in their presence.

5   Refer to medicines by their proper names. Never encourage children to take any medicine by calling it "candy," for later they may be tempted to eat it as a treat.

6   Clean out your medicine cabinet periodically. Get rid of old medicines by flushing them down the drain, rinsing the containers in water, and then discarding them. Do not put any container with its contents into a refuse can.

7   Keep handy the telephone numbers of your family doctor, local police, nearest hospital emergency room, and poison control center.

8   For some poisonings, first aid treatment can be given at home. Therefore, every household with children should have a one-ounce container of syrup of ipecac for inducing vomiting when this is called for. Also, activated charcoal should be kept on hand for first aid use; its label indicates when this type of treatment should be used, but it is wise to check with your physician.

POISONING BY INHALATION

Characteristics and Causes

The mortality from poisoning by gases and vapors is increasing. These fatalities are due chiefly to poisoning by carbon monoxide produced by the incomplete combustion of fuels used by standing motor vehicles, cooking stoves, and heating equipment. In chapter 11 on Fire, more details are given about the relationship between fire and deaths from carbon monoxide. The National Safety Council classifies deaths from carbon monoxide in fires under fire deaths rather than as deaths from poisoning by gases and vapors.

Carbon monoxide is odorless and tasteless. It is produced during the incomplete burning of any carbon-containing (organic) material. Furnaces, water heaters, refrigerators, and gasoline engines are the most common sources of CO poisoning. An automobile can produce enough CO in 15 to 30 minutes to saturate the car's interior or that of a small garage.[25] Gas, coal, or oil appliances produce CO when a flue or other ventilating system is blocked or malfunctioning so that insufficient air reaches the flame. Charcoal briquettes cause problems only when used in confined areas with inadequate ventilation, such as an enclosed tent, trailer, or room.

Effects

Carbon monoxide itself kills about 1300 people a year in the United States, though perhaps half of the nearly 8400 nontransport annual fire deaths result from carbon monoxide intoxication. Of the recorded deaths, only 10 percent occur on the streets and highways, whereas 60 percent take place in the home, and the remainder occur in recreational sites, on industrial premises, and in unspecified areas. In the home, accidents involving automobile exhaust claim 40 percent of the lives, CO from utility appliance sources 30 percent, and gas from furnaces and other gas-producing equipment the remaining 30 percent. At least

10,000 to 12,000 additional persons seek medical attention each year for carbon monoxide exposure.[26]

Carbon monoxide has a peculiar effect on the body that makes it especially dangerous. As already mentioned, carbon monoxide and red blood cells (hemoglobin) have an affinity for each other. The red blood cell will pick up carbon monoxide when it is present in preference to oxygen; the affinity for carbon monoxide is about 250 times greater than for oxygen. As the ability of the blood to pick up oxygen from the lungs and to carry it to the tissues of the body declines, health quickly becomes impaired and death may occur rapidly.

An automobile engine running in a closed garage can create a deadly atmosphere in just seven minutes. Automobiles with air conditioners have a much greater concentration of carbon monoxide than similar automobiles not so equipped. However, current modifications being made in automobile engines are markedly reducing the amount of carbon monoxide produced.[27]

Effects of various concentrations of carbon monoxide range from mild headache to death and are described briefly in Table 12–1. The recovery from carbon monoxide poisoning is often thought to be complete and little attention is paid in the literature to the neurological and psychiatric results of such occurrences.[28] Ample evidence does exist that the changes in brain cells that occur in carbon monoxide poisoning are similar to those of oxygen deprivation. Although it can be assumed that many victims survive with less severe brain damage, few medical cases have been reported.

Vulnerability

In the United States, males account for over 70 percent of all the deaths from accidental poisoning by gas or vapor. While such fatalities occur at

table 12–1   *Effects of Carbon Monoxide*

amount	effects
Up to 10 percent	No effect, no longlasting or chronic effects. Can be flushed from body with clean air
10 to 20 percent	headache
20 to 30 percent	headache and fatigue; impaired judgment
30 to 40 percent	headache and nausea
40 to 50 percent	collapse
50 to 60 percent	coma, convulsions
60 to 70 percent	respiratory failure, depressed heartbeat, and death

source: Richard E. Waite, "Monoxide Under Study," *Journal of Environmental Health*, September 1970, p. 180.

all ages, the death rate is very low in childhood, increases with age, and reaches its maximum at the advanced ages.[29]

Children usually fare less well than adults with CO poisoning. Women, because they are usually comparatively anemic, tend to fare less well than men. Inactivity tends to ward off the effects of carbon monoxide.[30] Exercise or hard labor can cause higher levels of carbon monoxide in the blood quite rapidly during short exposures.

Threat[31]

Deaths occur most frequently in late autumn and winter, reaching a peak in December or January when people make greater use of home heating facilities and are confined indoors.

The majority of the fatalities due to inhalation of poisonous gas or vapor occur in and about the home and the home garage. Other sites include vehicles parked on streets and highways, public buildings, and trailers and cabins such as those commonly used by hunters, fishermen, and campers.

Carbon monoxide poisoning is most apt to occur in automobiles that are defective because of deterioration, damage, or faulty design.[32] Rust is a major factor in damaging the exhaust system and creating holes in the body of the car (through which carbon monoxide can enter). Usually these holes are in the muffler and the floor of the car. Even a two-year-old car can have significant rust damage.

Parking inside a garage with the engine running, apparently to provide warmth, is a main factor. Many deaths involve persons who were sleeping inside a car, often because of previous drinking. Sleeping may have been caused by a combination of alcohol and carbon monoxide, without real intent to fall asleep. Many deaths also involve parking in remote areas for romantic purposes. In addition to parking deaths, drivers have also been overcome by carbon monoxide while the vehicles were in motion.

Countermeasures: Pre-Inhalation

Poisoning by gases and vapors is best avoided by proper installation and inspection of heating and other burning appliances.

Suggestions concerning the automobile include:

1   Run the automobile's engine as little as possible inside a garage, and then only with the garage doors open.
2   Always have plenty of fresh air in the car.

3 Have the entire exhaust system inspected for leaks, and have any leaks corrected.

4 Keep the car engine properly tuned to reduce the amount of carbon monoxide produced.

5 If holes are drilled in the fire wall between the engine and the passenger compartment to install new accessories, be sure they are sealed to prevent engine fumes from entering the car.

6 If the car has air vent intakes in the front, close them while waiting in line behind other vehicles.

7 Have good circulation around and under the car if running the engine while the car is standing still.

Prevention of deaths in automobiles from carbon monoxide, according to Baker et al., might be achieved by the following procedures:[33] (1) production of an engine or fuel that does not produce carbon monoxide; (2) use of exhaust emission control devices that reduce the concentration of carbon monoxide in exhaust gases; (3) better separation of exhaust gases from auto compartments; (4) use of rust-resistant materials and better ventilation systems for fresh air; (5) use of built-in sensors to detect carbon monoxide; and (6) better education and publicization of the problem.

INSECT BITES AND STINGS

Characteristics and Causes

Many types of arthropods have been implicated in severe hypersensitivity reactions. By far the most frequently reported severe hypersensitivity reactions are caused by Hymenoptera — the honeybee, wasp, hornet, and yellow jacket.[34]

The honeybee is believed to be the most common stinging insect. It is frequently encountered in lawns and meadows as it seeks clover blossoms, and is easily stepped upon by bare feet. It nests in hollows of dead trees and in man-made hives. It is the only species of Hymenoptera which leaves its stinger and venom sac attached to the victim.[35]

The yellow jacket is the next most common stinging insect. It is smaller than the honeybee, with a narrow waist and a blunt body. It builds its round, paperlike nest in the ground under logs or rocks.[36]

The wasp, which causes the second highest number of fatalities (after the bee), has a leaner, spindle-shaped body with an elongated waist. It builds honeycomb or mud nests under the eaves of buildings or in sheltered areas in trees or bushes. The hornet has a body contour similar to the yellow jacket's but it is larger. It builds its large, hanging, pear-shaped papier-mache hives in trees or bushes.[37]

The few fatal spider bites seen in the United States are attributable to the black widow or to the brown recluse spider. (The black widow is so called because of its color and the popular notion that the female devours the male after mating; actually, some say that this occurs only when all other food sources are gone.) For a long time the black widow (most familiar) was thought to be the only highly poisonous species of spider in North America. In the late 1950s reports began to appear about the bite of the brown recluse.[38]

The black widow is found throughout the United States and is usually recognizable by its jet black color, with an abdomen usually marked with orange or red spots in the shape of an hour glass. Only the female is dangerous.

The brown recluse spider is small with a brown body. Both sexes of this spider bear a dark-brown somewhat hourglass-shaped (or, as generally described, violin- or fiddle-shaped) marking on the united head and thorax. They are prevalent in the southern states from Texas to Florida and range into Georgia, Indiana, Illinois, Missouri, and Kansas. Because of their long life span and survivability in a wide range of temperatures, their geographical distribution is not limited and may be spreading.

Effects

In a study of fatalities resulting from poisonous bites and stings, Parrish reported that the Hymenoptera were responsible for about 50 percent.[39] Snakes accounted for 30 percent, spiders for 14 percent, scorpions and others for the remaining 6 percent.

In general, spider-bite victims usually live about 18 hours and snake-bite victims from 6 to 48 hours.[40] Hymenoptera sting victims usually die within an hour. These victims were allergic to the insect sting. Perhaps many sudden unexplained deaths occurring outdoors in the summer months may be the result of insect sting allergy.

Anaphylactic reactions from stings are the most common cause of death from venomous animals in the United States. Death resulting from injected venom of Hymenoptera is from respiratory obstruction caused by swelling of the vocal cords or by severe constriction and congestion of the bronchial tubes, and anaphylactic shock.[41]

The toxicity of the black widow's venom is probably greater than that of the snake venoms, but the spider injects only a minute amount of poison. The bite is ordinarily dangerous to life only in infants and victims of multiple bites. The venom causes various neurologic effects which still need researching.[42] The main effect is muscle spasm, usually starting in the bite area. Death in previously well individuals is unlikely, with recovery complete within a week.[43]

The bite of the brown recluse, which many now consider to be more dangerous than that of the black widow, usually does not hurt much. After several hours it becomes very painful, with a blister forming surrounded by a reddened area. Necrosis sets in after about two days, continuing to its full extent for up to a week.[44] From animal studies it is known that the venom injected by the brown recluse spider may cause the death of tissue and the destruction of red blood cells, and that it contains a chemical that permits its rapid spread through living tissue.[45]

Threat

In the United States the peak incidence of insect stings and spider bites occurs in summer, especially in August for spiders and the spring months for insects. Stinging by bees is most likely on bright, warm days, especially if they are interfered with while gathering nectar.

A strain of honeybees in Brazil is spreading and could reach Texas within 15 to 20 years. Swarms of these bees are especially dangerous. Some reports have indicated that swarming bees attack and sting even without provocation. Aggressiveness and nervousness are especially characteristic of this strain of bees. The slightest disturbance at or near a hive may set off a chain reaction that "explodes" within seconds, with entire bee colonies going out of control.[46]

Vulnerability

The proportion of males getting insect bites exceeds that of females up to 20 years of age. After 20 the number of females stung increases. Only a small percentage of children under the age of 12 report severe reactions. After the age of 30 years severe reactions are even higher.[47]

Acquiring insect hypersensitivity seems to be related closely to exposure to insect stings, especially in nonallergic individuals. Those individuals who are insect sting sensitive are especially vulnerable to the ill effects of stings and may suffer severe—even fatal—reactions. More adults than children have fatal reactions to stings. This may be because allergic reactions to insect stings are cumulative—the first sting sensitizes the victim and more stings cause increasingly severe reactions.

The stings or bites of poisonous spiders are more fatal to children than to adults. Even a small amount of the venom of a brown recluse spider or scorpion may have an immediate and deadly effect on a small child. Reactions to bites vary with individuals.

Countermeasures: Pre-Bite or -Sting

Persons especially susceptible to insect sting allergies should learn how to avoid unnecessary exposure to stings.[48] (It is estimated that 2 or 3 percent of the population is hypersensitive to bites and stings of insects.) Such a person should not live or work near commercial beehives. His home should have adequate screens on windows and doors. Flowering shrubs and fruit trees, which attract bees, should not be planted near the home, and care should be taken when one is in such areas. Wasp nests should be removed from eaves and bushes around the home. Food and refuse should be kept covered so that they do not attract insects. The susceptible person should not walk barefoot outdoors. Bees are said to be attracted to brightly colored, dark, and rough fabrics, as well as to strongly scented perfumes and powders. Some authorities advocate white, hard-finished clothing with a minimum of skin exposure. Commercially available topical insect repellents are not effective against bees, wasps, hornets, and yellow jackets. When a bee is around, swift movements should be avoided—a bee won't sting unless threatened.

SNAKEBITE POISONING

Characteristics and Causes

Poisonous snakes occur throughout most parts of the tropical and temperate zones of the world. They are more numerous in tropical or semitropical areas.

An average of ten deaths from snakebite[49] (less than one percent of those bitten by a poisonous snake) are reported annually in the United States, with over 6000 bitten.[50] Worldwide, deaths exceed 1000 according to one source;[51] but another source[52] reports over 40,000 deaths from snakebites every year—30,000 of them in Asia, mainly in India.

The dangerous snakes (only about 10 percent)[53] in the United States are all members of the pit viper family or coral snake family. Pit vipers—responsible for about 98 percent of venomous bites[54]—can be distinguished by the pit between the eye and nostril on each side of the head. The pit is a heat-sensitive device that aids in directing the snake in striking its victim. The venom from pit vipers reaches the victim through a bite. They inject their venom directly through two hypodermic needlelike fangs that have a hole down the middle and are connected to a venom reservoir. It is quite easy to identify a pit viper bite by the two fang marks (sometimes only one may be present) about ¼ to ½ inch apart. Some people have recommended that all pit vipers be captured and have their fangs removed. This would be a useless procedure since the fangs grow back.

The rattle attached to the tail will almost always identify a rattlesnake, but there are exceptions; in the young of some of the small rattlesnake species, the rattle may be overlooked. In pit vipers, elliptical pupils are another identification mark. Coral snakes have neither pits nor elliptical pupils, but can be distinguished by the broad rings of scarlet and black separated by yellow rings — "red next to yellow will kill a fellow." They have round pupils and a pair of short, erect fangs.

Effects

The venoms of different snakes produce their poisonous effects in different ways. For example, the coral snakes of this country inject powerful venoms that have a strong effect on nerve tissue (neurotoxic), but produce relatively little local tissue reaction. On the other hand, rattlesnakes inject venoms that contain powerful enzymes (hemotoxins) and cause extensive local tissue destruction by actually digesting the tissues into which they are injected. In addition, rattlesnake venom contains a hemorrhagic factor which has a destructive effect on the blood vessels themselves.

Many persons bitten by poisonous snakes have little or no envenomation; it usually comes as a surprise to learn that a poisonous snake was not poisonous (caused no ill effects). Many times a pit viper injects very little venom — and sometimes, none at all. The degree or severity of toxicity depends on these criteria:[55]

1   Age, size, and health of victim. A small child may have a severe reaction which doesn't endanger an adult.

2   Location, depth, and number of bites. A bite that penetrates a blood vessel can be highly toxic. A single, glancing stroke of the fangs is less dangerous than multiple or direct penetrating strokes of the fangs.

3   Duration of the bite. The longer the bite, the more venom injected. If a snake bites and hangs on for more than several seconds, then it may inject a large amount of venom.

4   The kind, size, and maturity of the snake. Most small, immature pit vipers do not produce sufficient venom to endanger an adult.

It usually takes several hours for the full effects of the venom of a snake to take effect because much of the venom is deposited in the tissues of the victim.

Threat

Most of the states having the highest bite rates per 100,000 population per year are in the southeast and southwest regions of the United States. States east of the Mississippi River with the highest rates are North Carolina, Georgia, West Virginia, Mississippi, and· South Carolina. The states west of the Mississippi River with the highest rates are Arkansas, Texas, Louisiana, Oklahoma, and Arizona.[56]

The most widely distributed poisonous snake in the United States is the rattlesnake, with 15 species.[57] One or more species of poisonous snakes are found in every state except Alaska, Maine, and Hawaii. (There are no snakes of any kind in Hawaii.) Large rattlesnakes are the most dangerous venomous snakes in the United States.

Copperheads inhabit the eastern United States from Massachusetts to Kansas southward to northern Florida and west to Texas.[58] Cottonmouths or water moccasins are found in aquatic habitats from southeastern Virginia through the southern lowlands up the Mississippi Valley to southern Illinois and west to central Texas.[59] They can bite a person while under water.

The American coral snakes are a group of some 40 to 50 species that attain their greatest number and variety in Mexico and northern South America, although they range from the southern United States to Uruguay. The better known United States coral snake is the North American coral snake which occurs from southeastern North Carolina through Florida and the Gulf States to central Texas and southward into Mexico. The smaller Arizona coral snake inhabits a limited region in southern Arizona, New Mexico, and Sonora.[60]

Snakebites are infrequent during the colder months of the year—November through March—when in general snakes are inactive or hibernating. Most bites (over 90 percent) occur from April through October. The peak months for snakebite accidents in the United States are July and August.[61] This striking seasonal distribution of bites coincides with the period when snakes are most abundant and active and when people have greater exposure because of outdoor occupations or recreation.

The majority of snakebite incidences occur between 6:00 A.M. and 9:00 P.M., which is the period when people are most active outdoors.[62]

Many species of poisonous snakes are nocturnal feeders, but people simply do not have as much exposure to the possibility of a bite during the hours after dark.

Most snakebite cases happened in the victim's own yards. Farm or ranch, near a lake, river, or other body of water, in the woods, and in a field away from the house are the other main locations of snakebite occurrences.[63]

Vulnerability[64]

More than 6000 persons are bitten by poisonous snakes in this country each year. The incidence of snakebite accidents is higher for males than for females.

Over half of the bites happen to persons less than 20 years of age. Children less than 5 years of age do not have an excessive bite rate as compared to young people aged 5 through 19 years of age. The lowest bite rate is for people 70 or more years of age. A popular myth is that children have excessively high fatality rates from snakebite accidents. This is not true. The greatest number of deaths from snakebites are found in adults aged 60 to 69 years.

Parrish lists the following as activities being participated in at the time of the bite: playing in own yards and elsewhere, working on a farm or ranch, handling a poisonous snake, hunting or fishing, and recreation other than hunting or fishing.

Countermeasures: Pre-Bite

1   Do not move when you hear a snake rattle. Snakes usually strike at moving objects.

2   In snake-infested areas wear shoes and other types of protection over legs (baggy pants) because more than half of all bites are on the lower part of the leg.

3   Avoid walking at night or in grass and underbrush. Do not climb rocky ledges without visual inspection.

4   Avoid the unnecessary handling of snakes and do not frighten others with snakes. A recently killed snake can strike and the separated head can inject venom even 15 minutes after the snake's death.

5   Do not sleep on the ground.

6   Be cautious around discarded lumber, debris, and firewood. Keep debris cleaned up. Don't attract mice and rats with garbage; they are the principle food supply for snakes.

7   When walking, be alert as to the intended path. Use a stick to poke clumps of grass and brush before walking through them.

8   Keep the grass, weeds, and brush cut so snakes cannot hide.

NOTES

[1]Howard M. Cann, Albert P. Iskrant, and Dorothy S. Neyman, "Epidemiologic Aspects of Poisoning Accidents," *American Journal of Public Health,* December 1960, p. 1915.

[2]Robert G. Scherz, "Prevention of Childhood Poisoning," *The Pediatric Clinics of North America* (Philadelphia: W. B. Saunders Co., August 1970), pp. 713–27.

[3]Robert H. Dreisbach, *Handbook of Poisoning* (Los Altos, Ca.: Lange Medical Publications, 1969).

[4]Dreisbach, *Handbook of Poisoning.*

[5]National Safety Council, *Accident Facts,* 1974, p. 7.

[6]Cann, Iskrant, and Neyman, "Poisoning Accidents," p. 1923.

[7]Robert M. Reece, "Childhood Lead Poisoning: A Preventable Disaster," *American Family Physician,* January 1974, pp. 136–37.

[8]Cann, Iskrant, and Neyman, "Poisoning Accidents," p. 1924.

[9]Raymond Sobel, "Traditional Safety Measures and Accidental Poisoning in Childhood," *Pediatrics,* November 1969, p. 811.

[10]Scherz, "Childhood Poisoning," p. 716.

[11]Charles Baltimore, Jr., and Roger J. Meyer, "A Study of Storage, Child Behavior Traits, and Mother's Knowledge of Toxicology in 52 Poisoned Families and 52 Comparison Families," *Pediatrics,* November 1969, p. 816.

[12]Robert G. Scherz, George H. Latham, and Carl E. Stracener, "Child-Resistant Containers Can Prevent Poisoning," *Pediatrics,* January 1969, p. 84.

[13]"Accidental Poisoning at a High Level," *Statistical Bulletin,* February 1968, p. 8.

[14]Cann, Iskrant, and Neyman, "Poisoning Accidents," p. 714.

[15]Scherz, Latham, and Stracener, "Child-Resistant Containers," p. 84.

[16]Henry L. Verhulst and John Crotty, "Poison Control Activities in the United States," *Journal of School Health,* February 1967, p. 50.

[17]Reece, "Childhood Lead Poisoning," p. 136.

[18]Michael C. Klein et al., "Lead Poisoning, Current Status of the Problem Facing Pediatricians," *American Journal of Disabled Children,* June 1974, pp. 805–7.

[19]Robert L. Fulwiler and Logan Wright, "Sequelae of Lead Poisoning in Children," *Oklahoma State Medical Association Journal,* September 1972, pp. 372–75.

[20]Ada and Frank Graham, "Lead Poisoning and the Suburban Child," *Today's Health,* March 1974, p. 39.

[21]Jay M. Arena, "The Peril in Plants," *Emergency Medicine,* February 1974, p. 221.

[22]Harry B. Andrews, "Salicylate Poisoning," *American Family Physician,* November 1973, p. 102.

[23]Joseph R. DiPalma, "Aspirin, Wonder Drug or Placebo?", *RN,* January 1974, pp. 55–62.

[24]Alan K. Done, "First Aid on the Home Front," *Emergency Medicine,* May 1974, p. 252.

[25]Alan K. Done, "Carbon Monoxide: The Silent Summons," *Emergency Medicine,* February 1973, p. 268.

[26]William Berman, "Carbon Monoxide . . . What It is, What It Does," *Traffic Safety,* August 1973, p. 10.

[27]Richard E. Waite, "Monoxide Under Study," *Journal of Environmental Health,* September 1970, p. 180.

[28]"Neurological Complications of Carbon Monoxide Poisoning," *Lancet,* January 13, 1968, p. 77.

[29]"Deaths Involving Accidental Gas Poisoning Increase," *Statistical Bulletin,* September 1968, p. 4.

[30]DONE, "Carbon Monoxide: The Silent Summons," p. 269.

[31]"Deaths Involving Accidental Gas Poisoning Increase," p. 5.

[32]SUSAN P. BAKER et al., "Fatal Unintentional Carbon Monoxide Poisoning in Motor Vehicles," *American Journal of Public Health,* November 1972, pp. 1463–67.

[33]Ibid.

[34]HENRY M. PARRISH, "Analysis of 460 Fatalities from Venomous Animals in the United States," *American Journal of the Medical Sciences,* February 1963, pp. 129–41.

[35]ROBERT E. ARNOLD, *What to Do About Bites and Stings of Venomous Animals,* 1973, p. 7.

[36]Ibid., p. 7.

[37]Ibid., p. 6.

[38]ALAN K. DONE, "The Bites of Bugs," *Emergency Medicine,* March 1973, p. 250.

[39]PARRISH, "460 Die of Snakebite in 10 Years."

[40]ARNOLD, "Bites and Stings of Venomous Animals," p. 5.

[41]MARY ANN PASSERO AND SUSAN C. DEES, "Allergy to Stings from Winged Things," *American Family Physicians,* June 1973, p. 75.

[42]DONE, "Bites of Bugs," p. 250.

[43]DREISBACH, *Handbook of Poisoning,* p. 372.

[44]DONE, "Bites of Bugs," p. 250.

[45]FALLS B. HERSHEY AND CARL E. AULENBACHER, "Surgical Treatment of Brown Spider Bites," *Annals of Surgery,* August 1969, pp. 300–308.

[46]CLAUDE A. FRAZIER, "Brazilian Honey Bee," *Annals of Allergy,* March 1974, pp. 146–50.

[47]PASSERO AND DEES, "Allergy to Stings," p. 76.

[48]Ibid., p. 77.

[49]DREISBACH, *Handbook of Poisoning,* p. 354.

[50]HENRY M. PARRISH, "Incidence of Treated Snakebites in the United States," *Public Health Reports,* March 1966, p. 269.

[51]DREISBACH, *Handbook of Poisoning,* p. 354.

[52]F. BODIN AND C. F. CHEINISSE, *Poisons* (New York: McGraw-Hill Book Company, 1970), p. 183.

[53]F. BOYS AND H. M. SMITH, *Poisonous Amphibians and Reptiles,* 1959, p. 41.

[54]"Snakebite: Poisonous Until Proven Otherwise," *Patient Care,* May 30, 1971, p. 76.

[55]"Quick Action to Save the Snake Bite Victim," *Patient Care,* June 1968, p. 55.

[56]PARRISH, "Incidence of Treated Snakebites," p. 272.

[57]SHERMAN A. MINTON, "Identification of Poisonous Snakes," in *Snake Venoms and Envenomation* (New York: M. Dekker, 1971), p. 9.

[58]Ibid., p. 10.

[59]Ibid., p. 11.

[60]Ibid., p. 12.

[61]PARRISH, "Incidence of Treated Snakebites," p. 273.

[62]Ibid., p. 275.

[63]HENRY M. PARRISH, JOHN GOLDNER, AND STANLEY L. SILBERG, "Comparison Between Snakebites in Children and Adults," *Pediatrics,* August 1965, p. 253.

[64]PARRISH, "Incidence of Treated Snakebites," p. 272.

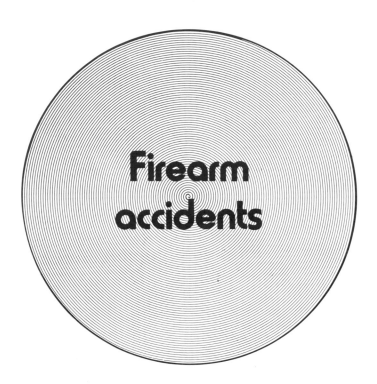

Firearm accidents

13 Guns are abundant in the United States. It is estimated that about half of all American homes have a firearm.[1] Regardless of the controversy during the past decade on the subject of firearms, individuals have developed strong opinions about the subject. But this fact remains—people still do own firearms.

Firearms are perhaps one of the most intriguing hazards. In the age group 1 to 24 years, shootings rank fourth after traffic accidents, drownings, and fires as causes of death. Firearm accidents are the sixth accidental cause of death in the United States. Some people shoot themselves, and some are shot by parents or other adults, but it seems likely that most are shot by their peers.

Much controversy has raged among television producers and their critics over the effects of the profuse portrayal of violence on television. Long before children have the advantage of formal schooling, they learn a wide variety of complex actions, including aggressive and dependent behaviors, group games, tricycle and bicycle riding, and sophisticated sentence structure. For example, young school children watched adults perform in different ways toward a Bobo doll. One group watched an adult hitting and saying aggressive things to the doll, another group watched adults behave more kindly toward the doll, and a third group didn't see any adult modeling cues at all. Even though these young children had no opportunity to practice or rehearse what they had seen, those seeing aggressive behavior instantly developed new forms of aggressive behavior. The premise is, then, that children seeing the use of guns on television will utilize them as a form of aggression when all does not go well for them. One study observed that an increase in gunshot wounds in children seems to be related to an increase in the number of guns.[2]

We could abolish privately owned firearms. No great dislocations in our economy would result from an absolute prohibition against firearms for private citizens. The only genuine costs involved would be the loss of opportunities for hunting and the costs of enforcement. The former could be circumvented by allowing hunters to rent hunting weapons and thus to keep the slaughter of humans by firearms almost entirely within their own ranks.

Certainly there will be portions of the population in the underworld or on its fringes who would probably keep firearms even if it were against the law. An enforcement of a law against private possession of firearms would probably be quite effective among ordinary, law-abiding citizens — those who keep revolvers in drawers against burglars — and this would mean that fatal accidents involving firearms would be drastically reduced. In particular, most of the 500 children (aged 5–14) killed annually as a result of shootings would be saved. The question to be put, then, is a straightforward one: does our society consider it a good bargain to trade the privilege of owning private firearms for the lives of 500 children each year? The answer to such a question can be interpreted only from what society actually does in this and in similar matters, not from what people say ought to be done.

The frightening aspect of the firearm accident problem is that many of these accidents occurred in a situation where there was no intention of doing any shooting at all. Most people think of hunting or target shooting when firearm accidents are mentioned. Most hunters spend just a few days a year in the field and the target shooters a day or two a month on the range, but the guns are kept in the home all year. Without question there is more firearm handling in the home than on the range and in the hunting field combined, yet the emphasis continues to be placed on range and hunter safety.

The problem of firearm safety in the home becomes more complex when the number of untrained people who have access to firearms is considered. In spite of the publicity firearms have received recently, they are not going to disappear.

The "quick draw" is attractive to some. This practice has no place in the home and if done in competition, only wax-loaded cartridges should be used.

EFFECTS

Bullet wounds may cause extensive and fatal damage.[3] In a penetrating wound there is an entry of the bullet, but no exit. In a perforating wound there is both an entry and exit point. The first effect of a high velocity missile is a "blowing-out" that causes inward bursting of soft tissue. A second effect is thermal (most bullets are hot when they penetrate). Another effect is the bounce phenomenon. Bullets sometimes hit hard tissue (e.g., rib, bone) and may bounce around in the body cavities and cause a great deal of damage to tissue and organs.[4] The extent of the injury is not governed by the size of the bullet entering the body, but rather by its speed and course of direction in the body and its point of entrance and exit. The damage is governed by the amount of energy imparted to the body. A bullet will continue to cause damage to all tissues that are in its path when passing through or before lodging in an organ or part of the body. When striking bone it may shatter fragments into adjoining tissues or organs, causing secondary damage. If the gun is in close contact with the skin, the expanding gases enter the tissues with explosive effects. The exit wound of a high velocity bullet is larger than the entrance wound. Intracranial, intrathoracic, and intra-abdominal hemorrhages are invariably present in gunshot wounds, depending on entrance and course of the bullet. The primary effect of intracranial and intrathoracic injuries is interference with the respiration or systemic circulation through anoxia. Bullets in the head or heart may be almost immediately incapacitating to the point of death or later may terminate fatally.

Shotgun wounds are different from those inflicted by other guns.[5] The nature of the injury is related primarily to the distance at which the shotgun is discharged. When the muzzle of the gun is about 20 feet or more distant from the victim (the maximum range of a shotgun is about 100 meters), the wound consists of many small superficial holes, each one of which is related to the entry of one pellet. The wound created is caused by the spray of pellets as they spread apart at the distance involved. Other parts of the shell and wadding fall away and are not involved in the injury. In head and neck wounds, the only significant damage is apt to occur as a result of eye penetration.

Shotguns discharged at close range produce massive destruction. The massive disruptive wounds resemble those of high velocity military weapons. Wounds are characterized by extensive destruction of soft tissue, by injuries to blood vessels and bone, and a 100 percent infection rate. At close range, the entire charge of the shotgun enters the wound, except for the brass base. All other shell fragments, wadding, and load of shot penetrate as a compact mass. However, even though much skin and flesh may be torn away, the victims who are brought to the hospital alive have an excellent chance of survival if breathing is secured and hemorrhage is controlled, providing there is no brain or spinal cord injury.

Reports indicate that the head (brain or skull injury) was affected in almost 50 percent of fatal firearm accidents. The second leading location of injury was the chest area (heart and lungs). The abdomen was the site of most of the remaining fatalities.

In one study the question about emotional effects was asked. The researchers found that a sizable number of the surviving children had from mild to severe long-range emotional effects and that many were having school difficulties since the accident.[6]

THREAT

Although firearm accident prevention programs often emphasize the inherent hazard to hunters in the field, about three-fifths of the estimated firearm accidental deaths in the United States result from mishaps in and about the home. Fatal home accidents appear to have little or no seasonal variation. Hunting fatalities are, of course, definitely related to the hunting seasons (usually the fall months).

Alaska, Mississippi, and Montana lead in accidental firearm death rates. Rhode Island, New Jersey, Massachusetts, and Connecticut have the lowest rates. The Rocky Mountain region has high rates, and this might be partially explained by the hunting opportunities along with the pro-gun attitude. The West was won with the gun, and guns have been noted to be very much a part of the culture in the western states (as evidenced by the rifle racks in many pickup trucks).

VULNERABILITY

Rabbit hunters have more accidents than deer hunters, and squirrel hunters are next in number of accidents. Though men are the primary victims in hunting accidents, it is the women who are getting shot in the home.

In children, males are more often involved. Almost one-third of all firearm deaths in the home involve children under 15 years of age. However, the highest death rate occurs in the 15–24 age grouping.

Alpenfels and Hayes cite the practice of giving to children as toys nonfunctioning models of tools used by adults.[7] These researchers indict the " 'play' gun which is pointed at both the imagined and real gi-ants of a child's world."

Inexperience is a dubious factor. Certainly it plays a role in many home accidents. However, the National Rifle Association reports that over two-thirds of the shooters have had three years or more experience in firearm usage prior to their accidents.

COUNTERMEASURES: PRE-SHOOTING

Prohibition of privately owned guns would greatly reduce the number of home accidents which befall children. Nevertheless, guns are such a part of the American culture (they are even specifically protected in the United States Constitution), that they will probably always be available.

The National Rifle Association sponsors two firearm safety courses: Home Firearm Safety and Hunter Safety. In hunting safety, the course is primarily trying to reach the new or young hunter. In some states it is a requirement that a young hunter take this course before he can qualify for a hunting license. In home firearm safety, the course is directed en-tirely to the adult (even those with no recreational interest in firearms).

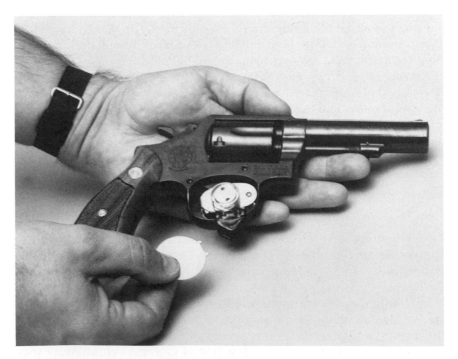

figure 13–1 Trigger lock. Photo courtesy of the National Safety Council.

Most children will be subjected to the handling of firearms whether or not they are doing the handling, so it is necessary that they too know the correct methods. They could be shot even though they are not handling the firearm. They must be able to detect a hazardous situation in order to be able to do something about it, or to know when to leave the area. The NRA Home Firearm Safety Course is not intended to interest children in firearms or shooting; its aim is to impress upon them that firearms do exist and that they should know the hazards that are involved.

The wearing of bright, prominently colored clothing while hunting does avert being shot, but it is interesting that a sizable number of hunting accidents still befall those wearing such apparel.

Guns should be stored completely unloaded (breech and magazine). The action should be closed and the gun uncocked. Storage of guns should be under lock and key with the ammunition stored separately and safely away from the gun(s) (see Figure 13–2).

Basic gun safety practices should be followed. Safe practices include: knowing the gun (determining if it's loaded, how the safety works, etc.), handling the gun properly (treating it as if it were loaded, always pointing the muzzle in a safe direction, keeping the finger outside the trigger guard, and keeping the action open when handling the gun), and accepting responsibility for observing safety rules (exercising self-control, not being a showoff, etc.).

Early training should include an awareness of what a firearm can do. A technique used to demonstrate the effects of a bullet is to fire a .22 hollow-point cartridge through a bar of soap. The effects are dramatic and leave the impression that the firearm can and does do damage.

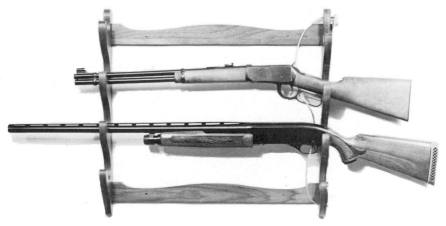

figure 13–2 Guns under a lock. Photo courtesy of the National Safety Council.

COUNTERMEASURES: SHOOTING

Firearms, especially those used in hunting, have some sort of a mechanical safety. This should never be considered a substitute for safe gun handling since it sometimes gives hunters a false confidence.

NOTES

[1]G. NEWTON AND F. ZIMRING, *Firearms and Violence in American Life*, National Commission on the Causes and Prevention of Violence (Washington, D.C., 1968), pp. 1–71.

[2]MARILYN HEINS et al., "Gunshot Wounds in Children," *American Journal of Public Health*, April 1974, pp. 326–30.

[3]BOK S. CHUNG AND RONALD L. KROME, "Bullet Wounds of the Face, Nature and Early Management," *Journal of the American College of Emergency Physicians*, March 1974, pp. 87–90.

[4]JOSEPH J. AMATO et al., "Vascular Injuries: An Experimental Study of High and Low Velocity Missile Wounds," *Archives of Surgery*, August 1970, pp. 167–74.

[5]MARK MAY et al., "Shotgun Wounds to the Head and Neck," *Archives of Otolaryngology*, December 1973, pp. 373–76.

[6]CHUNG AND KROME, "Bullet Wounds of the Face."

[7]ETHEL J. ALPENFELS AND ARTHUR B. HAYES, "Cultural Factors Affecting Accidents Among Children," in *Behavioral Approaches to Accident Research* (New York: Association for the Aid of Crippled Children, 1961), pp. 104–5.

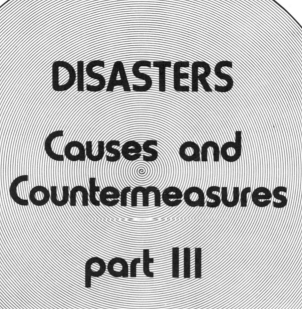

DISASTERS
Causes and Countermeasures
part III

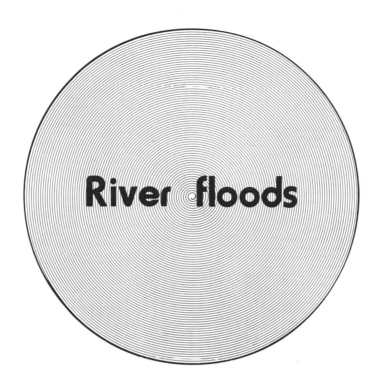

River floods

14 While flooding can occur from any accumulation or rise of water on land areas, this chapter treats only river floods. Flooding resulting from hurricanes, storm surges, and tsunamis is treated in other chapters.

In popular usage, "river flood" describes an overflow of water onto normally dry land. More professionally, hydrologists consider a river to be "in flood" when its waters have risen to an elevation (flood stage) at which damage can occur in the absence of protective works.[1] Floods and flooding are discussed below in the context of damage, actual or threatened.

CAUSES AND CHARACTERISTICS

A stream bed and the flood-plain lands adjacent to it are integral parts of every natural watercourse. The ordinary, intermittent overflow of the stream from its normal bed deposits sediment to form the adjacent flood plains, which act as a natural reservoir and temporary channel. Flooding occurs when excess water rises over lands that are not normally covered and are being used for human habitation or economic enterprise.

The predominant natural sources of excess water within the watersheds of a river are abnormally heavy rainfall or runoff from large accumulations of packed snow. Flooding from snowpack is caused by rising

263

temperatures, sometimes accompanied by rainfall, which melt the snow at an unusual rate.

A drastic increase in water runoff from watersheds is the all too common result of conditions brought about by both man and nature. Forest or brush fires destroy the ground cover so essential to drainage slopes. Man also denudes the watershed by cutting trees, by clearing land for agriculture or for industrial and residential development, or by failing to control the grazing of his herds.

A cause of serious flooding in the lower reaches of larger rivers is the concurrent arrival of flood crests from major tributaries. This condition was classically exemplified by frequent floods in the lower Mississippi River as a result of flood crests from two or more of the major tributaries — the Ohio River, the Tennessee–Cumberland complex, the Missouri River, and the Upper Mississippi.

Flooding can also occur when ice jams are formed and block the river flow. The ice jams are caused by atmospheric and current conditions that induce breakup of river ice but fail to clear the channel. Stoppages will cause flooding initially upstream and later downstream when the ice jam breaks.

Man's hydrologic structures can themselves lead to flooding. History is replete with disasters resulting from dam failures. Poor construction can have disastrous results, as certainly was the case in the 1963 failure of the Baldwin Hills Reservoir in Los Angeles County, California, which caused property damage in the millions of dollars.

Geophysical occurrences can trigger disastrous floods. Although such cases are infrequent, landslides have blocked channels to cause inundation of upstream areas. For example, Hebgen Lake, Montana, was created by a slide induced by a 1959 earthquake. Further dam failure caused by seismic activity is of particular concern, since the best dam sites are often in valleys created by early geologic upheavals in areas where such activity could well recur with disastrous effects.

EFFECTS

Primary Effects

The immediate or primary effects of floods are due to inundation and and the force of currents. (See Figure 14–1.) Residents and livestock of the area may be drowned, displaced, or injured by the flood waters and the current-borne debris. Swift currents and debris cause structural damage

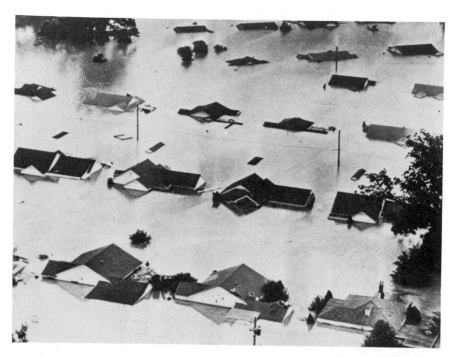

figure 14-1   Flood waters. Associated Press photograph from the American Red Cross.

to homes, buildings, roads, railroads, and bridges. Sanitary, power, water, and telephone installations are damaged and systems interrupted. Business inventories and personal belongings are lost or damaged. Crops and plants are carried away by currents or destroyed by inundation. Farms can lose stored feed, equipment, and buildings. The farmlands may be deeply eroded by new channels or lose areas of valuable topsoil and vegetation.

The dislocations and disruptions caused by floods can lead to hunger, disease, and costly deprivations for the affected populations. Many persons are left homeless when houses are made uninhabitable. Disruptions of transportation and communications can force evacuation of homes and separation of families. Health hazards are increased or created. Water may be contaminated through disruption of water and sanitary systems. Wild animals and snakes may be driven into inhabited areas; rats, when forced from their regular habitat, can cause particular health problems.

Secondary Effects

The force and depth of flood waters can cause disruptions and malfunctionings which become the proximate causes of further damage or hazard. For example, short-term pollution of a river could be caused by chemicals released by flood action on warehouses or other containers. Electrical fires can be caused by short circuits, and fire hazards are minimized or avoided by timely preventive measures. Nevertheless, the potential exists, and measures must be taken, sometimes with disruptive side effects.

Floods causing heavy property damage and the continuing disruptions of human activity may have many lingering results in the affected areas. Schools and businesses may remain closed, with consequent detriment to education, industry, commerce, and employment. Fields and pastures may lose productivity. Currents may silt up old channels and cut new ones, creating problems for navigation, or natural boundaries of rivers or flood plains may be altered, changing the pattern of future flooding. Fish and wildlife normally adjust to the flood itself.

THREAT

Floods can and do occur in almost any part of the United States. Certain areas such as the Pacific Northwest, the Rocky Mountain and Great Basin areas, and part of Southern California experience floods only during well-defined seasons. On the other hand, along the Southeastern and Gulf coasts, floods occur without any pronounced seasonal pattern.

Lastly, there are the areas in which a great flood may occur at any time of year but in which most floods occur during a fairly well-defined period of the year. These are in the Northeast and in the basins of the Ohio and upper Mississippi rivers, as well as the lower Mississippi.

Flash floods have occurred in almost every region of the United States. The areas most susceptible are the upper reaches of streams and creeks in regions that receive the torrential rains associated with the thunderstorms experienced most frequently in spring or summer.

Features of the Threat

The most important indices of a particular river as a flood threat are (1) the frequency and season of its floods, (2) the rate at which it rises and falls, and (3) the velocity and sediment load of its flood waters.

1. *Frequency and season*. The wet, mesothermal climatic areas of the Pacific Northwest and the arid and semiarid provinces of the Great Basin and Rocky Mountains experience floods usually as a result of spring snow melt. Major floods are infrequent, but there are frequent floods of lesser magnitude. The same frequency pattern applies to the semiarid, mesothermal areas of the Southern California Coast, but the flood season in these cases coincides with the winter rains.

As noted earlier, the areas that experience floods without seasonal restrictions are the humid, mesothermal climatic provinces of the Southeastern and Gulf coasts. Floods in the humid and subhumid, microthermal climatic areas of the Northeast and upper Ohio and Mississippi Basin are most frequent in winter and spring. The lower Mississippi is substantially influenced by the contributions of its upper basin and the Ohio Basin and, hence, is in turn likely to have its greatest floods during winter and spring. Nevertheless, these climatic areas may experience serious floods in any month of the year.

2. *Rate of rise and fall*. In a fast-rising flood, disruption may be severe but short lived, while a slow-rising and subsiding flood extends the period of inundation and disruption. At one extreme are the flash floods, characterized by the highest rate of rise and fall—that is, flood crests occur within a few hours and then fall rapidly. At the other extreme are the floods that continue for days in the great river basins. The lower Mississippi has sometimes exceeded flood stage for as long as 30 days.

3. *Velocity and sediment load*. The velocity of the flood water is also an important element of the threat. Velocity is determined by the streambed gradient and channel characteristics. The destructive effect is a function of these factors, together with the increase in volume of water and the type of debris swept along. The sediment carried in the flood may be a harmful deposit left after the waters subside; other areas, however, may be enriched by deposits of silt.

Record and Probability of Occurrence

Major flood conditions occur about every two to four years in the larger river basins of the Ohio, Missouri, upper Mississippi, and Columbia rivers. In contrast, the 1965 flood in the South Platte River near Denver, Colorado, was the first in over 30 years.

By analyzing records of stream flow and other hydrologic data, estimates can be made as to the probable frequency of occurrence of a flood of a given magnitude for a given river. For example, a flood might be referred to as a "ten-year flood," meaning that a flood of this magnitude is equaled or exceeded on the average of once in ten years. However, it is not possible to predict that such a flood will occur in any particular year.

VULNERABILITY

An estimated 50 million acres in the United States are subject to flooding. Although this is only 2.5 percent of the total land area, most of it is densely settled and is of high value.

People

Approximately 10 million people live in the significantly defined flood plains, and another 25 million nearby can be indirectly affected. For the United States in recent years, the average annual loss of life due to floods was 83.[2]

Property

As has been discussed earlier, property can be damaged in many ways by flood waters. Houses and other buildings vary in their vulnerability according to their siting and construction. Even those buildings that can withstand serious structural damage are vulnerable to extensive damage of exterior surface, furnishings, and contents.

Damage to transportation systems is particularly important in flood areas in that aid and recovery may depend on well-functioning systems. Roadbeds are vulnerable to scouring action (sidewash) and undermining if they run parallel to the flow, and to overflow if perpendicular. Even roadbeds well above the crest may be undermined by scouring and collapsed by slides. Bridge abutments are vulnerable to washout, causing collapse of the bridge structure, which itself is vulnerable to currents and current-borne debris. Airport runways, highways, and city streets can all suffer damage from immersion and can be rendered unusable for a time by water and deposits of mud and debris.

The currently accepted value for flood is $1 billion annually.[3]

Ecology

The animal and plant life of an area is relatively invulnerable to normal flooding. The existing ecological balance has already been affected, and indeed developed, by recurrent floods in vulnerable areas. Wildlife is mobile and adjusts readily to a temporarily changed environment.

Flash flooding can change the environment in sudden and lasting ways damaging to the ecology. In severe cases wildlife can be trapped and drowned, trees and vegetation can be washed away or be killed by water immersion, and hillsides can slide into valleys, leaving the underlying rock exposed.

COUNTERMEASURES: PREDICTION SYSTEMS

Sensors and Surveillance

Since the cause of river floods is the abnormal amount of water flowing into the river, the prediction of a flood is based on knowledge of the quantity of precipitation falling in the river drainage basin combined with an estimate of when and how much of this precipitation will find its way into the river (the runoff). The maximum quantity of precipitation for a given storm situation can be forecast with a fair amount of accuracy from meteorological and radar observations. However, forecasting accurately the quantity that will fall in a specific area is difficult.

Quantitative predictions of rainfall in an area are generally used not to forecast (since to do so would result in too many false alarms), but for two other purposes: to alert personnel involved in the flood forecasting process and, in areas subject to flash flooding, as the basis for warning of the possibility of such flooding.

The cooperative effort in the sensing and surveillance system is integrated by the National Weather Service (NWS), which by statute is solely responsible for the nation's public river and flood forecasting and warning program. In carrying out this program, the NWS offices responsible for flood forecasting receive data from NWS meteorological stations (including data from airborne and satellite sources) and weather radar surveillance stations throughout the country. Some 1500 river and 4000 rainfall member stations of the cooperative networks also feed information into the system. About 10 percent of the river and rainfall stations are automated and can be interrogated directly by the forecasting personnel. At the remaining 90 percent the measurements are read at the gauges by observers on a preestablished schedule (one to four times daily depending on prevailing conditions). Although the manual operation — staffed by private citizens who are paid nominal amounts — is relatively inexpensive and permits the gathering of additional data (such as actual weather, river conditions, or type of precipitation), it suffers from lack of continuous coverage, timeliness, and quick response.[4]

Early Warning

The amount of possible forewarning (the time between the issuance of the warning and the arrival of the flood at a given point) depends upon the causative occurrence, the distance of the given point from the area of the occurrence, and the speed with which the forecast can be prepared and the warning issued.

Thus, for floods caused by snowmelt, the forewarning time may be several months, since water content of the snow can be measured and a general prediction of future flood conditions made based on the expected runoff under meteorological conditions normally prevailing during the spring thaw. Such long-range predictions and warning of snowmelt floods have become standard practice, particularly in the Upper Mississippi Basin.

When rains of heavy intensity and extended duration occur in the upper reaches of a river system, flood warnings of several days to a week or more are possible for downstream areas. There are hundreds of communities located in the headwaters of streams, however, where flooding can occur within a few hours, or even minutes, after the occurrence of an intense storm. In areas subject to such flash floods, the warning time is minimal, and special measures and techniques must be used to prepare and disseminate warnings.

Types of Warnings

Using the organization described above, the typical progression of a flood warning or advisory is from the River Forecast Center to the River District Office, which in turn disseminates appropriate advisories or warnings to the general public and to agencies with particular operational or monitoring responsibilities. The warning information may be disseminated through all news media and through direct communication networks to most of the specialized agencies. Standardized types of flood warnings are as follows:

Flood Forecasts and Warnings.   These are issued as far in advance as conditions warrant. They include information on the crest stage expected, time of arrival of crest, and areas affected. They provide forecasts of peak discharge, maximum velocity, and dates when water levels will go above or below the flood stage. They are disseminated to specialized agencies and the general public as soon and as fast as possible.

Flash-Flood Warning.   These warnings are issued as far in advance as possible whenever meteorological and radar data indicate rainfall in amounts and intensity sufficient to create the potential for flash flooding. They are of necessity rather generalized warnings, specifying the expected time of occurrence and the areas that may be affected. They are disseminated to specialized agencies, community cooperatives, and the general public in the potentially affected areas.

COUNTERMEASURES: PREVENTION SYSTEMS

Disaster Avoidance

In the sense that an act of nature can be avoided by nullifying the damaging effects, engineering works and other control techniques provide the best measure of flood avoidance under normal conditions; however, there is always a chance that flood conditions could exceed the design criteria of the works and a disaster result. For this reason, such control methods are, for purposes of this discussion, considered as means of hazard reduction and are addressed below.

Measures can be taken to avoid many causes of failure of man-made structures, such as dams and levees, by application of adequate laws and regulations for construction of the structures and a system of proper inspection and maintenance. Particularly critical in this regard is the structural soundness of dams.

Weather modification may ultimately provide the means to eliminate the cause of floods, but it is in the future. There are two weather-modification methods that show promise of eventual success on the basis of existing data: the formation of high-level cirrus clouds to reduce the amount of radiation and retard the melting of the snowpack, and the heavy seeding of cumulus clouds with artificial ice nuclei to reduce total rainfall. Neither now nor in the near future will the "state of the art" afford a practical means of complete avoidance. However, developments in this field may provide, earlier, a means of lessening the magnitude of a flood and thus reducing the hazard.

Hazard Reduction

Since complete evacuation of the flood plain is infeasible, socially and economically, other measures must be used to reduce the hazardous effects.

Hazard reduction, or flood control, embodies those deliberate cost-effective measures taken to regulate the flow of flood waters and to reduce the economic impact of flooding. These measures can be broadly grouped into programs of (1) flood prevention and (2) flood-plain regulation.

Flood Prevention.   Flood prevention efforts are of two types: flood abatement and flood protection.

Flood Abatement. The objectives of flood abatement, commonly referred to as watershed management, are to regulate the runoff of water into the tributary streams and to control erosion to prevent debris and sediment from reaching the streams and eventually the larger rivers. The measures employed include the reforestation or reseeding of denuded areas, mechanical land treatment of slopes to reduce the grade or provide contour ditches or structures, construction of catchment basins for debris and sediment, clearing of debris and sediment in the upper streams, and creation of water-holding areas (small lakes and ponds behind simple earthen dams on smaller streams).

Some measures are funded entirely by the federal government, and others are cost-shared with state and local authorities, private organizations, or individuals. Still others are accomplished without federal support. In addition to the flood control benefit derived from such measures, most of them also produce economic and environmental benefits.

Flood Protection. Four major types of engineering works are in use for flood protection: levees and floodwalls (see Figure 14–2) as physical barriers against higher than normal water levels, channel improvements to increase the capacity of the channel to pass more water, channel diversion to provide a floodway around areas that require protection, and reservoirs to store water and release it gradually.

Flood-Plain Regulation.   This term is generally used to encompass flood-plain usage, floodproofing, and flood insurance. It represents a relatively recent concept in dealing with means to reduce flood losses.

Flood-plain usage entails the use of local ordinances to control usage of the flood plains by defining the types of development and construction permissible in the flood plain, within the framework of comprehensive urban planning, and by ensuring the most judicious use of the land compatible with the aim of minimizing flood damage.

Floodproofing encompasses design and layout of building, specification of materials, and such techniques as locating vulnerable equipment above maximum flood height and providing watertight emergency closures for lower-level openings. These features not only minimize the losses but, because of the added construction costs, often discourage use of flood-plain land for buildings.

An outstanding example of local flood-plain regulation is the Golden Triangle area of Pittsburgh, Pennsylvania. This area is at the confluence of the Allegheny and Monongahela rivers, which join there to form the

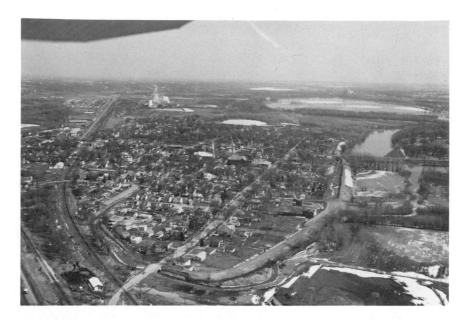

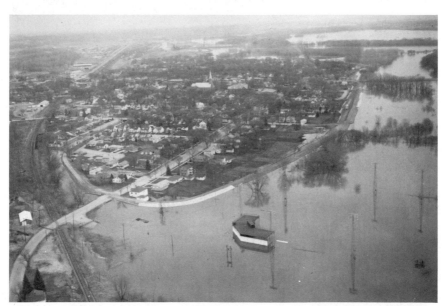

figure 14–2 Minnesota River, before and after. These pictures illustrate the protection afforded parts of Chaska, Minn. by a dike during the 1969 flood. Photos courtesy of U.S. Army Corps of Engineers, St. Paul District.

Ohio River. The "Point" area of the Triangle was severely flooded in 1936 to depths of nine feet. If the 1936 flood (a "200-year" flood) were to recur, the water level at the Point would be reduced ten feet by reservoirs which have since been constructed upstream. By local regulations construction has been limited to areas with an elevation at least one foot above this reduced level, and floodproofing is now required for the ground floors of all buildings as an added protection. The lower area of the Point, which is still subject to damage from the "200-year" flood, has been purchased by the state and converted into a public park.

Flood insurance, as underwritten by the federal government, encourages local communities to regulate their flood-plain development by making such regulations a prerequisite for insurance eligibility.

The main problem in instituting flood-plain management measures is the delineation of the flood plain in terms of expected future flooding on the basis of such factors as expected frequency and maximum height. The Corps of Engineers, on request of local communities, prepares flood-plain information studies which describe the flood hazard for the area and suggest regulatory and nonregulatory measures to reduce flood losses.

SUGGESTED INSTRUCTIONS

General Information and Definitions

The National Oceanic and Atmospheric Administration (NOAA), through its Weather Service's River Forecast Centers and River District offices, issues *flood forecasts and warnings* when rainfall is enough to cause rivers to overflow their banks and when melting snow may combine with rainfall to produce similar effects.

Flood warnings are forecasts of impending floods, and are distributed to the public by radio and television and through local government emergency forces. The warning message tells the expected severity of flooding (minor, moderate, or major), the affected river, and when and where flooding will begin. Careful preparations and prompt response will reduce property loss and ensure personal safety.

Flash flood warnings are the most urgent type of flood warning issued, and are also transmitted to the public over radio, television, and by other signals (e.g., sirens) established by local government to meet local needs.

Suggested Flood Safety Instructions

before the flood:

1   Find out how many feet your property is above or below possible flood levels so when predicted flood levels are broadcast, you can determine if you may be flooded. Also ask for the location of the nearest safe area.

2   Keep a stock of food which requires little cooking and no refrigeration; electric power may be interrupted.

3   Keep a portable radio, emergency cooking equipment, lights, and flashlights in working order.

4   Keep first aid and critical medical supplies (prescription drugs, insulin, etc.) at hand.

5   Keep your automobile fueled; if electric power is cut off, filling stations may not be able to operate pumps for several days.

6   Keep materials like sandbags, plywood, plastic sheeting, and lumber handy for emergency waterproofing.

when you receive a flood warning:

1   Store drinking water in closed, clean containers; water service may be interrupted.

2   If flooding is likely, and time permits, move essential items and furniture to upper floors of your house.

3   If forced or advised to leave your home, move to a safe area *before* access is cut off by flood water.

4   Cut off all electric circuits at the fuse panel or disconnect all electrical appliances. Shut off the water service and gas valves in your home.

during the flood:

1   Avoid areas subject to sudden flooding.

2   Do not attempt to cross a flowing stream where water is above your knees.

3   Do not attempt to drive over a flooded road. You can be stranded and trapped.

4   If your vehicle stalls, abandon it immediately and seek higher ground. Many people drown while trying to rescue their car.

after the flood:

1   Do not use fresh food that has come in contact with flood waters.

2   Test drinking water for potability; wells should be pumped out and the water tested before drinking.

3   Do not visit disaster area; your presence will probably hamper rescue and other emergency operations.

4   Do not handle live electrical equipment in wet areas; electrical equipment should be checked and dried before returning to service.

5   Use flashlights, not lanterns or torches, to examine buildings; flammables may be inside.

6   Report broken utility lines to police, fire, or other appropriate authorities.

7   Keep tuned to your radio or TV stations for advice and instructions of your local government on: where to go to obtain necessary medical care in your area; where to go for emergency assistance such as housing, clothing, and food; and ways to help yourself and your community recover from the emergency.

NOTES

[1]GILBERT F. WHITE, *Human Adjustment to Floods* (Chicago: University of Chicago Press, 1945), p. 37.

[2]*Climatological Data, National Summary, 1970,* U.S. Department of Commerce, National Oceanic and Atmospheric Administration (NOAA), Environmental Data Service (Asheville, N.C.: 1971), p. 94.

[3]*A Plan for Improving the National River and Flood Forecast and Warning Service,* U.S. Department of Commerce (Silver Spring, Md.: Office of Hydrology, December 1969), p. 13.

[4]MARSHALL M. RICHARDS, "Making Flood Warnings More Timely," paper presented at the Meeting of Experts on Flood Mitigation. Venice, Italy, October 1970, contained in *Flood Experts Meeting, U.S. Background Papers* (Tab D), NATO Committee on the Challenges of Modern Society.

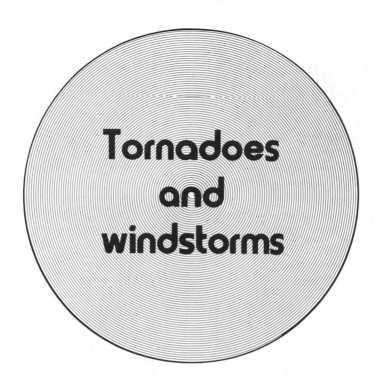

Tornadoes and windstorms

CAUSES AND CHARACTERISTICS

15 Tornadoes are local atmospheric storms of short duration formed of winds rotating at very high speeds, usually in a counterclockwise direction. To the observer these storms are visible as a vortex, a whirlpoollike column of winds rotating about a hollow cavity in which centrifugal forces produce a partial vacuum. As condensation occurs around the vortex, a pale cloud appears—the familiar and frightening tornado funnel. Air surrounding the funnel is also part of the tornado vortex. As the storm moves along the ground, this outer ring of rotating winds becomes dark with dust and debris, which may eventually darken the entire funnel. It is from the twisting spiral updraft that tornadoes have been dubbed "twisters." (See Figure 15-1.)

Windstorms refer to the damaging effect of winds caused by fast-moving frontal passages, thunderstorms, and squall lines that do not produce tornadoes. Windstorm causes, characteristics, and effects are similar to those of a tornado, except that they lack the extreme violent action and noticeable funnel. Since both of these natural hazards possess these similarities and produce widespread damage and loss of life, they are treated as one for the purpose of this study unless otherwise indicated.

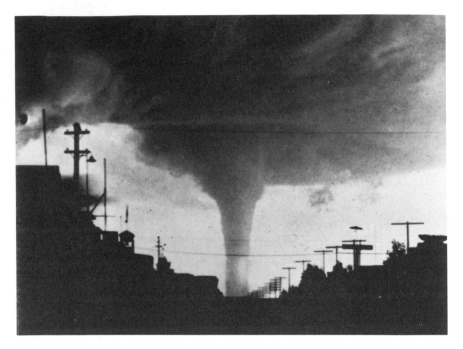

figure 15–1 Tornadoes are most likely to be wholesale killers when they are least expected. Photo courtesy of the Environmental Science Services Administration.

Tornado formation requires the presence of layers of air with contrasting characteristics of temperature, moisture, density, and wind flow. Complicated energy transformations, which are not fully understood, produce the tornado vortex. Many theories have been advanced as to the type of energy transformation necessary to generate a tornado. The two most frequently quoted ascribe tornado generation to either the effect of thermally induced rotary circulations or the mechanical effect of converging rotary winds.

Tornado formation attributed to the thermal effect is the result of forces set up by the imbalance created when cool air overrides warm air. The imbalance is compensated by rapid upward convection from the lower layers of warm air which become a rotary flow and form the tornado vortex.

If the mechanical effect prevails, slowly rotating air currents are constrained by external forces. These constraints cause the radius of rotation to lessen, thus increasing the speed of rotation (in the same way that an ice skater increases his speed of rotation by drawing in his arms). Ultimately, the converging, accelerating, rotating winds form the tornado vortex.

Currently, scientists seem to agree that neither process generates tornadoes independently. It is more probable that tornadoes are produced by the combined effects of both thermal and mechanical forces, with one or the other being the stronger generating agent or the triggering mechanism.

These small but severe storms form several thousand feet above the earth's surface, usually during warm, humid, unsettled weather, and in conjunction with a squall line of severe thunderstorms. Sometimes a series of two or more tornadoes is associated with a parent thunderstorm. As the thunderstorm or squall line moves, tornadoes may form at intervals along its path, travel for a few miles, and then dissipate. The forward speed of tornadoes has been observed to range from almost no motion to 70 miles per hour.

Tornado funnels appear as an extension of the dark, heavy cumulonimbus clouds of thunderstorms and stretch downward toward the ground. On the average, tornado paths are only an eighth of a mile wide and are seldom more than ten miles long. However, there have been spectacular instances in which tornadoes have caused heavy destruction along paths more than a mile wide and almost 300 miles long. A tornado traveled 293 miles across the states of Illinois and Indiana on May 26, 1917, and lasted 7 hours and 20 minutes. Its forward speed was 40 miles per hour, an average figure for tornadoes.[1] One of the more than 50 tornadoes that ripped through the Mississippi Delta on February 21, 1971, traveled for 159 miles. Its speed was 55 miles per hour.[2]

If the same atmospheric conditions occur over a large body of water, the vortex phenomenon is referred to as a "waterspout." Instead of the dust and debris found over land, the funnel cloud usually consists of water spray. (See Figure 15–2.)

EFFECTS

If there is some question as to cause and formation of tornadoes, there certainly is none on the destructive effects of these violent storms. The dark funnel of a tornado can destroy solid buildings, make a deadly missile of a piece of straw, uproot large trees, and hurl people and animals for hundreds of yards. Tornadoes do their destructive work through the combined action of their strong rotary winds, flying debris, and the partial vacuum in the center of the vortex. As a tornado passes over a building, the winds twist and rip at the outside walls, while the reduced pressure in the tornado's eye causes explosive pressure difference between the inside and outside of the building. Walls collapse or topple outward, windows explode, and the resulting debris is driven through the air in a dangerous barrage. Heavy objects, such as machinery and railroad cars, are lifted and carried by the wind for considerable distances. In 1931, for example, a tornado in Minnesota carried a rail-

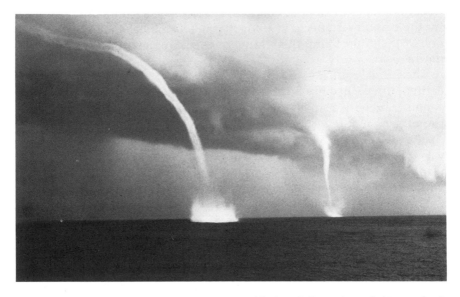

figure 15–2   Waterspouts. Photo courtesy National Oceanic and Atmospheric Administration.

road coach (weighing 83 tons, with 117 passengers aboard) some 80 feet through the air before dropping it in a ditch.[3]

Although the life of a tornado is short and its destructive path relatively small, this type of storm has caused considerable destruction of property and a heavy loss of life, especially in densely populated areas. The actual loss to the United States economy from the effects of tornadoes is quite high, and the costs in human suffering and loss of life are immeasurable.

One of the most destructive series of tornadoes occurred on April 3, 1974, when more than 100 tornadoes ripped through 11 states in the South and Midwest, causing 318 deaths in the United States and eight deaths in Canada.[4]

THREAT

Record

Tornadoes have been reported in areas outside the United States but only very infrequently. In the United States they have occurred in all 50 states, with no season being free of them. Normally, the number of tornadoes is at its lowest in the United States during December and January and at its peak in May. The months of greatest total frequency are

April, May, and June. (See Figure 15–3.) In February, when tornado activity begins to increase, maximum frequency occurs over the Central Gulf states. During March, the area of maximum frequency moves eastward to the Southeast Atlantic states, where tornado occurrence reaches a peak in April. During May, it moves to the Southern Plains states, and, in June, northward to the Northern Plains and Great Lakes areas and even as far east as western New York State. The reason for these shifts is the increasing penetration of warm, moist air from the south into the continental land mass, while contrasting cool, dry air surges in from the north and northwest. Tornadoes are generated with greatest frequency where these air masses meet and collide.

Although records of tornadoes in the United States have been kept for a long time, a reliable statistical history of these disturbances dates back only to 1953, the year in which the U.S. Department of Commerce began its tornado forecasting efforts. For example, from 1916 through 1952, fewer than 300 tornadoes were reported in any one year. In 1953, however, more than 437 tornadoes were observed and reported, and the number has never fallen below that level for any one year since then. From 1953 through 1970, an average of 642 tornadoes per year occurred in the United States, about half of them during April, May, and June. For the same period, the annual average number of tornado days — days on which one or more tornadoes were reported — was 159. Average annual frequency by states for this period ranges from 104 tornadoes in Texas to less than three in most of the Northeastern and Far Western states. Figure 15–4 shows the tornado incidence for each of the 50 states by number of occurrences and number of deaths during the 1953–1970 period.

Loss of life and property from windstorms has also been considerable. For example, in the United States the death figure attributable to this phenomenon closely approximates total deaths from tornadoes. It is interesting to note that approximately 20 percent of the total deaths resulting from windstorms occurred in one year, 1928.

Probability

Tornadoes may occur at any hour of the day or night but, because of the meteorological combinations that create them, they form most readily during the warmest hours of the day. The greatest number of tornadoes — 82 percent of the total — occur between noon and midnight, and the greatest single concentration — 23 percent of the total activity — falls between 4:00 and 6:00 P.M.

The mathematical chance that a specific location will be struck by a tornado in any one year is quite small. For example, the probability of a

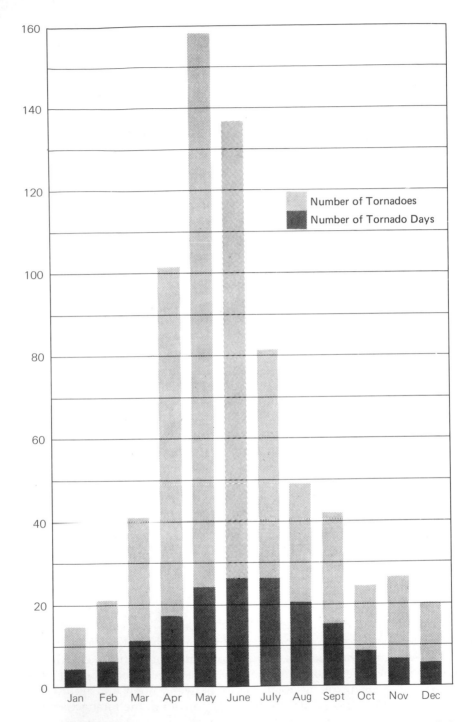

figure 15–3 Average number of tornadoes and tornado days each month in the United States (based on 12,739 tornadoes that occurred from 1956–1973).

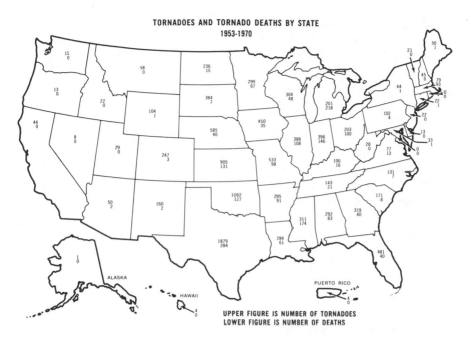

TORNADOES AND TORNADO DEATHS BY STATE
1953-1970

UPPER FIGURE IS NUMBER OF TORNADOES
LOWER FIGURE IS NUMBER OF DEATHS

figure 15–4 Tornadoes and tornado deaths by state, 1953–1970. Upper figure is number of tornadoes; lower figure is number of deaths.

tornado striking a given point in the area most frequently subject to tornadoes is about once in 350 years. In the Far Western states, the probability is close to zero. However, tornadoes have provided many statistical exceptions. Oklahoma City has been struck by tornadoes 26 times since 1892. Baldwyn, Mississippi, was struck twice by tornadoes during a 25-minute period on March 16, 1942. A third of Irving, Kansas, was left in ruins by two tornadoes which occurred 45 minutes apart on May 30, 1879. Austin, Texas, had two tornadoes in rapid succession on May 4, 1922, and Codell, Kansas, was struck on the same date—May 20—in three consecutive years: 1916, 1917, and 1918.[5]

More tornadoes occurred in 1967 than in any prior year of record for the United States; in 44 states, 912 tornadoes killed 116 persons and caused property damage in the millions of dollars.

Information on the numbers and area distribution of windstorms is not included in the regular climatological statistics.

VULNERABILITY

The relative vulnerability of people, property, the economy, and the ecology to the effects and damage attributed to tornadoes is far-reaching but at times somewhat difficult to separate. All are adversely affected but to different degrees and in different ways.

People are highly vulnerable. Often with little or no warning and in a matter of seconds, a tornado can transform a thriving street in a community into a ruin. Death and injury result from such causes as the disintegration or collapse of buildings brought about by the extreme pressure differential, debris driven by the high winds, flash flooding resulting from the associated heavy downpour, and electrocution caused by fallen utility lines.

As previously mentioned, the greatest damage to property results from both the force of the high winds and the effects of the extreme pressure differentials. Each aggravates the losses caused by the other. The combined effect often transforms a wooden building into a pile of rubble. Reinforced structures sustain damage to a lesser, but nonetheless significant, degree. Overhead power and telephone lines are cut and poles snapped. Mature trees in residential areas, parks, and forest lands are often snapped in two or uprooted. Crops, livestock, and farm dwellings bear the brunt of the tornadoes in rural areas.

Since a tornado is short-lived and usually affects a narrow path, the losses to the economy are seldom as heavy as those caused by other natural hazards, such as hurricanes and floods. They can, however, be very severe locally. This is especially true when a tornado strikes a densely populated area. Here the cleanup, repair, and recovery actions necessary to rehabilitate the affected area are usually costly and can absorb the primary efforts of government agencies and private citizens for days.

The ecological damage that results from a tornado is rather difficult to assess accurately, mainly because most of those effects are latent or gradual. Because the area affected is usually small, however, this damage is limited.

COUNTERMEASURES: PREDICTION SYSTEMS

Sensors and Surveillance

New or better technological countermeasures in the detection and surveillance of severe storms are required in order to prevent or lessen the ravages incurred. Over the years, the National Weather Service, tasked by the Congress with severe weather surveillance, has employed a variety of means and techniques in trying to accomplish this goal. In tornado-prone areas, observational units gather information on the development, formation, detection, and existence of tornadoes. Ground-based radar units (some of which are also used in hurricane surveillance) are used to help detect and study the intensity and movement of these storms. In the last decade, earth-orbiting satellites have provided weather pictures of areas beyond the range of ground radar. Despite the integrated use of all these means, certain gaps continue to exist, specifically in detection and surveillance; because tornadoes are small and short-lived, they may not be detected (except in rare instances) by conventional weather-observing networks.

As an aid in solving this problem, networks of storm reporters — spotters consisting of thousands of public-spirited citizens and organizations — are established throughout the tornado belt. These spotters, trained in recognizing the characteristics of severe thunderstorms and tornadoes, are alerted to the possibility of dangerous weather through tornado watches issued by the National Weather Service.

When a watch is in effect, spotters keep on the alert and notify by phone the nearest National Weather Service Office (or a Community Warning Center where one is established) as soon as a tornado or severe thunderstorm is sighted, describing the type of storm, its location, intensity, and direction of movement.

At the National Weather Service Office, the spotters' reports are plotted usually on a radar screen. Thus, the radar operator can relate the reports to the radar echoes accompanying the severe weather. By this means, the National Weather Service Office can quickly determine the direction and rate of movement of the tornado or severe thunderstorm, alert other spotters to the existence or threat of tornadoes, and determine which areas should be given immediate warnings.

This system is also used to follow the further progress of the storm cloud or clouds and to watch for additional tornadoes or severe thunderstorms. More than one may strike an area at the same time. Unless reports are continuously received, collated, and evaluated, therefore, confusion may develop as to the location and direction of the threatening condition.

Early Warning

The National Weather Service has five basic methods for disseminating its warnings of tornadoes and severe thunderstorms to the general public:

The Broadcast Industry. The networks of AM–FM radio and TV stations covering the United States provide a very effective means of reaching a large section of the population endangered by these severe disturbances. Recent statistics, in fact, show that in emergency conditions about 90 percent of the total population of an area can be quickly alerted.[6] The broadcast industry has shown excellent cooperation in discharging this public service function.

NOAA Weather Wire Circuits.   The National Weather Service leases circuits to every community of appreciable size in 28 states (and eventually will provide coverage for all 50 states). Newspapers, broadcast media, and other interested parties can have terminal receivers connected to these circuits for a modest monthly service charge. Thus National Weather Service is linked to the broadcast industry and to communities. In addition, it can, through these same circuits, activate special devices to alert subscribers to be on the watch for a tornado. (In addition to tornado forecasting and warning, these circuits are used for forecasting and warning of other weather phenomena.)

Special Radio Weather Warning System.   The National Weather Service also operates a special warning transmission facility broadcasting continuously on VHF–FM frequencies 162.40 and 162.55 megahertz. Individuals and agencies having suitable receivers may obtain warning of tornadoes and severe thunderstorms by this means. The equipment also has the capability to activate receivers in schools, hospitals, government offices, factories, and other establishments within a transmitting range of about 50 miles.

Telephone Network.   The National Weather Service also relies on commercial telephone service to distribute its warnings to local designated civil defense agencies, law enforcement agencies, and other organizations which in turn can quickly relay messages to the affected communities.

Local Siren Systems.   These are used as an aid in the tornado warning process.

All these means of communication are essential to the National Weather Service's capability to effect early warning of impending tornadoes.

COUNTERMEASURES: PREVENTION SYSTEMS

Disaster Avoidance

Avoidance of a tornado, especially in the tornado belt, is virtually impossible. The best means to mitigate its effects, therefore, is to help prepare people for this natural hazard. A campaign to educate the public on characteristics, effects, and perils of tornadoes and severe storms and on safety rules to follow will considerably reduce injuries and the loss of life. Over the years, the National Weather Service has published and distributed brochures, pamphlets, and films emphasizing these points. Its personnel have given lectures and conducted seminars on the subject.

The effectiveness of this campaign can be greatly reinforced by a Tornado Plan. Certain communities, working in conjunction with their civil defense agencies, have formulated and initiated such plans, which become operational on notification from the National Weather Service or when threatening conditions approach.

Hazard Reduction

The extremely high winds, overpressure, heavy rains, and hail associated with tornadoes and severe thunderstorms are the major causes of the resulting damage to human life and property. At present, there is no known method of totally eliminating these hazards. However, certain recommended safety rules can be followed which should reduce or lessen the perils to individuals.

It is particularly important to realize that a ring of hills around an area does *not* protect it from a tornado, despite popular belief. Some of the worst hit areas, such as Worcester, Massachusetts, have had a ring of hills on the side from which the tornado came.

Structures can be protected only by being designed to withstand the high winds and pressure differentials associated with tornadoes. Local building codes in areas of heavy tornado incidence should be suitably revised to achieve this goal. Mobile homes present a special problem because of their vulnerability to overturning during strong winds. They should be firmly anchored with cables.

SUGGESTED INSTRUCTIONS

General Information

The tornado is a violent local storm with whirling winds of tremendous speed. It appears as a rotating, funnel-shaped cloud which extends toward the ground from the base of a thundercloud. It varies from gray to black in color. The tornado spins like a top and may sound like the roaring of an airplane or locomotive. These small, short-lived storms are the most violent of all atmospheric phenomena and, over a small area, the most destructive.

Tornado *WATCH* — means tornadoes are expected to develop

Tornado *WARNING* — means a tornado has actually been sighted or indicated on radar

Warnings

The National Weather Service issues severe weather warnings to the public over radio and TV stations.

Examples of General Announcements

Radio and television stations will broadcast the latest severe weather warnings and tornado watch information.

Knowing what to do when a tornado is approaching may mean the difference between life and death. If you see any revolving, funnel-shaped clouds on a cloudy day, report them by telephone immediately to the local police department, sheriff's office, or National Weather Service office. But do not use the phone to get information and advice — depend on radio or TV as indicated above.

Examples of Tornado Safety Rules

When a *tornado watch* is announced:

1   Keep your radio or television on and listen for the latest Weather Service warnings and advisories. If power fails, use portable battery radio or your car radio.

2   Keep watching the sky, especially to the south and southwest. (When a tornado watch is announced during the approach of a *hurricane*, however, keep in mind that the tornado may move from an easterly direction.)

When a *tornado warning* is announced:

1   Your best protection is an underground shelter or cave, or a substantial steel-framed or reinforced concrete building. (If none is available, take refuge in other places as indicated below.)

2   If your home has no basement, take cover under heavy furniture on the ground floor in the center of the house, or in a small room on the ground floor that is away from outside walls and windows. (As a last resort, go outside to a neaby ditch, excavation, culvert, or ravine.)

3   Doors and windows on the sides of your house away from the tornado may be left open to help reduce damage to the building, but stay away from them to avoid flying debris.

4   Do not remain in a trailer or mobile home if a tornado is approaching. Take cover elsewhere.

5   If advised that you are likely to be in the path of a tornado, and if time permits, electricity and fuel lines should be cut off.

6   If you are outside in open country, drive away from the tornado's path, at a right angle to it. If there isn't time to do this — or if you are walking — take cover and lie flat in the nearest depression, such as a ditch, culvert, excavation, or ravine.

7   *Schools*   If the school building is of good steel-reinforced construction, stay inside away from the windows and remain near an inside wall on the lower floors if possible.

8   *Avoid auditoriums and gymnasiums* with large, poorly supported roofs.

9   In rural schools that do not have reinforced construction, move school-children and teachers to a ravine or ditch if storm shelters are not available.

10   *Factories and Industrial Plants*   When possible, shut off electrical circuits and fuel lines if a tornado approaches the plant. Workers should be moved to sections offering the best possible protection, in accordance with advance plans.

11   *Shopping Centers*   Go to a designated shelter area (NOT to your parked car).

12   *Office Buildings*   Go to an interior hallway on the lowest floor, or to a designated shelter area. Stay away from windows.

Examples of Announcements Concerning Safety Measures After the Passage of the Tornado

1   Use extreme caution in entering or working in buildings that may have been damaged or weakened by the disaster, as they may collapse without warning. Also, there may be gas leaks or electrical short circuits.

2   Don't take lanterns, torches, or lighted cigarettes into buildings that have been damaged by a natural disaster, since there may be leaking gas lines or flammable material present.

3   Stay away from fallen or damaged electric wires — they may still be dangerous.

4   Check for leaking gas pipes in your home. Do this by smell — *don't use matches or candles.* If you smell gas, do this: (a) Open all windows and doors; (b) Turn off the main gas valve at the meter; (c) Leave the house immediately; (d) Notify the gas company or the police or fire department; (e) Don't reenter the house until you are told it is safe to do so.

5   If any of your electrical appliances are wet, first turn off the main power switch in your house, then unplug the wet appliance, dry it out, reconnect, and finally, turn on the main power switch. (Caution: Don't do any of these things while you are wet or standing in water.) If fuses blow when the electric power is restored, turn off the main power switch immediately and inspect for short circuits in your home wiring, appliances, and equipment.

6   Check your food and water supplies before using them. Foods that require refrigeration may be spoiled if electric power has been off for some time.

7   Stay away from disaster areas. Sightseeing could interfere with first aid or rescue work, and may be dangerous as well.

8   Don't drive unless necessary and, if you must, drive with caution. Watch for hazards to yourself and others, and report them to local police or fire departments.

9   Report broken sewer or water mains to the Water Department.

10   Keep tuned to your radio or TV stations for advice and instructions of your local government on: where to go to obtain necessary medical care in your area; where to go for necessary emergency assistance for housing, clothing, food, etc.; and ways to help yourself and your community recover from the emergency.

NOTES

[1]*Tornado,* U. S. Department of Commerce, National Oceanic and Atmospheric Administration (NOAA) (Washington, D.C.: U.S. Government Printing Office, 1970).

[2]*Mississippi Delta Tornadoes of February 21, 1971,* Natural Disaster Survey Report 71–2, U. S. Department of Commerce, NOAA (Washington, D.C.: U.S. Government Printing Office, July 1971), pp. iii, 5.

[3]*Tornado.*

[4]Metropolitan Life Insurance Company, *Statistical Bulletin,* January 1975, p. 6.

[5]*Tornado.*

[6]*Summary Report of the Warning Working Group,* Office of Telecommunications Policy (Washington, D.C.: U.S. Government Printing Office, September 1971), p. 9 and Annex H, p. 9.

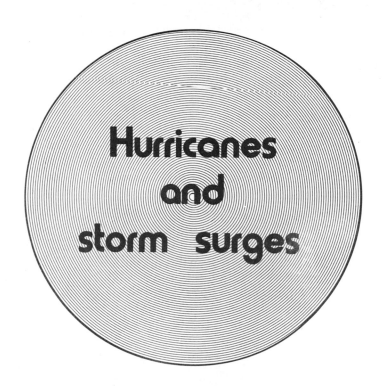

Hurricanes and storm surges

CAUSES AND CHARACTERISTICS

16 "There is still no exact understanding of the triggering mechanism involved in hurricane generation. . . ."[1] The conditions needed to produce hurricane circulation, however, and the relationships between the hurricane itself and the surrounding atmospheric processes have been defined. Hurricanes are tropical cyclones, formed in the atmosphere over warm ocean areas, in which winds reach speeds of 74 miles per hour or more and blow in a large spiral around a relatively calm center—the so-called eye of the hurricane. Hurricanes can be compared to giant whirlwinds in which air moves in a large, tightening spiral about a center of extreme low pressure. This circulation is counterclockwise in the Northern Hemisphere and clockwise in the Southern Hemisphere.

These storms, as they occur in different oceans and hemispheres, bear names given locally: *baguio* in the Philippines, *cyclone* in the Indian Ocean, *typhoon* in the Pacific. In our hemisphere, the name for this type of storm is *hurricane*. Some people erroneously refer to tornadoes as cyclones, but that term should never be applied to a tornado, twister, or waterspout.

It appears that the current practice of naming hurricanes with girls' names began during World War II and has been the official National

Weather Service policy since 1953. The National Weather Service prepared a list of four sets of tropical cyclone names in alphabetical order for the Gulf of Mexico, Carribean, and Atlantic Ocean areas. Names beginning with Q, U, X, Y, and Z were not included because of their scarcity. A separate set of names is used each year, beginning with the first name in each set. Although each set is used again every four years, names used for major hurricanes—like 1965's Betsy—are retired for at least ten years and another name is substituted. The record number of Atlantic hurricanes in a single season is 21.

Typhoons and Pacific hurricanes have also been feminized. In the eastern North Pacific, the alphabetical listing of names is prepared in sets of four, and designations are cycled from year to year. In the central and western North Pacific, the practice differs because of the high incidence of tropical cyclones. The four sets prepared for typhoons originating there are not cycled annually; instead, all names are used consecutively, regardless of the year—for example, if the past typhoon season ended with Phyllis then the next season would begin with typhoon Rita, both from the same set of names.

The hurricane is unique in both structure and strength (see Figure 16–1). On the average, the area that contains winds with speeds of at least 74 miles per hour covers some 100 miles in diameter, while gale-force winds—winds of over 40 miles per hour—extend over an area 400 miles in diameter.[2] Its spiral is marked by heavy cloud bands, some containing very heavy rains and some only light rains or no rain at all. These spiral bands, composed of cumulus and cumulonimbus clouds, rise until condensing water vapor is swept off as ice-crystal wisps of cirrus clouds. Thunderstorm electrical activity is observed in these bands as lightning.

In the lower few thousand feet, moist air flows into the system and is carried upward by ascending columns of air near the center. The size of the hurricane and the intensity of its winds decrease with altitude. The cyclonic circulation is gradually replaced above 40,000 feet by high altitude winds in the opposite direction (anticyclonic) circulating about a center hundreds of miles away. These high altitude winds act as a suction-pump exhaust system for the hurricane's heat engine, which is fueled by the warm water over which it forms. At lower levels, where the hurricane is most intense, winds on the rim of the storm follow a wide spiral pattern, like the slower currents around the edge of a whirlpool. Like those currents, the winds accelerate as they approach the center of the vortex. The outer band has light winds (perhaps 30 miles per hour) at the rim of the storm; within 30 miles of the center, however, winds may exceed 150 miles per hour.

Hurricane winds are produced, as are all winds, by differences in atmospheric pressure. The pressure gradient — the rate of pressure change with distance — produced in hurricanes is the most severe in the atmosphere, excepting only the pressure change across the narrow funnel of a tornado. In the hurricane, winds move toward the low pressure area in the warm, comparatively calm core. There converging air currents are drawn upward by a combination of convection, the mechanical thrusting of the converging currents, and the suction action of high altitude circulations. This spiral is marked by thick cloud walls curling inward toward the storm center, releasing heavy precipitation and enormous quantities of heat energy.

At the center, surrounded by a band in which this strong vertical circulation is greatest, is the core — the eye of the hurricane. The eye, like

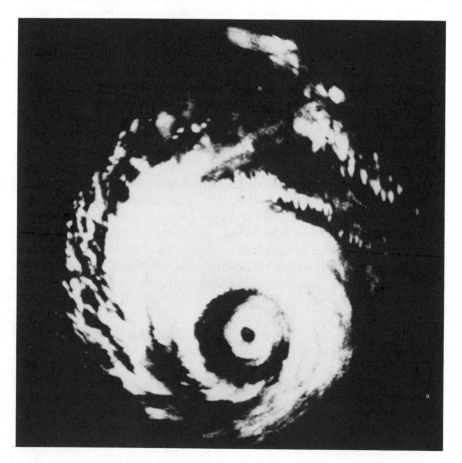

figure 16–1 Hurricane Beulah, 1967, as seen on the radarscope at Brownsville, Texas. Photo courtesy National Oceanic and Atmospheric Administration.

the spiral rainbands, is unique to the hurricane; no other atmospheric phenomenon has this virtually calm core. On the average, eye diameter is about 14 miles, although diameters of 25 miles are not unusual. Inward, from the heated tower of maximum winds and cumulonimbus clouds, winds diminish rapidly to something less than 15 miles per hour in the eye; at the opposite wall, winds increase again, but come from the opposite direction because of the cyclonic circulation of the storm.

While this is the description of a typical hurricane, hurricanes do have individual characteristics which may or may not conform to those just described. Extreme variability and instability prevail within each storm system. Pressure and temperature gradients change rather slowly while the storm is over warm ocean water but may fluctuate wildly across the storm as the hurricane develops its erratic life in the face of forces (such as cooler air and rough terrain) which will ultimately destroy it.

If it is an August storm, its average life expectancy is 12 days; if a July or November storm, it lives an average of 8 days. While a hurricane lives, the generation of energy within its circulation is immense. There is as yet no satisfactory way of modifying or controlling a hurricane; it remains one of nature's most awesome activities.

EFFECTS

Over the years, the toll in lives exacted by hurricanes has diminished encouragingly. In the United States this reduction has resulted primarily from the timely warnings given to the people living along the coasts. Damage to fixed property, however, continues to mount as areas affected by hurricanes undergo further extensive economic development. (See Figure 16–2.) Most of the death and destruction associated with hurricanes is caused by wind, flood-producing rains, and—most lethal of all—storm surges.

Wind.   As winds increase in velocity, horizontal pressure against structures mounts with the square of wind velocity, so that a tenfold increase in wind speed increases the wind-created force a hundredfold. For example, a 25-mile-per-hour wind causes pressure of about 2 pounds per square foot; a wind of 200 miles per hour causes pressure of about 220 pounds per square foot (all with respect to a flat surface). For most structures, such an added force is sufficient to cause failure. Hurricanes may also produce a destructive effect by lowering the atmospheric pressure outside a closed structure sufficiently to cause normal pressure inside to explode outward and collapse the building. Tall structures like radio towers, buffeted by gusting hurricane-force winds, may oscillate until structural failure occurs.

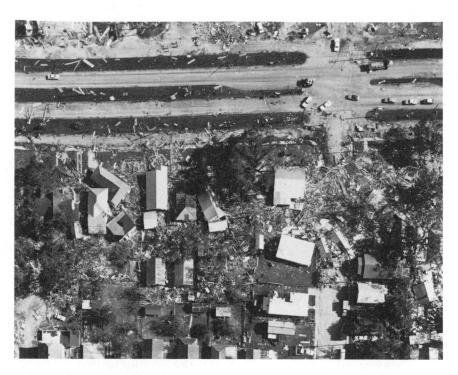

figure 16–2 Even with timely warning, hurricanes can leave death and destruction behind. This is a portion of Biloxi, Miss. after Hurricane Camille struck, 1969. Camille killed more than 255 people. Photo courtesy National Oceanic and Atmospheric Administration.

Floods.   Floods produced by hurricane rainfall usually are more destructive than the winds associated with hurricanes. The typical hurricane brings 6 to 12 inches of rainfall to the area it crosses, often in a few hours. The resulting floods produce great damage and loss of life, particularly in mountainous areas.

The winds from Hurricane Diane (1955), for example, caused little damage as they moved onto the continent. Long after the winds had subsided, however, floods produced by rainfall in Pennsylvania, New York, and New England killed 200 persons and cost an estimated $700 million in damage.

Another example was Hurricane Camille in August 1969. Two days after this severe storm had wrecked the Louisiana–Mississippi coastline, its remnants dumped record-breaking amounts of rainfall in the mountains of western Virginia. The resultant flash floods claimed over 100 lives and caused more than $100 million in damages.

Storm Surges.   The hurricane's worst killer comes from wind-driven waters, as the following examples show: more than 6000 persons perished in Galveston in 1900; some 2000 persons drowned in Florida in 1928 when the waters of Lake Okeechobee were literally blown out of their shallow basin; and about 380 drowned when Hurricane Audrey struck Louisiana in June 1957.

Over the deep ocean, waves generated by hurricane-force winds may reach heights of 50 feet or more. Beneath the storm center, the ocean surface is drawn upward (like water in a giant straw) a foot or so above normal by reduced atmospheric pressure. This creates large swells on the ocean's surface. Thus, a hurricane's presence may be detected well in advance of its arrival on land by sea swells emanating from the storm.

As the storm crosses the Continental Shelf and moves toward the coast, mean water level may rise 15 feet or more. Behind the storm center, offshore hurricane-force winds may cause a decrease in mean water level, setting up strong currents. The advancing storm surge is superimposed on normal astronomical tides and, in turn, wind waves are superimposed on the surge. This buildup of water level can produce severe flooding in coastal areas, particularly when the storm surge coincides with normal high tides.

Much of the United States's densely populated coastline along the Atlantic and Gulf coasts lies less than 10 feet above mean sea level. It is therefore highly susceptible to various forms of storm surge damage. Surge heights along flat coasts can bring catastrophe. A surge forced up a narrow channel, such as a riverbed, may appear as a wall of water— incorrectly called a "tidal wave"—engulfing everything in its passage. Extended pounding by giant waves of water weighing some 1700 pounds per cubic yard can demolish any structure not specifically designed to withstand such forces. Currents, set up along the coast by storm-surge water heights, and the combined wind and wave actions erode foundations and cause buildings to topple. Waves and currents severely erode beaches and highways and other manmade objects through prolonged pounding. In confined harbors, damage to shipping may be very extensive. Estuarine and bayou areas can become polluted and thus endanger the public health.

THREAT

Record

Most hurricanes form in a belt between 8 degrees and 15 degrees north and south from the Equator. Within this zone, the most likely areas of formation are those in which the surface water temperature is high, such as the Caribbean Sea. All hurricanes begin at sea as tropical disturbances and tend to dissipate over land. The general classification for all such occurrences is "tropical cyclone." During the early days of meteorology, many tropical cyclones must have occurred in the oceans without being reported. In recent years, however, improved reporting procedures have provided more complete records of occurrences. The average annual death toll for the United States was 107, while estimated damage averaged approximately $142 million annually.

The North Atlantic, Caribbean Sea, and Gulf of Mexico areas produce the hurricanes that ultimately affect the Gulf and East coasts of the United States. The months of most frequent hurricane occurrence in the North Atlantic and adjacent waters are August, September, and October.

Probability

Along the Atlantic and Gulf coasts, the normal hurricane season extends from June through November. Early in the season the Caribbean and the Gulf of Mexico are the principal areas of origin. In July and August this center shifts eastward, and by September it spreads from the Bahamas southeastward to the Lesser Antilles and eastward to the Cape Verde Islands off the west coast of Africa. After mid-September the major points of origin shift back to the western Caribbean and the Gulf of Mexico. During an "average" year, one can expect fewer than eight tropical cyclones, of which about five would develop into hurricanes.

VULNERABILITY

As in other weather-related disasters, the vulnerability to hurricane damage of people, property, the economy, and the ecology is far-reaching. Each is adversely affected to different degrees and in different ways.

People are usually the most vulnerable to the ravages of hurricanes during the initial phase. Death and injury attributed to this natural hazard usually result from flying debris, drowning caused by the flooding of lowlands from the storm surge and excessive rainfall, and electrocution because of downed utility lines.

Damage to property is caused by high wind, rain, and flooding. Winds uproot trees and shrubs and also do physical damage to the roofs of residential, commercial, and industrial structures. As a result, rain enters the building and aggravates the damage. Flooding destroys crops, livestock, personal possessions, and real property. After the high waters recede, they leave behind a mud silt residue, which adds to the damage and the rehabilitation costs. Along coastal waterways, storm surges are also responsible for beach erosion and the undermining and collapse of waterfront property.

The preparation required in boarding up residences and business establishments for the onslaught of a hurricane, as well as the dismantling process, is costly. Further, the issuance of hurricane warnings results in the closure of many business and community activities, with resultant loss of income.

The vulnerability of the general economy and the ecology of areas affected by hurricanes has not been subjected to systematic study. The impact, however, is significant.

COUNTERMEASURES: PREDICTION SYSTEMS

Sensors and Surveillance

From the first discovery of an initial tropical disturbance in the easterly trade-wind belt, a hurricane is kept under surveillance by a variety of sensing devices and observation systems. First, there is the network of continental and island weather stations reporting surface and upper air data. Ships and aircraft crossing the tropical ocean areas provide supplementary information. More recently, weather surveillance satellites have been added which provide more timely data on hurricane activity covering wider areas. These systems provide the meteorologists of NOAA's National Weather Service (NWS) the information necessary to monitor the weather in general and hurricanes in particular.

In addition, hurricane reconnaissance flights are conducted by the U.S. Navy, the U.S. Air Force, and NOAA's Research Flight Facility. Acting as the long-range eyes of the hurricane warning system, these flights reconnoiter the potentially hazardous areas.

As the disturbance intensifies and moves toward land, a radar fence extending from Brownsville, Texas, to Brunswick, Maine, tracks and monitors its speed and movement. With this information a landfall point can be determined.[3]

While the storm is being tracked, a watch is kept on tidal heights in the path of the storm for corroborating indications. A network of tide gauges located along the coastal areas measures the swells that precede storm surges during the final approach and passage of a hurricane. National Weather Service offices in the coastal regions can monitor changes in local water level—an important element in forecasting the arrival and destructive potential of storm surges and hurricane-driven waves. Once the hurricane is over land, the network of weather-reporting stations, volunteer spotters, law enforcement agencies, and land-based radar systems assumes the role in monitoring the position, speed, direction, and other essential characteristics of the storm.

Early Warning

The responsibility for general hurricane early warning rests with the director of the National Hurricane Center. Local warning responsibility, however, is assigned to seven designated NWS offices (Hurricane Warning Offices) — at Miami, New Orleans, Washington, Boston, San Juan, San Francisco, and Honolulu. In addition, supplemental forecasts are issued by local NWS Forecast Offices and contain detailed information on conditions expected to affect the local area for which they have forecast responsibility.

Meteorologists of the National Hurricane Center continuously monitor basic weather data for evidence of tropical disturbance formation by noting changes in the pressure, wind, cloud, and rainfall characteristics. Once the disturbance is confirmed, attention is focused on determining whether the system will intensify, remain the same, or dissipate. If intensification occurs, a prediction of the path, speed, and direction of the storm is made. Hurricane "watches" (when a hurricane poses a threat) are issued at least 36 hours before the storm is expected to affect an area. Hurricane "warnings" refine the watch area and signify that hurricane conditions are imminent. These warnings are usually issued to allow residents at least 12 hours of daylight to take protective action and plan for evacuation. As the hurricane moves closer to land, "advisories" are issued every six hours, with intermediate "bulletins" every two or three hours.

Warnings in the Pacific

The incidence of tropical cyclones in the Pacific is some three times what it is in the Atlantic. But the easterly trade winds work favorably in the Pacific, and very rarely — twice a year on the average — do tropical storms or hurricanes strike along the western coastline of Mexico.[4]

At Hurricane Warning Offices in San Francisco and Honolulu, the same watch is kept for the same destructive storms, and warning is given to ships and coastlines in their paths.

Communications

The Hurricane Warning Offices and the National Hurricane Center are linked by normal National Weather Service communications and by a special internal teletypewriter circuit. This system is activated from June 1 through November 30 for the primary purpose of collecting and disseminating hurricane-related data and coordinating the actions of the Hurricane Warning Offices. Thus, the products of the hurricane forecasters go directly to all NWS Forecast Offices, interested local governments, law enforcement agencies, and other emergency forces (e.g., the Coast Guard and Red Cross). In addition, these systems serve the mass-news media, through which the general public is informed.

As the emergency develops, the public in areas threatened by a hurricane is given two types of information: one relates to storm location and movement (speed and direction), wind force, height of storm surge and potential flooding, rainfall forecast, time of onset, and identification of recommended sections to be evacuated; the other advises people to take stock of their preparedness requirements, keep abreast of the latest advisories and bulletins, be ready for quick action, and take the precautions necessary to protect life and property.

The efficiency of the warning system is such that virtually 100 percent of hurricane deaths are now preventable in the United States.

COUNTERMEASURES: PREVENTION SYSTEMS

Disaster Avoidance

For the permanent inhabitants of certain areas of the continental United States, notably the Gulf and East coasts, there is as yet no practical way to avoid a hurricane. Public education and research currently offer the most useful ways to meet this inevitable threat: research should help reveal more fully the nature of hurricanes, and public information programs will continue to teach precautionary measures.

The National Weather Service conducts a continuing public education program along the Gulf and Atlantic coasts. The program consists of distributing information brochures and pamphlets and making radio-TV spot announcements on hurricane preparedness. In addition, meetings to explain the effects and ravages of hurricanes are organized with local governments, disaster agencies, the news media, and the general public.

The National Weather Service also conducts research into the physics of hurricanes—the causes of their generation and the forces that drive them. During the last several decades, experiments have sought ways of modifying hurricanes by reducing their destructive forces. The first effort was made in 1947 under *Project Cirrus*, when 80 pounds of dry ice were dispersed into a moderately strong hurricane. Since 1962, experiments have been carried out almost every year. The results have been promising, but much work remains before real benefit can be seen from these hurricane modification programs.

Concurrently, research to improve forecasting models and techniques is being conducted in an attempt to produce more accurate and timely forecasts. Continuous programs are conducted to improve the accuracy and efficiency of the observing and communications networks.

Hazard Reduction

Certain safety rules can be followed which should reduce the perils to human life. Anyone living in areas frequently affected by hurricanes should enter each hurricane season with emergency supplies. Before arrival of a hurricane, windows should be boarded or protected with storm shutters, outdoor objects secured or placed under shelter, automobiles fueled to permit rapid evacuation, and the progress and position of the storm closely monitored. Suitable shelter—preferably on high ground—should be sought. During the storm, people should remain indoors until notified that the hurricane has passed and that it is safe to go outdoors. Local authorities should designate carefully selected evacuation routes for residents of low-lying areas and beach communities.

The protection of property can be improved substantially by replacing substandard building codes with updated and improved versions designed to ensure that structures will withstand the forces associated with hurricanes. Comprehensive preparedness plans, periodically updated, can aid residents of affected areas in countering the more severe consequences of destructive storms.

SUGGESTED INSTRUCTIONS

General Information—Warnings

The National Weather Service issues warnings when hurricanes are approaching the United States mainland.

A hurricane watch means a hurricane *may* threaten an area within 24 hours. A hurricane watch is *not* a hurricane warning, but a first alert for emergency forces and the general public in prospectively threatened areas. When your area is under a hurricane watch, you should continue normal activities, but stay tuned to radio or television for all Weather Service advisories.

A hurricane warning becomes part of advisories when a hurricane is expected to strike an area within 24 hours. Advisories containing hurricane warnings include an assessment of flood danger in coastal and inland areas, small-craft warnings, gale warnings for the storm's periphery, estimated storm effects, and recommended emergency procedures.

Other issued warnings are:

1   *Small-craft warning.* When a hurricane moves within a few hundred miles of the coast, advisories warn small-craft operators to take precautions and not to venture into the open ocean.

2   *Gale warning.* When winds of 38–55 miles per hour (33–48 knots) are expected, a gale warning is added to the advisory message.

3   *Storm warning.* When winds of 55–74 miles per hour (48–64 knots) are expected, a storm warning is added to the advisory message.

Gale and storm warnings describe the coastal area affected by the warning, the time during which the warning will apply, and the expected intensity of the disturbance. *When storm warnings are part of a tropical cyclone advisory, they may change to hurricane warnings if the storm continues along the coast.* Radio and television will broadcast latest hurricane advisories.

Precautionary Measures—After Warning and Prior to Hurricane

1   Keep your radio or television on and listen for the latest Weather Service warnings and advisories. When a hurricane approaches, also listen for *tornado* watches and warnings. (See "Suggested Instructions" for tornadoes, page 287.) If power fails, use portable battery radio or your car radio. Check your battery-powered equipment. Your radio may be your only link with the world outside the hurricane, and emergency cooking facilities and flashlights will be essential if utility services are interrupted.

2   Plan your time before the storm arrives. Waiting until the "last minute" might mean you'll be marooned.

3   Leave beaches or other low-lying areas that may be swept by high tides. Leave early; don't run the risk of being marooned.

4   Moor your boat securely before the storm arrives, or move it to a designated safe area. When your boat is moored, leave it, and don't return once the wind and waves are up.

5   Board up windows or protect them with storm shutters or tape. Danger to small windows is mainly from wind-driven debris. Larger windows may be broken by wind pressure.

6   Secure outdoor objects that might be blown away or uprooted. Garbage cans, garden tools, toys, signs, porch furniture, and a number of other harmless items become missiles of destruction in hurricane winds. Anchor them or store them inside before the storm strikes.

7   Store drinking water in clean, closed containers, such as jugs, bottles, and cooking utensils. Your town's water supply may be contaminated by flooding or damaged by the hurricane.

8   Keep your car fueled. Service stations may be inoperable for several days after the storm strikes because of flooding or interrupted electrical power.

9   Unless advised to evacuate, stay at home if your house is sturdy and on high ground. If it is not or if you live in a mobile home, move to a designated shelter and stay there until the storm is over.

10   Remain indoors during the hurricane. Travel is extremely dangerous when winds and tides are whipping through your area.

11   Beware the "eye" of the hurricane. If the calm storm center passes directly overhead, there will be a lull in the wind lasting from a few minutes to half an hour or more. Stay in a safe place unless emergency repairs are absolutely necessary. Remember, at the other side of the "eye" the winds rise very rapidly to hurricane force, and come from the opposite direction.

Evacuation

If you are warned to evacuate your home temporarily and move to another location (including predesignated hurricane shelters), there are certain things to remember and do. Here are the most important ones.

Follow the Instructions and Advice of Local Authorities.   If you are told to evacuate, do so promptly. If you are instructed to move to a certain location, go there—don't go anywhere else. If certain travel routes are specified or recommended, use those routes rather than trying to find short cuts of your own. If you are told to shut off your water, gas, or electric service before leaving home, do so. Also find out from the radio or TV where emergency housing and mass feeding stations are located, in case you need to use them.

Secure Your Home Before Leaving.   If you have time, and if you have not received other instructions from the local authorities, you should lock your house doors and windows. Park your car in the garage, carport, or driveway, close windows, and lock the car (unless you are driving to your new temporary location).

Travel with Care.   If the local authorities are arranging transportation for you, precautions will be taken for your safety. But if you are walking or driving your own car to another location, keep in mind these things:

1   Leave early enough so as not to be marooned by flooded roads, fallen trees, and wires.

2   Make sure you have enough gasoline in your car.

3   Follow recommended routes.

4   As you travel, keep listening to the radio for additional information and instructions from your local government.

Safety Measures — After Passage of Hurricane

1   Remain in shelters until informed by those in charge that you may return to your home.

2   Keep tuned to your radio or TV stations for advice and instructions of your local government on: where to go to obtain necessary medical care in your area; where to go for necessary emergency assistance for housing, clothing, food, etc.; and ways to help yourself and your community recover from the emergency.

3   Use extreme caution in entering or working in buildings that may have been damaged or weakened by the disaster; they may collapse without warning. Also, there may be gas leaks or electrical short circuits.

4   Don't take lanterns, torches, or lighted cigarettes into buildings that have been damaged by a hurricane; there may be leaking gas lines or flammable material present. Use battery-powered flashlights, spots, etc., if available.

5   Stay away from fallen or damaged electric wires, which may still be dangerous. Notify the power company or the police or the fire department.

6   Check for leaking gas pipes in your home. Do this by smell—don't use matches or candles. If you smell gas, do this: (a) open all windows and doors; (b) turn off the main gas valve at the meter; (c) leave the house immediately; (d) notify the gas company or the police; (e) don't reenter the house until you are told it is safe to do so.

7   If any of your electrical appliances are wet, first turn off the main power switch in your house, then unplug the wet appliance, dry it out, reconnect it, and finally, turn on the main power switch. (Caution: Don't do any of these things while you are wet or standing in water.) If fuses blow when the electric power is restored, turn off the main power switch again and then inspect for short circuits in your home wiring, appliances, and equipment.

8   Check your food and water supplies before using them. Foods that require refrigeration may be spoiled if electric power has been off for some time. Also, do not use fresh food that has come in contact with flood waters.

9   Stay away from disaster areas. Sightseeing could interfere with first aid or rescue work, and may be dangerous as well.

10   Don't drive unless necessary, but if you must, drive with caution. Watch for hazards to yourself and others, and report them to local police or fire departments.

11   Report broken sewer or water mains to the water department.

Remember: Hurricanes moving inland can cause severe flooding. Stay away from river banks and streams until all potential flooding is past.

NOTES

[1]*Hurricane — The Greatest Storm on Earth,* U.S. Department of Commerce, National Oceanic and Atmospheric Administration (NOAA) (Washington, D.C.: U.S. Government Printing Office, 1971), p. 10.

[2]Ibid., p. 12.

[3]ROBERT H. SIMPSON, "Hurricane: Yes or No," NOAA, U.S. Department of Commerce (Washington, D. C.: U.S. Government Printing Office, July 1971), p. 15.

[4]*Hurricane — The Greatest Storm on Earth,* p. 23.

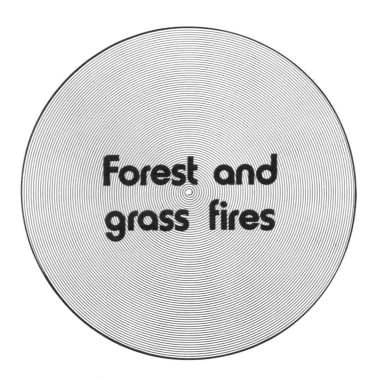

Forest and grass fires

17 **Man-Made.** Man is responsible for 65 percent of all the forest and grass fires* occurring throughout the United States. Arsonists and debris burners are responsible for about 21 and 16 percent, respectively. The United States has over 30,000 fires annually.

Natural. While accounting for about 35 percent of the fires over the entire United States, lightning is the leading cause of forest fires in the western part of the country.

Factors Influencing Forest and Grass Fires. Seven major factors that influence fire behavior and burning characteristics can be grouped under the general headings of *fuels, weather,* and *topography* (see Figure 17–1). Because of the variety and changing condition of burnable fuels in the forests and grasslands, the degree of flammability will tend to fluctuate. Four weather factors—precipitation, relative humidity, temperature, and winds—influence forest and grass fire behavior, chiefly

*Includes all wildland fires (such as brush and tundra).

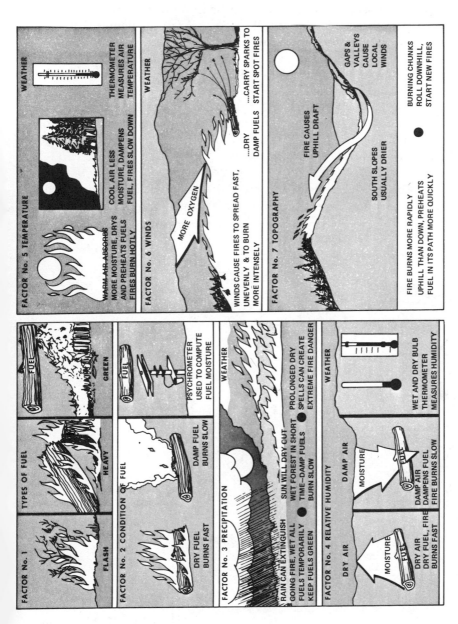

figure 17-1 Major factors influencing fires. From U.S. Forest Service, *Manual for Forest Fire Fighters.*

because of their effect upon burnable fuels. Topography has a decided effect upon fire behavior in that fire burns more intensely and rapidly uphill because the fire causes uphill drafts that fan the flames. This advancing flow of heat also more quickly heats and ignites the materials above the flames.

The daily cycle of burning—the fire day—is fairly consistent and must be considered in predicting fire behavior. The fire day begins in mid-morning about 10 o'clock and continues on through the day and night until the same time the following day. During this time, many of the previously mentioned seven factors come into play to influence fire behavior (see Figure 17–2).

Kinds of Fire. In terms of the natural area affected, conflagrations may be described as forest, brush, or grass fires—although any single

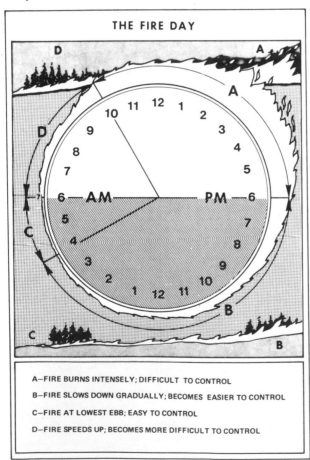

THE FIRE DAY

A—FIRE BURNS INTENSELY; DIFFICULT TO CONTROL

B—FIRE SLOWS DOWN GRADUALLY; BECOMES EASIER TO CONTROL

C—FIRE AT LOWEST EBB; EASY TO CONTROL

D—FIRE SPEEDS UP; BECOMES MORE DIFFICULT TO CONTROL

figure 17–2 The fire day. From U.S. Forest Service, *Manual for Forest Fire Fighters.*

disaster may involve more than one of these different areas. Woodland blazes are further characterized, according to place of origin within the forest, as surface, duff, crown, spot, or tree fires (see Figure 17–3).

Surface Fire. The surface fire is the most common fire in eastern woodlands. It usually runs through the flash fuels that litter the forest floor. The surface is generally fast burning and quite hot, and it is easily influenced by wind action. However, under normal conditions it is fairly easy to control.

Duff Fire. The duff fire, or underground fire, is usually the result of a surface fire. It burns deep into the accumulated leaf litter or peat called "duff" and may smolder to a depth of several feet. The burning is slow but the heat, being confined, is intense, and it dries out the fuel in its path, enabling the duff fire to burn into areas thought too damp to support combustion. Decayed logs and stumps buried in duff help to spread and prolong the fire. A duff fire may smolder for days with little show of smoke or flames, and for this reason it is particularly dangerous. The duff fire usually occurs after prolonged dry spells or during dry summers and is difficult to handle, for it must be dug out, trenched down to mineral soil, or flooded out with water.

Crown Fire. The crown fire occurs when fire sweeps through the foliage, leaves, and needles of trees, large bushes, or dense brush. It is more common in dense stands of evergreens, and in most eastern states is usually restricted to pine plantations or oak thickets. Crown fires are supported only by the large amount of fuel burning on the surface. They are generally controlled by separating the fuel from the fire or by attacking the fire in areas where the amount of surface fuel is not sufficient to support a crown fire.

Spot Fire. Spot fires are nearly always the result of sparks or embers being carried ahead of a large going fire where they ignite new fires. These small "spots" may burn until they join together or are overrun by the larger fire. They are particularly dangerous, since they can cross a fire line sometimes for a mile in advance of a going fire.

Tree Fire. Tree fires are fairly common in most states and are usually detected and extinguished before they have time to spread to the surface. These fires may be caused by lightning or by persons smoking out bees or game. If a tree fire is too far advanced, the tree is usually felled and the fire extinguished with dirt or water. Otherwise, water from a spray tank is used to put out the fire.

Brush Fire. A typical example is the chaparral fire which rages periodically in California. Chaparral, a dry form of fuel, is composed of chamise, manganite, and scrub oak. These flash fuels offer easy ignition and are consumed rapidly and completely by combustion. Brush fires

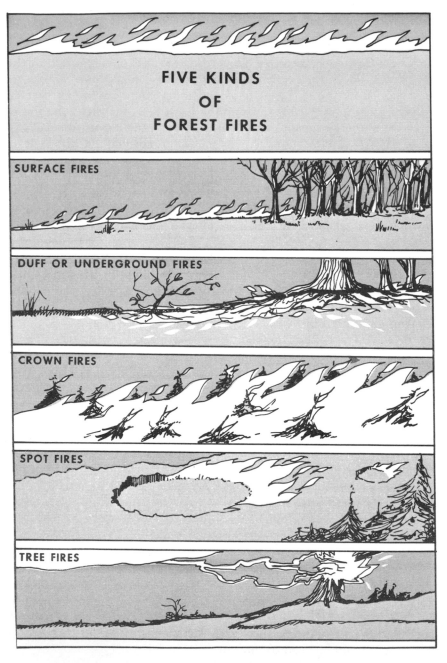

figure 17–3 Kinds of forest fires. From U.S. Forest Service, *Manual for Forest Fire Fighters.*

are difficult to control because of the intense heat generated and the rapidity with which they consume any available ground fuels (see Figure 17–4).

Grass Fire. This type of fire is most dangerous when the grass is in a dried or "cured" state. Although grass can grow to heights in excess of six feet, it still has the burning behavior of a flash ground fuel. Heavy grass fuel burning ahead of a high wind can develop into a dangerous menace because of its heat, speed of travel, and power to roll over barriers.

EFFECTS

Primary Effects

Loss of life, although not usually as high as in other disasters, is a too-frequent tragedy in most fire disasters. Many businesses are forced to cease operations, communications and electric power systems are dis-

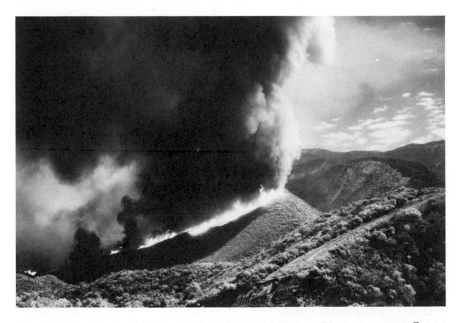

figure 17–4   Brush fire, Los Padres National Forest. Photo courtesy Forest Service, USDA; photo taken by F.E. Dunham.

rupted, and the losses in recreation and travel activities are incalculable. Private residences are often destroyed in forest and brush fires. Of national significance is the complete destruction of valuable resources such as timber, grass, wildlife habitat, and scenic vistas.

These effects are illustrated in disastrous fires which have occurred in the United States. Some examples:

1 The greatest single fire disaster this country has ever known, in terms of lives and property lost, occurred in eastern Wisconsin in 1871. The Peshtigo fire burned over 1¼ million acres and killed 1500 people.

2 The Tillamook fire in Oregon in 1933 killed as much timber (10.5 billion board feet) as had been cut in the entire United States during the previous year. Some 300,000 acres, mostly virgin timber, were destroyed.

3 In the Maine fire in 1941, which burned over 200,000 acres, 15 lives were lost, more than 1200 homes were destroyed, and property loss was estimated at $30 million.

4 In Southern California during a one-month period of critical fire weather in 1970, 1260 fires burned more than 600,000 acres, killed 14 people, destroyed some 900 homes and other structures, and generated a potential for an aftermath of erosion, floods, and mudslides.

Secondary Effects

In addition to the immediate damage from fire, there are secondary effects (see Figure 17–5) which may be of long-term duration:
Small trees are destroyed and large trees suffer damage that may result in disease and insect infestation.

Capacity of reservoirs is sharply reduced through siltation caused by soil erosion. For example, the Gibraltar Reservoir of the City of Santa Barbara, California, lost 50 percent of its capacity in approximately 25 years.

Large amounts of debris from forest fires collect where heavy rains carry it to water basins. Los Angeles County scheduled removal of 18 million cubic yards of debris from San Gabriel Dam No. 1, much of it due to the Polecat Canyon fire in 1960. Removal costs were estimated at $1.25 to $2.00 per cubic yard ($25 to $30 million).

Following a fire of slightly over 5000 acres, the Montrose flood of March 23, 1934, which occurred in Los Angeles County, resulted in the loss of 34 lives and $5 million in other damages. In adjacent unburned areas there was no evidence of increased soil erosion or excessive water runoff.

Wildland grass fires cause severe damage to range lands. Not only is

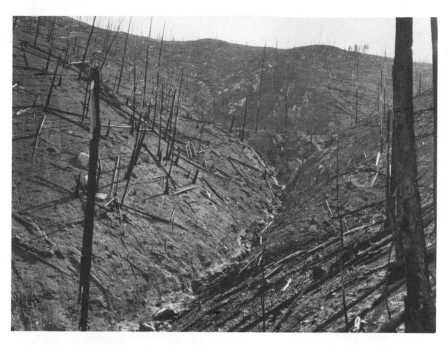

figure 17–5   Burned over area. Photo courtesy Forest Service, USDA; photo taken by A.R. Croft.

much of the vegetation removed, but the heat from range fires also dries out the root systems and quite frequently lays the soil bare.

Barren soils are subject to wind and water erosion, which in turn causes flooding and pollution of the air and water. Successive burns bring about severe erosion, which delays natural regeneration. In extreme instances the soils become sterile.

Rangeland fires, which destroy vegetative cover, adversely affect food supplies for domestic animals, wildlife, birds, and microorganisms (see Figure 17–6).

THREAT

The factors contributing to a high-danger threat in any part of the country involve the hazardous combination of ground fuels, weather, and people. In the East, the normal fire seasons are spring and fall, while weather conditions may cause them to extend through the summer and winter months. In the West, the normal fire-danger period develops during the dry summer months. This whole pattern can be materially

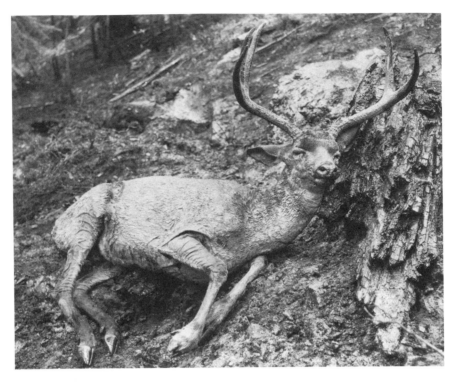

figure 17–6 Fire kills. Photo courtesy U.S. Forest Service; photo taken by L.D. Bailey.

altered by changes in weather and burnable forest fuels. A drought or a prolonged dry spell threatens a continuous fire-potential situation until sufficient precipitation occurs.

VULNERABILITY

In the United States, with an area in excess of two billion acres, more than half is in forest and grasslands. The remaining area consists of 500 million acres of cities, highways, and water areas and some 500 million acres of farmlands and small wooded lots, usually lying outside of city limits.

Fuels in the woodlands are varied in kind, quality, amount, and degree of flammability. As the deciduous trees lose their leaves in the fall of the year, ample ground fuel is provided for serious fires, until winter conditions make the fuel less flammable. One of the greatest dangers occurs in the spring, when the leafless trees allow the full sweep of drying winds. In coniferous forests the accumulation of needle fuels is a gradual process, but when dry, these fuels can produce an almost explosive force. The hazardous combination of fuels, weather, and people can quickly transform a static area to one of dynamic force.

People and Property

Real estate and residential losses run high when rural forest and grass fires reach the conflagration stage and invade urban areas. With the continuing migration of people and the extension of urban and suburban areas into woodlands and grassland fringes, the chances of a conflagration with major losses are increasing significantly.

Economy

Timber destruction, with subsequent growth losses, constitutes a substantial impact on increasingly valuable lumber resources. High-quality hardwoods for furniture manufacturing come from the northern forests and provide a variety of products in the building industry. Pines of the South provide building materials and an ever-increasing supply of raw products for the pulp mills. The western timber also provides plywood, particle board, and pulpwood, plus miscellaneous other lumber supplies. If forest resource losses are not kept within reasonable bounds, reforestation projects may not be able to meet increasing demands for timber products.

COUNTERMEASURES: PREDICTION SYSTEMS

Sensors and Surveillance

The key to efficient fire control is early detection. Lookout towers and aircraft are the backbone of the fire detection system. The tower is particularly valuable in areas of many man-caused fires which require constant surveillance. These fixed observation posts are manned during the fire seasons and are often supported by both aircraft and reports from local citizens. Fire control agencies are making increased use of aircraft for fire detection and mapping, including the use of infrared systems which can sense fires at night and through dense smoke. Air surveillance provided by commercial and private aircraft daily crisscrossing the nation is also an important component of the warning system.

In addition to the customary visual sighting, the Forest Service is now using an airborne multispectral infrared (heat-detecting) scanning system, which permits thousands of square miles to be covered rapidly. Also, a low resolution infrared fire spotter, in low-flying aircraft, is being used to locate fires and hot spots when smoke is not visible.

The weather satellites can provide a valuable platform for frequent fire monitoring of nearly all areas of the earth.

Forecasts

The Fire Weather Service provides a nationwide forecast and advisory service for forest and range management interests covering a wide variety of activities. Information from twice daily forecasts is used in computing predictions of fire danger for the forest and range areas and in planning of fire suppression tactics.

Danger Ratings

Fire Danger Ratings delineate the general areas where conditions of fuel and weather warrant constant fire surveillance activities. Fire danger ratings are used in determining the strength and positioning of fire control forces and in making decisions to restrict, close, or open commercial and recreational areas, to shut down logging operations, and to reschedule hunting seasons.

COUNTERMEASURES: PREVENTION SYSTEMS

Disaster Avoidance

The most significant individual contribution in the prevention of forest and grass fires is an educational and enforcement program to reduce drastically the number of man-caused fires. Education of people encompasses a broad spectrum of activity to which all protection agencies and many private organizations have directed strong efforts.

The "Smokey Bear" program, which carries a message directly to the people, is probably the most widespread and best known of the prevention programs. "Smokey" first appeared as the symbol of forest fire prevention in 1945, portraying a natural symbol with emotional appeal to forestry, civic, and youth organizations, conservation societies, and sportsman clubs. It is estimated that the "Smokey Bear" program has saved the United States more than $10 billion through the prevention of resource losses.[1]

Despite this prevention message, most fires are still caused by man. The most acute problem exists with the people living or working in or near forested areas. The prevention program involves person-to-person contact, good fire laws, strong law enforcement, and support of the courts, as well as education about the damaging effects to natural resources and to people themselves.

Hazard Reduction

People and Property.   In many states the steady movement of people into areas of critical fire hazard has added tremendous burdens on the protection agencies. This movement subjects people and their property to the hazards of both fire and flood disasters. Some action has been taken by states and countries in fire prevention measures governing development and construction, such as the establishment of hazardous fire boundaries. Also, the United States Department of Agriculture is conducting research to convert areas of highly flammable fuels to less flammable species and to improve firebreaks, fuel disposal methods other than prescribed burning, and methods of eliminating the most resistant woody species of ground cover.

Brush Conversion or Modification.   Of the many fire hazard reduction measures under consideration by federal and state agencies, the modification of highly flammable fuel areas near population centers deserves mention.

In an effort to prevent future disasters, federal, state, and local agencies and organizations have suggested possible courses of action to reduce the brush fire hazards and to improve the ecology of affected areas:[2]

1   Analyze flood and erosion potential, together with appropriate remedial measures.

2   Investigate the efficiency of various methods of reseeding (more effective planting of grasses to replace brush).

3   Establish green belts—to include properly planted and irrigated public rights of way for highways, power lines, and aqueducts—as natural fire breaks to protect urbanized areas.

4   Determine appropriate redevelopment of areas to best accommodate plants, wildlife, and recreation.

5   Relocate power lines.

6   Reorder water priorities, and investigate the potentialities of effluent (treated sewage) irrigation.

Lightning Modification.   United States Forest Service experiments extending over the past two decades indicate a possible 66 percent reduction in cloud-to-ground lightning by massively seeding clouds with silver iodide nuclei, delivered from special airborne ramjet-type generators.

Firefighting Systems.   The development of extensive road and trail systems and the use of tractors, plows, trenchers, aircraft, and infrared air-mapping units have been combined to form an efficient fire suppression capability. The firefighting team is composed of professionals from federal, state, and local agencies, plus private contractor personnel.

The vital factor of an effective fire suppression program is early detection, followed by a swift initial attack. Procedures vary with topography, nature of the plant life in the affected areas, and weather conditions. Generally, fires are first contained by constructing a holding line at the head of the spreading fire. This operation is accomplished by bulldozing, hand raking, or plowing to mineral soil. At this stage, water, chemicals, earth, and back-firing can be used to extinguish fires. Air tankers have proved to be invaluable in attacking fires early and preventing their spread by dropping chemical retardants, pending the arrival of ground firefighters or smokejumpers. The rapid deployment of air tankers or helicopters, followed quickly by ground-support personnel, is an initial attack technique effective in preventing small fires from becoming major conflagrations.

The deployment of the needed resources is changed seasonally, with concentrations in the East during the spring and fall (sometimes extending through the winter months in the deep South), and the West during the dry summer months.

SUGGESTED INSTRUCTIONS

General Information

Forest fires can occur at any time of the year but mostly occur during long, dry hot spells. Most forest fires are caused by human carelessness, negligence, or ignorance. Forest fire prevention, therefore, is mainly a problem of creating a better understanding of the importance of forests, an awareness of the danger of fire in the woods, and a sense of personal responsibility to safeguard the forests from damage.

Warnings

Though forest fires can start without warning, the federal and state governments maintain a system of watch towers or surveillance aircraft manned by the U.S. Forest Service and the State Forest Services to ensure that the location of fires can be determined, warnings issued, and necessary emergency actions taken.

In Case a Forest Fire Threatens

1   Keep posted on the progress of the fire by listening to radio and television broadcasts.

2   Knowing what to do when a forest fire threatens may mean the difference between life and death. If you see such a threat, report it immediately by phone to the local police department, fire department, or fire warden. Do *not* use the phone to get information and advice—depend on radio or TV for this.

3   If you are burning debris for cleanup, such as "woods-burning" in the South, immediately stop.

4   Put out all fires in the home and other structures.

5   If in the woods, put out camp fires.

6   Make certain your own property is clear of combustibles, particularly brush that is hazardous to your home or other structures.

7   Hook up garden hoses and check out your water supply for possible "wetting down" of roofs if sparks from the forest fire threaten.

8   If time permits and it is required, remove and clear away flammable vegetation up to 30 feet on each side of your home or other structure (this is an extension of Step 6).

9   Close all windows (cover if possible), remove combustibles near windows and other openings, protect and secure stock and pet animals.

10   After your own home is prepared, be ready to assist in constructing community firebreaks *if* asked to do so.

11   If area evacuation is called for, get full information on exit routes and relocation areas.

If Your Community Is Involved in a Forest Fire

1   Cooperate with authorities. Keep posted on the progress of the fire by listening to radio and television broadcasts.

2   Follow evacuation directions.

3   *Do not use firefighting entrance routes.* These are reserved for Emergency Services only.

4   Assist in community firefighting operations if you are between stipulated ages and able-bodied. All others keep clear of fire area.

5   Make certain you are under the supervision of a designated firefighter. Follow his instructions since he knows how the fire is being fought and where you will be of most value to the operation.

6   Follow safety precautions to prevent getting trapped. Ground winds and fuels are tricky. Follow instructions. Keep informed. Know where the fire is in relation to you. Know your escape route. Keep calm. Maintain communication with your supervisor. *(Don't go it alone!)* Make sure you understand instructions.

NOTES

[1]"Smokey's Record," pamphlet (revised 1970), State Foresters in cooperation with the U.S. Forest Service.

[2]*A Consideration of Certain Environmental Implications of the September 1970 Fires in San Diego County and Suggested Studies,* Century III Institute (October 7, 1970).

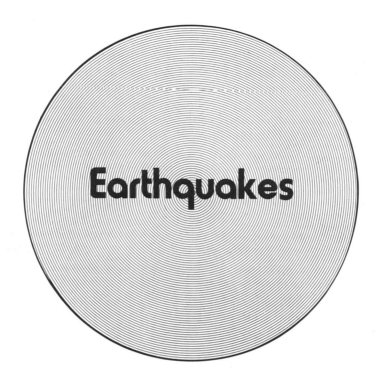

Earthquakes

CAUSES AND CHARACTERISTICS

18 The "solid" earth is acted upon by the periodic forces of the solar system producing stresses and movement of the earth's surface. Also, in geologic time there is shifting of the earth's axis, as indicated by wandering of the magnetic poles. Recent evidence indicates that the material from the upper mantle is welling up along the mid-Atlantic ridge and causing the movement of large areas of the earth's surface called "plates." These plates are thought to interact in one of three ways: spreading where new crust is formed, subduction where one plate plunges under another, or fault action where two plates rub.

This theory of plate tectonics, as a cause of earthquakes, has gained wide acceptance in the past several years.* It attempts to reconcile evidence of geology, seismicity, gravity, and geomagnetics. The most positive evidence of its validity is provided by seismicity, specifically, the occurrence of earthquake belts which outline the large plates and give a measure of the kind and amount of movement occurring at the interface

*Tectonics is a branch of geology concerned with structure, especially with folding and faulting.

of the blocks they define. As the blocks move relative to one another, stresses form and accumulate until a fracture or abrupt slippage occurs. This resultant release of stress, usually occurring within a few cubic kilometers of the earth's crust, is called an earthquake.

The relatively small portion of the crust at which the stresses are relieved by movement is the focus of an earthquake. From this point, mechanical energy is propagated in the form of waves which radiate from the focus in all directions through the body of the earth. When this energy arrives at the surface of the earth, sometimes from as deep as 700 kilometers, it forms secondary surface waves of longer periods. The frequency and amplitude of the vibrations thus produced at points on the earth's surface, and hence the severity of the earthquake, depend on the amount of mechanical energy released at the focus, the distance and depth of the focus, and the structural properties of the rock or soil on or near the surface of the earth at the point of observation.

The duration of most earthquake tremors is expressed in seconds. For example, the 1933 Long Beach, California, earthquake lasted seven seconds, whereas the 1906 quake in San Francisco extended over forty seconds.

EFFECTS

A large earthquake is one of nature's most devastating phenomena. The energy released by a magnitude 8.5 earthquake on the Richter scale is equivalent to 12,000 times the energy released by the Hiroshima nuclear bomb. While these cataclysms have their foci well below the earth's surface, cities have been destroyed and thousands of lives lost in a few seconds as the result of great earthquakes of the past.

Primary Effects

The onset of a large earthquake is initially signaled by a deep rumbling or by disturbed air making a rushing sound, followed by a series of violent motions in the ground. The surroundings seem to disintegrate. Often the ground fissures, and there can be large permanent displacements—21 feet horizontally in San Francisco in 1906 and 47 feet vertically at Yakutat Bay in 1899. (Figure 18–1 shows an example of vertical displacement.) Buildings, bridges, dams, tunnels, or other rigid structures are sheared in two or collapse when subjected to this movement. Vibrations are sometimes so severe that large trees are snapped off or uprooted. People standing have been knocked down and their legs broken by the sudden lateral accelerations.

As the vibrations continue, structures with different frequency-

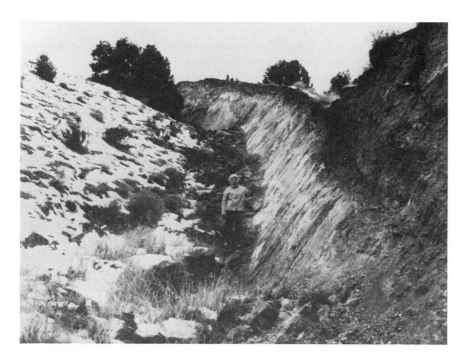

figure 18–1 Earthquake of December 16, 1954. Vertical displacement at Fairview Peak, Nevada. NOAA/Environmental Data Service photo.

response characteristics are set in motion. Sometimes resonant motion results. This is particularly destructive, since the amplitude of the vibrations increases (theoretically without limits) and usually structural failure occurs. Adjacent buildings of different frequency response can vibrate out of phase and pound each other to pieces. In any event, if the elastic strength of the structure is exceeded, cracking, spalling, and — often — complete collapse result. Water tanks, bridges, the walls of high-rise buildings, are especially vulnerable to vibrational motion. The walls of high-rise buildings without adequate lateral bracing frequently fall outward, allowing the floors to cascade one on top of the other, crushing the occupants between them. In the poorer countries, where mud brick and adobe are used extensively in construction, collapse is often total even to the point of returning the bricks to dust.

Water in tanks, ponds, and rivers is frequently thrown from its confines. In lakes, an oscillation known as "seiching" occurs, in which the water surges from one end to the other, reaching great heights and overflowing the banks. In the 1964 earthquake in Alaska, for example, water rose six feet at Memphis, Tennessee, 5000 miles from the center, as a result of this type of action.

Secondary Effects

Often as destructive as the earthquake itself are the resulting secondary effects such as landslides, fires, tsunamis, and floods.

Landslides are especially damaging, and often account for the majority of the lives lost. The 1970 earthquake in Peru is a case in point. The total number of deaths was in excess of 70,000, with 50,000 injured. Of those killed, 40,000 were swept away by a landslide which fell 12,000 feet down the side of Mt. Huascaran. It roared through Yungay and Raurachirca at 200 miles per hour, leaving only a raw scar where these villages had been.

The fire damage frequently increases because of the loss of firefighting equipment destroyed by the quake and the breaking of the water mains essential to firefighting. Blocked access highways can hinder the arrival of outside help. This type of secondary effect is well illustrated by the San Francisco earthquake of 1906, in which only approximately 20 percent of the half billion dollars in damage was estimated to have been due to the earthquake, while the remainder was caused by the fire, which was out of control for several days. One of the greatest disasters of all times, the Kwanto, Japan, earthquake in 1923, also resulted from large fire losses. Almost 40 percent of the dead perished in a

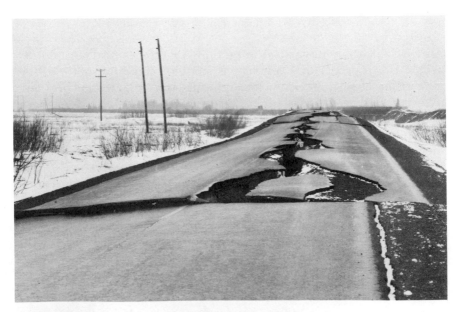

figure 18–2 Earthquake damage, Anchorage to Seward Highway. U.S. Army photograph.

firestorm that engulfed an open place where people had gathered in a futile attempt to escape the conflagration.

Other secondary effects include the disruption of electric power and gas service, which further contributes to fire damage. Also, highways and rail systems are frequently put out of service, presenting special difficulties to rescue and relief workers.

Tsunamis (seismic sea waves) are also often secondary effects of earthquakes. They are a unique phenomenon, however, and are treated in another chapter.

THREAT

Record

It is estimated that several million earthquakes occur annually throughout the world. They range from minor tremors that are barely perceptible to catastrophic shocks. Most earthquakes originate beneath the sea, where they cause little concern unless tsunamis are generated. Such waves occasionally cause damage and loss of life thousands of miles away, as well as near the earthquake origin. Approximately 700 shocks each year may be classed as strong, that is, capable of causing considerable damage in the areas where they occur (Richter scale magnitude of 5.5 or greater).

The National Oceanic and Atmospheric Administration's National Earthquake Information Center, with the cooperation of many foreign and domestic agencies, locates each of these larger shocks within a few hours. Annual epicenter maps that pinpoint earthquake locations are produced. They show the existence of certain well-defined seismic belts stretching over large areas of the world, and the persistence of the overall pattern for any selected period of time. Figure 18–3 shows the general location of the world seismic belts.

The world's greatest seismic belt is known as the Circum-Pacific Belt. It includes the entire rim of the Pacific Ocean from the Tonga and Fiji Islands through the Philippine and Ryukyu Islands, Japan, the Aleutian Islands, southern Alaska, and the Pacific coast of the United States and Central and South America. A second major belt, known as the Alpide, extends westward from New Guinea, through the Himalayas, across the southern portion of Eurasia, through the Mediterranean, and to the Azores in the Atlantic Ocean. The third major belt extends from northern Siberia across the Arctic Ocean to Spitsbergen and then southward along the mid-Atlantic ridge to the Antarctic Ocean in the south; it then

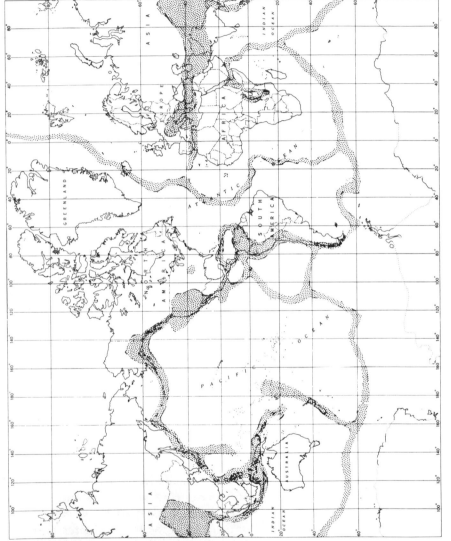

figure 18-3   Major seismic belts of the world. NOAA/Environmental Data Service photo.

continues around the southern tip of Africa into the central Indian Ocean. There are also many minor belts, such as that looping eastward from the Pacific through Mexico, the West Indies (including the Windward Islands), and those countries bordering the southern shores of the Caribbean Sea.

Earthquakes in these well-defined belts are to be expected, but great shocks also occur occasionally in areas outside the belts. Examples of such areas in this country are southeastern Missouri and the Charleston, South Carolina, region. However, many years usually elapse between destructive shocks in these atypical regions. The cities of the Pacific coast are therefore not alone in their vulnerability to destructive earthquakes, for the potential threat also exists in many areas ordinarily considered to be only moderately seismic. As a matter of fact, there is recorded seismic activity in all regions of the United States.

Probability

The areas of heaviest activity are known and well defined. However, the capability does not now exist to predict the time of earthquake occurrence in a given area. NOAA seismologists have developed a seismic risk map for the United States that characterizes the earthquake risk in terms of zones. When more precise data are available, this map can be used in developing local building codes and determining local insurance rates. The map can also be used by seismological engineers to develop more effective construction criteria. (See Figure 18–4.)

VULNERABILITY

People

Earthquake-prone areas include some of the most densely populated regions in the world, such as Japan, the western United States, and the shores of the Mediterranean Sea. It is estimated that over 500 million persons could well suffer damage to their property, while a significant proportion of them are in danger of losing their lives in severe earthquakes. In areas of the world where minimum control of construction and design is exercised, death tolls often reach staggering numbers (see Table 18–1).

The loss of life in the United States has been relatively light, considering the number of destructive earthquakes that have occurred (see Table 18–2). This is due in part to better than usual construction prac-

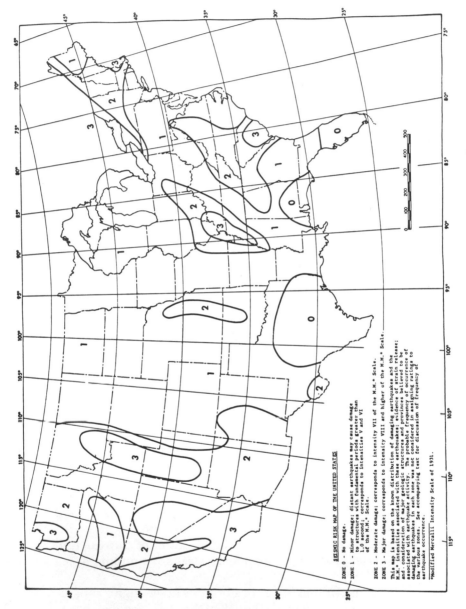

SEISMIC RISK MAP OF THE UNITED STATES

ZONE 0 - No damage.

ZONE 1 - Minor damage; distant earthquakes may cause damage
to structures with fundamental periods greater than
1.0 second; corresponds to intensities V and VI
of the M.M.* Scale.

ZONE 2 - Moderate damage; corresponds to intensity VII of the M.M.* Scale.

ZONE 3 - Major damage; corresponds to intensity VIII and higher of the M.M.* Scale.

This map is based on the known distribution of damaging earthquakes and the
M.M.* intensities associated with these earthquakes; evidence of strain release; and
consideration of major geologic structures and provinces believed to be
associated with earthquake activity. The probable frequency of occurrence of
damaging earthquakes in each zone was not considered in assigning ratings to
the various zones. See accompanying text for discussion of frequency of
earthquake occurrence.

*Modified Mercalli Intensity Scale of 1931.

figure 18-4   Seismic risk map of the United States. S.T. Algermissen, USGS photo.

328

table 18–1   *Major Recorded Earthquakes — NOAA.*

year	locality	deaths
856	Greece, Corinth	45,000
1038	China, Shansi	23,000
1057	China, Chihli	25,000
1268	Asia Minor, Silicia	60,000
1290	China, Chihli	100,000
1293	Japan, Kamakura	30,000
1531	Portugal, Lisbon	30,000
1556	China, Shensi	830,000
1667	Caucasia, Shemaka	80,000
1693	Italy, Catania	60,000
1737	India, Calcutta	300,000
1755	Northern Persia	40,000
1755	Portugal, Lisbon	60,000
1759	Lebanon, Baalbek	30,000
1783	Italy, Calabria	50,000
1797	Ecuador, Quito	41,000
1811	U.S., New Madrid, Mo.	Several
1819	India, Cutch	1543
1822	Asia Minor, Aleppo	22,000
1828	Japan, Echigo (Honshu)	30,000
1868	Peru and Ecuador	25,000
1875	Venezuela and Colombia	16,000
1886	U.S., Charleston, S.C.	60
1896	Japan, Sea Wave, Sanriku Coast	22,000
1897	India, Assam	1542
1905	India, Kangra	20,000
1906	U.S., San Francisco, Calif.	700
1906	Chile, Valparaiso	1500
1908	Italy, Messina	75,000
1915	Italy, Avezzano	29,970
1920	China, Kansu	180,000
1923	Japan, Tokyo-Yokohama	143,000
1932	China, Kansu	70,000
1935	Pakistan, Quetta	60,000
1939	Chile, Chillan	30,000
1939	Turkey, Erzincan	23,000
1946	Eastern Turkey	1300
1946	Japan, Honshu	2000
1948	Japan, Fukui	5131
1949	Ecuador, Pelileo	6000
1950	India, Assam	1500
1953	Northwestern Turkey	1200
1954	Algeria, Orleansville	1657
1956	Northern Afghanistan	2000
1957	Northern Iran	2500
1957	Outer Mongolia	1200
1957	Western Iran	2000
1960	Morocco, Agadir	12,000
1960	Southern Chile	5700
1962	Northwestern Iran	10,000
1963	Yugoslavia, Skopje	1100
1964	Southern Alaska	131
1965	Chile, El Cobre	400
1966	Eastern Turkey	2529
1967	Venezuela, Caracas	236
1968	Northeastern Iran	11,588
1970	Western Turkey	1086
1970	Northern Peru	66,794

table **18–2**   *Lives Lost in Major U.S. Earthquakes*

year	locality	lives lost
1811	New Madrid, Mo.	Several
1812	New Madrid, Mo.	Several
1812	San·Juan Capistrano, Calif.	40
1868	Hayward, Calif.	30
1872	Owens Valley, Calif.	27
1886	Charleston, S.C.	60
1899	San Jacinto, Calif.	6
1906	San Francisco, Calif.	700
1915	Imperial Valley, Calif.	6
1918	Puerto Rico (tsunami from earthquake in Mona Passage	116
1925	Santa Barbara, Calif.	13
1926	Santa Barbara, Calif.	1
1932	Humboldt County, Calif.	1
1933	Long Beach, Calif.	115
1934	Kosmo, Utah	2
1935	Helena, Mont.	4
1940	Imperial Valley, Calif.	9
1946	Hawaii (tsunami from earthquake in Aleutians)	173
1949	Puget Sound, Wash.	8
1952	Kern County, Calif.	14
1954	Eureka-Arcata, Calif.	1
1955	Oakland, Calif.	1
1958	Khantaak Island and Lituya Bay, Alaska	5
1959	Hebgen Lake, Mont.	28
1960	Hilo, Hawaii (tsunami from earthquake off Chile coast)	61
1964	Prince William Sound, Alaska (tsunami)	131
1965	Puget Sound, Wash.	7
1971	San Fernando, Calif.	65

source: *Earthquake Investigation in the United States* (Rev. 1969), U.S. Department of Commerce: OEP data used for 1971 earthquake.

tices, but more to fortuitous circumstances, such as the majority of the people having been in relatively safe places at the time of the earthquake. For example, the loss of life in the 1971 San Fernando quake would have been much greater had it occurred several hours later, when the freeways would have been crowded with the normal rush hour traffic.

Much effort has been made to educate the public, in the United States and other countries, to be cognizant of the need for proper construction and to instruct them in the proper actions to be taken during and after an earthquake. It is hoped that this knowledge will lessen the vulnerability of people to earthquakes.

Property

Property loss covers nearly every type of structure and includes damage to highways, waterways, transmission lines, sewers and underground pipelines, and railways. In some instances, land itself is lost through subsidence of large areas, erosion, and slide action. Such a loss occurred in the Turnagain Heights area of Anchorage as a result of the Alaskan earthquake of 1964, where an entire subdivision slid from its original site toward Turnagain Arm.

In many areas, construction standards are low and casualty rates are correspondingly high. Earthquakes, however, have shown that modern structures (such as those in Agadir, Morocco) and even construction designed specifically to resist earthquakes (such as that in Caracas, Venezuela, and San Fernando, California) often suffer irreparable damage or complete destruction.

Economy

Earthquakes have drastic short- and long-term economic effects. Short-term effects include the loss of merchandise through breakage and spoilage; the disruption of commerce in the face of interruptions in transport, communications, and other services; the shutdown of shops and factories; and the loss of revenue due to the disruption of public utilities and transportation services. Merchandising and production firms are often closed from several days to several weeks, even in areas not directly damaged, because of disruptions in the labor force such as cleanup and rehabilitation efforts, the lack of transportation, and physical or emotional problems.

Long-term economic loss results from the actual destruction of property. Reconstruction priorities vary according to local demands. Generally, temporary housing and life-support activities come first, closely followed by restoration of utilities, highways, railroads, and other support services. Restoration and rebuilding of individual dwellings and repair and reconstruction of small shops and businesses often take months and can result in serious loss to individuals.

Ecology

Violent earthquakes, such as those in Montana (1959), Alaska (1964), and Peru (1970), cause major changes in the physical environment, which in turn alter the ecology drastically and leave scars that may take years to erase. The chief changes are due to inundation, both transient and permanent, and large landslides. Except for minor reinforcement in road and railway cuts to ensure slope stability, and the construction of breakwaters to lessen the danger of inundations, very little can be done to adjust to these changes. In addition, large forest areas are often destroyed, with trees uprooted, snapped off, or shaken so severely that they eventually die.

COUNTERMEASURES: PREDICTION SYSTEMS

Sensors

The monitoring of seismic activity first became systematized during the final decade of the nineteenth century. For the next 30 years, seismological monitoring efforts concentrated on gathering information of a purely scientific nature. The endeavor encompassed data on the structure of the entire earth, and any earthquake of note was recorded on a large proportion of the seismograph stations of the world. International cooperation and data exchange were extensive from the outset.

Seismometers and strong-motion seismographs are the sensors used in earthquake surveillance.

Seismometers.   Seismometers, basically, are carefully constructed pendulums. When the ground vibrates, the pendulum mass tends to remain stationary, and a measurable differential motion results between the mass and the base of the instrument.

Strong-Motion Seismographs.   Unlike sensitive seismographs that operate 24 hours a day and record distant earthquakes, strong-motion seismographs remain idle until triggered into operation by local earth motion.

Seismoscopes.   Within the past few years, strong-motion seismographs in Alaska and California have been supplemented by relatively low-cost seismoscopes.

Surveillance Systems

At present, there are more than 500 active seismograph stations operating continuously throughout the world, under the control of government agencies, institutions of higher learning, and private groups. In addition, several times as many temporary seismographs are in operation at any given time, being used for specific studies.

There are generally three types of earthquake surveillance: worldwide seismography, local seismic recording, and strong-motion seismography.

COUNTERMEASURES: PREVENTION SYSTEMS

Disaster Avoidance.   At present and for the foreseeable future, the possibility of preventing earthquakes is extremely remote. The discovery of the correlation between deep-well waste disposal at the Rocky Mountain Arsenal and the minor earthquake activity in the nearby Durham, Colorado, area has led to the Rangely, Colorado, experiment, being conducted by the U.S. Geological Survey. Results to date have indicated that it is possible to "unlock" interfaces between rock strata by pumping fluid under pressure down a bore hole so that it is forced between the layers. Whether this lubricating action can be applied to areas of shallow earthquake activity to dissipate stresses gradually by causing many microtremors is indeed problematical. However, it provides a very fertile area for research in the immediate future.

Hazard Reduction.   Much of the disastrous effect of earthquakes can be mitigated in the long run. Seismology will provide more reliable and definitive data on the probable location and probability of occurrence of future earthquakes. This information must be used in determining proper population distribution and location and strength of structures of all types. Places where people gather (schools, theaters, halls of all types) must be situated in the safest practicable areas with respect to earthquake dangers. Similar consideration will have to be given to vital support services (hospitals, fire stations, and emergency centers). Furthermore, critical interchanges and concentration points for public utilities, transportation, and communications must be subjected to these same stringent criteria and provided with a backup and bypass capability. In dealing with gathering places and support services, construction criteria should be very conservative, with lifesaving considerations overshadowing economic concern.

Less critical structures should be treated less stringently, and in these cases construction criteria can include greater concessions to economic considerations. Construction with increased lateral bracing, and banning construction across active faults and in areas of unstable slopes, can be very helpful and are being incorporated into many building codes in California. Refinement and widespread acceptance of these types of regulations can make a significant contribution to hazard reduction in other parts of the country.

The science of engineering seismology makes practical use of the knowledge gained from monitoring the behavior of structures during earthquakes. Better building designs based on knowledge of earthquake-induced stress, and taking into account economic considerations, are being developed.

SUGGESTED INSTRUCTIONS

Safety Rules

The actual earth movement of an earthquake is seldom a direct cause of death or injury. However, this movement causes collapse of buildings and other structures. Most casualties result from:

1   Falling bricks and plaster.
2   Splintering glass.
3   Toppling furniture, collapsing walls, falling pictures and mirrors.
4   Rock slides on mountains and hillsides.
5   Fallen power lines.
6   Sea waves generated by earthquakes.
7   Fire caused by broken gas lines and spillage of gasoline and other flammables—a danger that may be aggravated by lack of water due to broken mains.
8   Drastic human actions because of panic. (This rarely happens.)

The following are items to consider before, during, and after an earthquake.

Before an Earthquake

Check for earthquake hazards. Bolt down or provide other strong support for water heaters and other gas appliances. Much fire damage has resulted from toppled appliances and broken gas lines caused by earthquakes. Place large and heavy objects on lower shelves of closets and storage areas. Brace or anchor high or top-heavy objects. Wire or anchor overhead fixtures. Do not stack glassware or crystal; slight shaking will topple it.

In new construction, follow building codes or other sound practices to reduce earthquake hazards. Build on solid ground or dig down to bedrock when laying foundations. Avoid fill and sedimentary areas as much as possible and do not build below dams that might be destroyed, severely damaged, or breached.

During an Earthquake

Remain calm. Think through the consequence of any action you plan to take. Try to reassure others.

If indoors, watch for falling plaster, bricks, light fixtures, and other objects. Watch out for high bookcases, china cabinets, shelves, and other furniture that might slide or topple. Stay away from windows, mirrors and chimneys. If in danger, get under a table, desk, or bed; in a corner away from windows; or in a strong doorway. Encourage others to follow your example. Do not run outside. Don't use candles, matches, or other open flames during the tremor. Douse all fires.

If outside, avoid high buildings, walls, power poles, and other objects that could fall. Do not run through streets. If surrounded by buildings, take shelter in the nearest strong one. If possible, move to an open area away from all hazards. If in an automobile, stop in the safest place available, preferably an open area. Stop as quickly as safety permits, but stay in the vehicle for the shelter it offers.

After an Earthquake

1   Check for injuries. Do not attempt to move seriously injured persons unless they are in immediate danger of further injury.

2   Check for fires.

3   Wear shoes in all areas near debris or broken glass.

4   Check utility lines and appliances for damage. If gas leaks exist, shut off the main gas valve. Shut off electrical power if there is damage to wiring. Do not use matches or lighters until it has been established that there are no gas leaks.

5   Do not turn light switches on and off. This creates sparks that can ignite gas from broken lines.

6   Clean up spilled medicines, drugs, and other potentially harmful materials immediately.

7   Draw a moderate quantity of water in case service should be disrupted. Do not draw a large quantity as this could interfere with firefighting. If water is off, emergency water may be obtained from hot water heaters, toilet tanks, melted ice cubes, and water packed in canned vegetables. If water pipes are damaged, shut off water supply at main valve.

8   Check to see that sewage lines are intact before permitting continued flushing of toilets.

9   Do not eat or drink anything from open containers near shattered glass, as

glass contamination may exist. Only if their use is essential should liquids be strained through many folds of a clean handkerchief or cloth.

10   Check chimneys for cracks and damage. Unnoticed damage could lead to a fire. The initial check should be made from a distance. Approach chimneys with great caution.

11   Check closets and storage shelf areas. Open closet and cupboard doors carefully to guard against objects falling.

12   Check individual house or apartment building for structural damage and if deemed necessary evacuate your family until competent authority declares it safe to return. Stay out of severely damaged buildings; aftershocks can shake them down.

13   Do not heed or spread rumors. They often do great harm following disasters. Stay off the telephone, except to report an emergency. Turn on your radio and/or television to get the latest emergency bulletins.

14   Do not go sightseeing immediately, particularly in beach and waterfront areas where sea waves could strike, or in areas where buildings have collapsed or where electric wires may be down but still alive. Keep the streets clear for passage of emergency vehicles. Be prepared for additional earthquake shocks.

15   Respond to requests for assistance from police, firefighting, and relief organizations, but do not go into damaged areas unless your assistance has been requested. Cooperate fully with local authorities.

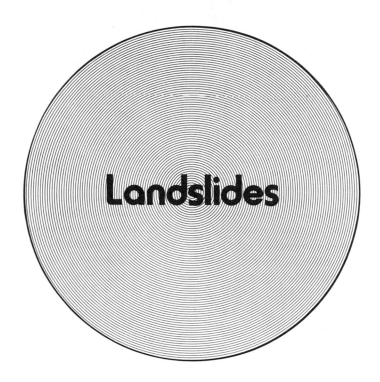

Landslides

CAUSES AND CHARACTERISTICS

19 Landslides can be categorized according to their causative factors. In actuality, landslides often occur from a combination of the causes described here and combine several types of slide action.

Slow Erosion. Water, freezing and thawing, and wind erosion gradually wear away supporting materials and cause two types of slides: rock falls, where overhanging material drops to the valley floor without disturbing material in between; and avalanches, where dry material sweeps down a mountain, gathering momentum and masses of loose debris as it progresses.

Water. Heavy rains frequently cause marginally stable slopes to give way to two forms of slides: as avalanches, taking out surface material below the main failure zone; and mud flows or slumps, with the material becoming liquefied and flowing downward, usually from a tilted basin-shaped area, leaving a scarped depression at the upper end and an outflow over the surface below, where it comes to rest.

Often, slopes stabilized by vegetation are denuded by forest or brush fires, as found in Southern California. The scarred areas lose their capacity for holding mosture and, during the following rainy season, the rainfall can turn hundreds of slopes into rivers of mud.

Glacial Action.   Advancing glaciers frequently displace supporting material along the valley walls and, as they melt, ice support is removed from the slopes above them. Landslides and mud flows result, with the latter particularly in stream deltas.

Earthquake.   Landslides are one of the secondary effects of earthquakes (see Figure 19–1). The seismic vibrations cause landslides of two types: in one type, material is shaken loose and forms an avalanche, as in the case of the Hebgen, Montana, earthquake in 1959; in the other type, the particles of the soil act as a liquid, causing ground failure and slumping over wide areas, as occurred in the Van Norman Dam as a result of the San Fernando earthquake in 1971. This latter effect is evident even in level terrain, where buildings actually sink into the ground because of the loss of bearing capacity of the affected soil.

Engineering Defects.   In some instances, man-made highways and railroad cuts or embankments traverse the toe of a slide area, in which case the upslope material becomes unstable and susceptible to slides.

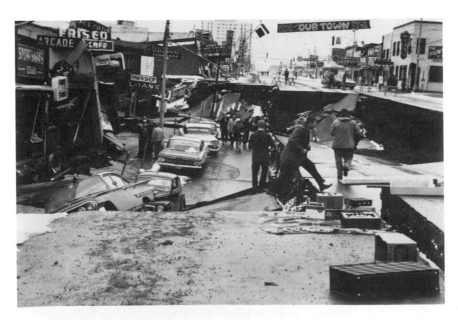

figure 19–1 Landslide caused by earthquake in Anchorage, Alaska. Photo courtesy U.S. Department of the Interior, Geological Survey.

This situation also occurs in excavations for dams, bridge abutments, and buildings. If the slope stability has been miscalculated, erosion or heavy rains trigger very destructive slides (see Figure 19–2).

EFFECTS

Primary Effects

Landslides involve great amounts of material which move at tremendous velocity and are deposited on otherwise undisturbed ground when they come to rest. Everything in the path of a large slide is destroyed. Where soil liquefaction occurs, bizarre effects are encountered. On relatively gradual slopes, foundation material can lose its bearing strength and an entire subdivision or village may shift downslope; deep cuts and depressions are often formed, and buildings are tilted, are torn asunder, or settle into the ground.

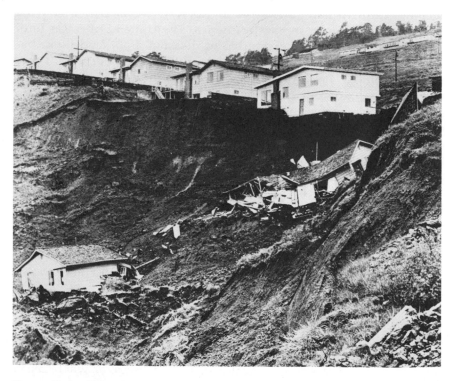

figure 19–2 Urbanization increases vulnerability to damage from natural disasters, such as landslide. Photo courtesy U.S. Department of the Interior, Geological Survey.

Secondary Effects

Additional damage is caused by the air blast which precedes and, to some degree, extends laterally from the sliding material. Reports of persons having their clothes torn off and being seriously injured by the air blast alone are numerous in the histories of large avalanches.[1] Another secondary effect of landslides is the formation of water waves when slides terminate in lakes or inlets. In one such instance, a slide formed a wave more than 1700 feet high when it dropped in Lituya Bay, Alaska, after an earthquake in July 1958.

THREAT

Record and Probability of Occurrence

The danger of landslides is ever present in all mountainous countries, such as Northern Italy, Switzerland, Norway, Nepal, Tibet, and the countries of the Andes in South America. The United States was until recently considered less susceptible to disasters from landslides, because most of its mountainous areas are not heavily populated. However, the potential danger of such occurrences in this country was emphasized by the Madison Canyon, Montana, slide of 1959. As a secondary effect of the Hebgen Lake earthquake, the face of Mt. Madison fell to the Madison River Canyon below and filled it to a depth of 400 feet, forming Earthquake Lake, which is five miles long. Buried in the slide are at least 19 bodies of persons who had been camping in the area at the time of the quake. In all, 28 people were killed.[2]

During the 1964 Alaska earthquake, the soil liquefaction problem was forcefully brought to the attention of engineers and the general public by the destruction in the Turnagain Arm area of Anchorage. It is now recognized that similar conditions exist in other metropolitan areas where buildings rest on extensive water-soaked landfill or relatively unstable clay slopes, such as the cities around San Francisco Bay and Puget Sound.

Very little systematic study has been made of the historic distribution and potential occurrence of landslides. Slope, precipitation, and geologic conditions are the primary factors considered in identifying landslide risk. Available data indicate that slides are not common on slopes less than 5 degrees or greater than 35 degrees, or where mean annual precipitation is less than 10 inches.

A historical summary of landslides that have occurred in the United States is presented in Table 19–1.

table 19–1 *Landslides of the United States—From U.S. Geological Survey. The Number of Slides and the Damage Per Slide Have Increased, and Will Continue to Increase, as Construction and Development Expand into Susceptible Areas*

type slide	major areas	number of historical slides	approx. per 100 sq. mi.	frequency per 40,000 sq. mi.	est. prop. damage (million $ adjusted to 1971 values)	recorded deaths
rockslide & rockfall	White, Blue Ridge, Great Smoky, Rocky Mtns., & Appalachian Plateau	Several hundred	—	1 per 10 yrs.	30	42
rockslump & rockfall	Widespread in Central & West U.S.; prevalent in Colo. Plateau, Wyo., Mont., Southern Calif., Oreg., & Wash.	Several thousand	Av. 10 per yr. hill areas; 1 per yr. plateaus	100 per yr. hill areas; 10 per yr. plateau areas	325	188
	Appalachian Plateau	Several thousand	1 per 10 yrs.	70 per yr.	350 (mainly in highway & railroad damage)	20
	Calif. Coast Ranges Northern Rockies	Several hundred	1 per 10 yrs.	10 per yr.	30	—
slump	Maine, Conn. Riv. Valley, Hudson Valley, Chicago, Red Riv., Puget Sound, Mont. glac. lakes, Alaska	About 70	1 per 100 yrs.	1 per yr.	140	103
	Long Island, Md., Va., Ala., S. Dak., Wyo., Mont., Colo.	Several hundred	1 per 50 yrs.	1 per yr.	30 (mainly to highways & foundations)	—
	Mississippi & Missouri Valleys, eastern Washington & southern Idaho	Several hundred	1 per 10 yrs.	1 per yr.	2	—
	Appalachian Piedmont	About 100	—	1 per yr.	less than 1	—
debris flow & mudflow	White, Adirondack, & Appalachian Mountains	Several hundred	1 group slides, 10+ per group, per 100 yrs. in White Mtns. & N.C.	1 group slides, 10+ per group, per 15 yrs.	100	89

VULNERABILITY

People

Persons living in areas of substantially sloping ground (6 degrees to 35 degrees), especially in mountain valleys that have heavy snow or rainfall, are especially vulnerable to landslides. The danger is greater if the area also has a history of seismic activity. Persons living on the alluvial bench of plateaus along the seacoast in seismic areas are also very much exposed to the danger of mud flows and ground liquefaction.

Property

Property located on the slide area or in its path cannot be protected from the destructive forces of a landslide, particularly one caused by an earthquake. Such slides occur infrequently in populated areas but, when they do, they are even more destructive to property situated in their limited path than are tsunamis.

Economy

Reliable estimates as to how much landslides cost are difficult to obtain. It is estimated, however, that the average yearly cost of landslides in the continental United States runs into millions of dollars. For example, $20 million was spent over a 20-year period for fill in Grand Coulee Dam to correct damage from landslides and avoid further damage. In a 27-state survey of slide damage to highways, 10 states reported damage between $100,000 and $1 million. The direct cost to repair damage to equipment and freight and to compensate for loss of revenue can increase this amount appreciably.[3] Occasionally, a slide strikes a water, gas, or electric utility installation or a dam, or diverts a stream, causing interruption to public facilities. This type of occurrence can have significant economic impact on the affected region.

The economic loss created by landslides in critical areas is normally related to the volume of material involved, but this is not necessarily so in all instances. For example, a slump of 10,000 yards on a highway can be as costly in creating traffic delays and accidents as one much larger. The only difference would be in the additional cost of removing a larger volume of material.

The most destructive and costly slides are those which occur in soil or unconsolidated material (rock fragments, loess, sand, or silt), because of the tremendous masses of material involved, the large areas covered, and the high frequency of occurrence of such slides. Lateral spreading of dikes in Holland, a rock fragment flow at Elm, Switzerland, mud flows in the Quebec Province of Canada, the slumps affecting highway and railroad fills, and sand and silt flows of coastal areas are typical examples of these destructive slides.

Estimates of property damage and deaths from landslides in the United States are shown in Table 19–1.

Ecology

Ecological processes are completely destroyed in any of the slide actions, whether abrupt or long term. The areas affected are very limited in size, however, even for the largest disruption, and the surrounding balance is maintained essentially intact. The exception: where a stream is dammed or diverted, the resulting ecological changes can be significant. These changes can be helpful in some cases, such as in providing needed water resources for the local fauna and flora.

COUNTERMEASURES: PREDICTION SYSTEMS

Sensors and Surveillance

There are sensors used in seismic surveillance that have equal applicability in early detection and surveillance of potential landslides. They are not, however, being used in a systematic way. Similarly, rainfall, temperature, and seismic data, all significant for evaluation of possible landslide susceptibility of an area, are not being collated and analyzed with this objective in mind.

Surveillance by track and highway maintenance crews and by forest rangers is the present method of monitoring suspect areas. Unfavorable soil conditions noted visually and preliminary bulging and spalling are indicators of the need for remedial action and warning.

Early Warning

Based on current technology, the degree of danger can be noted, but little definitive information as to the time of occurrence can be given. Early warning for the vast majority of landslides is therefore not possible. Of course, for long-term slumping, the onset can be recognized and preventive measures instituted.

COUNTERMEASURES: PREVENTION SYSTEMS

Disaster Avoidance

New facilities can be protected from landslide danger by a combination of actions.

First, the susceptibility to slides of any parcel of land on which a facility is to be located must be determined accurately. On highly susceptible land, appropriate zoning laws and other building limitations can be used to control the construction practices in the potentially dangerous areas. The laying of rights of way for dams, bridge abutments, and watersheds should be done with special consideration of the landslide characteristics of the area.

If unavoidable landslide risk must be taken, good engineering practice can do much to reduce danger. Methods of slide prevention include removal of unstable materials, selection of a safe slope factor in excavation, provision for both surface drainage and subsurface drainage between the overburdened material and bedrock, and the installation of retaining walls, bulkheads, pilings, and tie rods.

Many of these methods are used in combination. Before a road embankment is constructed, for example, the unstable material should be removed and firm material shaped for drainage and restraining contours. Cut slopes constructed with benches or berms are preferable to a uniform slope. A horizontal surface drain can be placed at the foot of each embankment in the terraced series as further insurance against possible slides.

In areas where landslides are expected but for various reasons the above methods of prevention are not practical, it may be possible to construct debris basins to catch the bulk of the slide material without damage to improved areas. When such debris basins become full, the material can be removed to provide space to handle future landslides. As the result of 1970 and 1971 brush fires and of the 1971 earthquake, some projects of this nature were undertaken in Southern California.

Hazard Reduction

With present knowledge, only some slight mitigation of slide hazards is feasible. Susceptible areas must be identified, if at all possible. The probable path can then be left as open park, thereby reducing the danger to structures and also lessening population density. If highways, railways, or aqueducts must traverse unstable areas in which control of earth slumps is not possible, such areas can be bridged, allowing the

movement to continue without disturbing the artery, albeit at a substantial increase in cost.

NOTES

[1]SAMUEL W. MATTHEW, "The Night the Mountains Moved," *National Geographic,* Vol. 117,
No. 3 (March 1960), 334.

[2]Ibid.

[3]EDWIN B. ECKEL, ED., *Landslides and Engineering Practices,* Publication 544 (Washington,
D.C.: National Academy of Sciences—National Research Council, 1958), pp. 6–7.

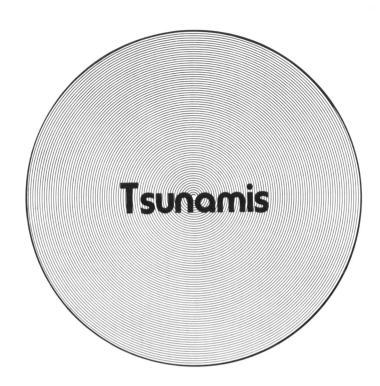

Tsunamis

CAUSES AND CHARACTERISTICS

20 A tsunami* is a train of long ocean waves impulsively generated by earthquakes or submarine disturbances. The magnitude of the forces involved is quite large. The energy released by earthquakes can be several times greater than that of the largest nuclear explosions. Earthquakes of such magnitude occur frequently beneath the sea, particularly along shorelines of the Pacific Ocean area. While only a small percentage of these generate tsunamis, a tsunami can rival or even surpass an earthquake in its destructive force.

Tsunami waves are relatively rare phenomena, neither completely understood by scientists nor fully appreciated by the inhabitants of vulnerable coastlines. Tsunamis are generally confined to the Pacific Basin and the Pacific littoral. Historically, a tsunami of major proportions has struck the United States or its Pacific possessions on the average of every eight years, based on occurrences and damage since 1946. (Records of damage to the United States prior to that time are incomplete, but the incidence within the Pacific Basin supports this expectation.)

*From Japanese, "harbor wave."

Tsunami waves are extremely destructive to life and property. They may impact as the result of an earthquake as distant as the opposite shore of the Pacific, or strike in the immediate epicenter region, as in Alaska in 1964. (The term "tidal wave" is misleading since a tsunami has nothing to do with the tides. Tides are used to indicate a warning.)

Tsunamis may have amplitudes of a foot or less in deep water and in the open ocean may not be detectable. When they enter shallow water along a coast, however, they are slowed to less than 40 miles per hour, and much of their energy is converted to wave heights of up to 100 feet or greater.

These waves are believed to originate as vertically displaced columns of ocean water. Seismic or volcanic alterations of the ocean floor may cause tsunamis by imparting vertical movement to water. It has also been postulated that submarine avalanches on the slopes of the Pacific trenches produce tsunamis. Some investigators believe that long-period ground waves, which sometimes accompany large earthquakes, are possible tsunami generators. Deformation of the sea floor as these ground waves travel across it could possibly generate reinforced water waves by setting up resonant oscillations of trench water, with consequent displacements at the surface of the sea.

In any event, the nature of the relationship between seismic or volcanic disturbances and tsunamis is not well defined. Tsunami amplitude is a function of earthquake magnitude and depth of origin; of water depth in the region of tsunami generation; of extent, direction, and velocity of changes to the earth's crust; and of efficiency of energy transfer from the earth's crust to sea water. The specific effect upon tsunamis of these independent factors, however, is not fully understood.

No definite correlation has been possible between the configuration of specific regions of the ocean floor and tsunami configuration in those regions. It is not completely clear, for example, why tsunami waves may be of negligible size at one point along a coast and of much larger proportions at other coastal points nearby. Nor is it possible to predict whether the destructive component of a tsunami will lie in its powerful surge across a beach, or in a gradual rising of sea level followed by a rapid draining back to the sea.

Thus, it is impossible to say with any certainty what size a tsunami will assume at specific locations or how it will accomplish its destructive work. However, it is known that the speed of tsunamis varies with water depth. This relationship permits prediction of tsunami arrival times at all points in the Pacific Ocean area. While understanding of the physics of tsunamis is limited, knowledge of their destructive potential is not.

EFFECTS

The effects of these waves on the coastal areas of the Pacific are characterized by maximum destructive force at the water's edge. Damage further inland is potentially high, even though the force of the wave has
diminished, because of the floating debris that batters the inland installations. Ships moored in harbors often are swamped and sunk or left
battered and stranded high on the shore. Breakwaters and piers collapse, sometimes because of scouring actions that sweep away their
foundation material and sometimes because of the sheer impact of the
waves. Railroad yards and oil tank farms situated near the waterfront
are particularly vulnerable. Oil fires frequently result and are spread by
the waves.

THREAT

Record

Tsunamis are phenomena generally restricted to the Pacific Ocean. Although there have been authenticated tsunamis in the Atlantic and Indian oceans, these are rare and are often only local disturbances. The
chief reason for lesser tsunami activity in the Atlantic and Indian oceans
is the small number of really large earthquakes in these oceans; the seismic belts traverse these ocean areas rather than follow the coastline as
they do in the Pacific. Since 1900 in the Pacific area, 181 tsunamis have
been recorded; 34 caused damage near the source only and 9 were destructive both locally and distantly. Local waves generated by earthquake action on water in confined areas are sometimes called tsunamis
but do not have their true characteristics. They can, however, be very
destructive and reach great heights.

Probability

As with earthquake prediction in general, only the projection of the historical trend can be used to determine the probability of future tsunami
occurrences and effects. It is known that some areas such as the Aleutian Islands, Hawaii, Chile, and Japan are especially susceptible to tsunami inundation.

It is recognized that the set of conditions under which a wave will be
generated can vary only within a narrow range; that is, the epicenter,
depth of focus, magnitude, and ocean-bottom configuration must be in
just the right combination for a tsunami to occur. This fact makes the
prediction of a tsunami, once an earthquake is detected, an attainable

goal, perhaps in the near future. But much research still remains to be done for the determination of precise probabilities of occurrence.

VULNERABILITY

People

In disasters caused by earthquakes that generate tsunamis, landslides, and other serious secondary effects, the tsunami can be the greatest hazard to human life. Tsunamis, major and local, took the most lives in the Alaskan earthquake of 1964, while landslides caused the most damage. In 1960, the people of Hilo, Hawaii, suffered 61 dead and 282 injured from a tsunami of distant origin, an earthquake in Chile.

Tentative standards for hazard areas on Pacific coasts define the potential danger areas as those within one mile of the coast that are lower than 50 feet above sea level for tsunamis of distant origin and lower than 100 feet above sea level for tsunamis of local origin.[1]

The number of endangered persons in a threatened area obviously depends heavily on the efficiency of warning and evacuation. Minutes count, since a tsunami can travel at speeds in excess of 600 miles per hour in the open sea and at the relatively slower speed of about 40 miles per hour only on reaching shallow water.

Property

The characteristic destructive force of a tsunami is clearly a danger of disastrous proportions to property. Fixed property in the vulnerable littoral and movable property that is caught there are equally endangered. Ships in harbor, the harbor and dockside facilities, railroad yards and rolling stock, tank farms, and bridges are all examples of durable property that can be heavily damaged or destroyed.

Economy

Tsunamis cause such devastation that the affected areas are generally left devoid of all housing and vital services, except for a narrow fringe at the edge of the wave action where damage may be less severe. Port facilities, fishing fleets, and public utilities are frequently the backbone of the economy of the affected areas, and these are the very resources which generally receive the most severe damage. Until debris can be cleared, wharves and piers rebuilt, railroad yards and tank farms reestablished, utilities restored, and the fishing fleets reconstituted, communities may find themselves without fuel, food, and employment. Wherever water transport is a vital means of supply, disruption of coastal systems can have far-reaching economic effects.

Ecology

Tsunamis rank with avalanches in the thoroughness with which they disrupt the ecological balance. Their effects are especially disastrous to fish, mollusks, shore plants, and marine and land organisms in a narrow zone along the littoral.

COUNTERMEASURES: PREDICTION SYSTEMS

The prediction of tsunami generation is even more difficult than the prediction of earthquakes. Not only must the earthquake potential for a given area be predicted, but also the consequent potential for tsunami generation. However, because of the difference in velocity between earthquake waves (20,000 mph) and tsunamis (600 mph), it is possible to locate an earthquake once it has occurred, to analyze its potential for generating a tsunami, and to issue warnings in time for protective measures to be taken.

Seismic vibrations traverse the interior of the earth at great speeds and can reach any point on the globe in a maximum of 20 minutes. This speed of propagation permits seismologists to locate the sources of tsunami generation in less than an hour. Early warning of tsunamis is technically feasible through integrated monitoring of the seismic and sea-level activity of the Pacific Basin.

At seismograph stations, earthquake waves that travel through the earth and across its surface are picked up and translated into electrical signals, which deflect the seismograph's recording arm sufficiently to record the earthquake's "signature." From this signature, or seismogram, seismologists can determine the approximate magnitude of the earthquake and also the surface distance between the seismograph station and the source of the disturbance.

COUNTERMEASURES: PREVENTION SYSTEMS

Disaster Avoidance

The forces involved in a tsunami cannot be controlled. The most that can be accomplished, therefore, is to reduce the hazard prior to its onslaught.

Hazard Reduction

Tsunami hazard reduction is of lesser scope than the same task involving other types of natural disasters (e.g., hurricanes and earthquakes), because the affected area is usually limited to about one mile inland from the coast.

An accurate delineation of areas that might be subject to inundation is essential for source emergency planning and zoning. By proper regulation, schools, hospitals, public buildings, emergency control centers, and places where people usually gather in large numbers can be built outside the danger limit and still be accessible for general use. In addition, engineering designs can be employed in construction of breakwaters, docks, and shore facilities to improve their capability to withstand or divert the forces of the waves, and buildings can be designed so that damage to the lower floor would not jeopardize the integrity of the whole structure. Other feasible longer-term measures include situating tank farms above the danger line and providing them with cutoff devices in pipelines coming from the waterfront. Railway terminals can be augmented with a general holding area out of the danger zone to reduce the concentration of rolling stock on the piers and shoreline loading spurs.

If warning is received early enough (two to five hours), hasty preventive action can be taken: people can be evacuated, ships can clear harbors or seek a safer anchorage, planes and rolling stock can be moved, buildings can be closed, shuttered, and sandbagged.

Comprehensive educational programs to keep the public informed of the nature of the danger and of steps to be taken for personal protection have been proven especially important. Paradoxically, the very warning that can sometimes be given of a tsunami may cause people to endanger themselves to watch such a spectacular event. The likelihood of multiple tsunamis must always be kept in mind. In the tsunamis of May 1960, the third and fourth waves striking the Chilean coast were higher than the first or second in some places. Many people died because they returned to the coast too quickly.

Early warning coupled with education of the affected populations, proper zoning, and suitable structural design can aid in reducing the disastrous effect of this natural hazard.

NOTE

[1]Coast and Geodetic Survey, 1965.

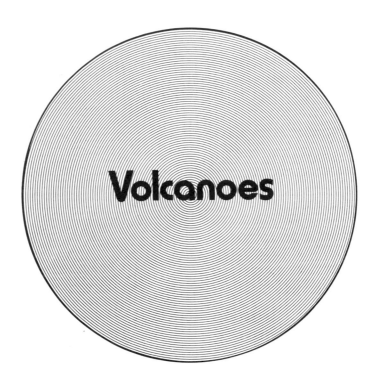

Volcanoes

CAUSES AND CHARACTERISTICS

21 Worldwide, volcanoes are a very rare but very potent menace. Active volcanoes are few in number, and the areas near most are sparsely populated. Most of the largest eruptions have occurred in uninhabited areas, such as the Valley of Ten Thousand Smokes (1912) and Bezymianny, Kamchatka (1956). But, as one authority on volcanoes points out, such an eruption in a densely populated area would produce "a catastrophe of unheard-of proportions."[1]

Volcanic activity results in a number of different phenomena. There are, for example, the effects of ground water heated by molten material (magma). Geysers and hot springs are caused by this heating process. When the emission of superheated sulfurous steam occurs, the geysers are called solfataras. Those that are cooler and nonsulfurous are called fumaroles. There are also other types of gas emissions from vents and fissures. In addition, solid material such as scoriae (cinders), bits of lava, and ashes are ejected into the atmosphere. The flow of lava down the volcano slopes often accompanies spectacular and violent eruptions.[2] (See Figure 21-1.)

The underlying cause for the formation of molten material (magma) is the process of orogenesis (mountain building). Shifting rocks are forced to great depths, where increased temperature and pressure cause them to dissolve and be converted to magma. Once formed, these

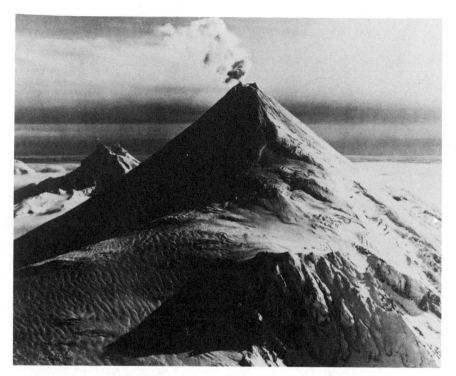

figure 21-1 Shishaldin Volcano, an imposing composite cone, towers 9372 feet above mean sea level on Unimak Island in the Aleutian Chain. Photo courtesy U.S. Department of the Interior, Geological Survey.

magma exert pressure on the surrounding solid material. If this material has fissures running towards the surfaces, the molten material surges upward.[3] The rise of lava to the surface from depths of tens to hundreds of miles is the ultimate cause of volcanoes. Much of this material is deposited close to the vent or vents from which it is ejected and, in time, forms a hill or mountain—a volcano (see Figure 21-2). Such mountains are being formed all the time. In 1943, Paricutin developed in a cornfield in Mexico. In most cases, volcanic eruptions occur at the sites of pre-existing volcanic cones.

EFFECTS

Primary Effects

There are three chief dangers posed by volcanic eruptions: lava flows, airborne clouds of volcanic debris, and pyroclastic rocks and flows.

Lava flows are the most familiar product of volcanic eruptions. They

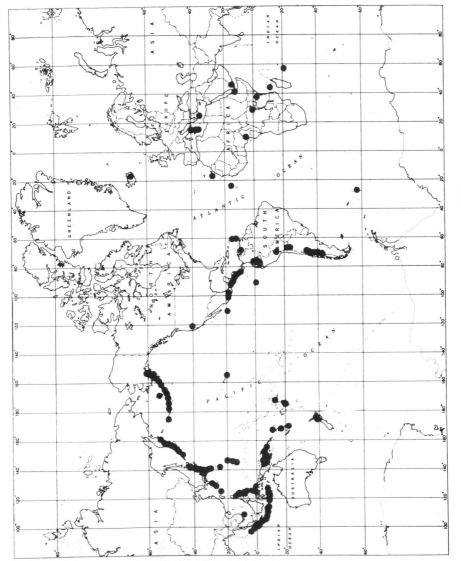

figure 21-2 Location of volcanoes which have erupted since 1900.

are essentially the overflow of magmatic material from the lava lake in the crater of the volcano or an associated vent. (See Figure 21–3.) Lava flows can be nonexplosive (effusive) or explosive (eruptive). Suboceanic volcanoes usually are the effusive type. Those on islands and continental land masses are generally eruptive. However, some variations can be expected for nearly every volcano.

In the case of an effusive volcano, the lava flow is relatively rapid near the source, where the lava is very hot, but farther from the source it cools, becoming covered with a viscous skin which slows and eventually stops the flow.[4]

Lava flows produced by an eruption are generally preceded by ejection of cinders and lava fragments, followed by a quiescent period when collapsed material from the crater walls temporarily blocks the opening. Then, after a short interval, a violent eruption occurs, producing lava fountains as much as a half mile high. Lava flows formed in this manner are very fluid and travel very rapidly. For example, an eruption of Vesuvius in 1779 caused a river of lava 65 feet wide, which traveled at 25–30 feet per second.[5]

Airborne ash from volcanoes contains cinders and pyroclastic rocks. Pyroclastic rocks are formed by the rapid expansion of gas in the lava, which shatters the solid material, or by the explosion of steam when

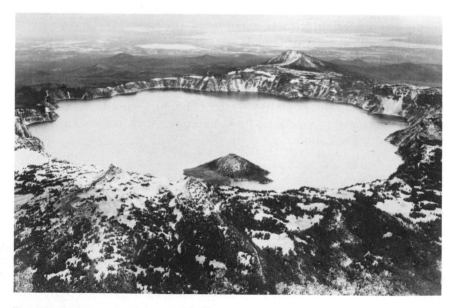

figure 21–3 Crater Lake, Oregon. Photo courtesy U.S. Department of the Interior, Geological Survey.

lava runs into the sea. These materials are blown into the air, where they remain suspended for long periods but eventually fall back to earth.

There are also pyroclastic flows that occur when solid particles suspended in a gas behave like a liquid. The resulting fluid ash moves with great speed, even over a gentle slope.[6] It deposits material very rapidly to form ignimbrite sheets, rock layers that may be as much as 1600 feet thick. The Katmai, Alaska, eruption in 1912 produced 300 million cubic feet of ignimbrite in 60 hours. Yellowstone Park is an area of broad ignimbrite sheets. In the Lamar River area of the park there are 27 distinct forests buried, one on top of another, by successive pyroclastic deposits.

In the Pacific Northwest, the Cascade Volcanoes have had a long history of lava flows. They also have a potential for producing choking clouds of fine ash over vast areas, suffocating or severely affecting the breathing of people located within 10 to 20 miles of the volcano. Dozens of ash layers from the Cascade Volcanoes have been recognized and mapped recently by members of the U.S. Geological Survey (USGS). The debris from the 6600-year-old eruption at Crater Lake was showered in a layer more than six inches deep over much of central Oregon. If similar eruptions were to take place today and the wind happened to be blowing in an adverse direction, Mt. Rainier or Mt. Hood could shower a layer of debris more than six inches deep over downtown Seattle or Portland. In such an eventuality, the loss of life and property would, of course, be enormous.[7]

Of far graver danger in the Cascades is the possibility of large-scale eruptions that produce pyroclastic flows. They travel downslope along the ground at speeds up to 80 miles an hour and are capable of traveling tens of miles from their volcano. Crater Lake, for example, was a source of large volumes of pyroclastic flow material which traveled nearly 50 miles from the volcano.

Secondary Effects

Secondary effects of volcanic activities vary in origin and type, but all present significant potential dangers. The large volume of loose ejecta that is scattered on slopes near active volcanoes is highly susceptible to rapid erosion by heavy rains. In addition, the crumbly debris that makes up much of a volcanic mound is highly unstable and can be josteled loose — especially during periods of local earthquake activity. The sudden downslope movement of this material, regardless of its origin, can produce debris flows which in many ways are the most dangerous threat posed by volcanoes.

The sudden release of glacial meltwater from the northeast slopes of Mt. Rainier, for example, formed a gigantic mud flow that traveled 45 miles down the valley of the White River before spreading out on the Puget Sound lowland over an area 30 miles long and 3 to 5 miles wide.[8] Numerous other debris flows have been identified in this area.

Small or intermediate-size steam explosions, not related directly to a volcanic eruption, can also dislodge large volumes of fragmented material, which can become a part of debris flows.

THREAT

Record

Despite their rarity, volcanoes have on occasion been enormously destructive. Among the worst in recorded history were these:[9]

Vesuvius, A.D. 79, which destroyed Pompeii (burying it until rediscovery in 1595) and killed 16,000

Skaptar Jokull, Iceland, 1783, which killed 10,000 people, most of the island's livestock, and even crops in Scotland 1000 kilometers away

Tamboro, Indonesia, 1815, by which 12,000 perished directly and up to 70,000 because of famine following destruction of the crops

Mt. Pelée, Martinique, 1902, whose pyroclastic flows completely destroyed the city of St. Pierre in a matter of minutes, killing all but two of its 30,000 inhabitants

La Soufriere, St. Vincent, also 1902, which took 2000 lives and caused the extinction of the Carib Indians

Kelut, Indonesia, 1909, killing 5500 people

Mt. Lamington, Papua, 1951, with 6000 fatalities

Mt. Agung, Bali, Indonesia, 1963, killing 1500

Villarica, Chile, 1963–64, which forced 30,000 to evacuate their homes

Taal, the Philippines, 1965, claiming 500 lives

Figure 21–2 portrays the geographic location of the world's active volcanoes, and Table 21–1 summarizes the percentage of active volcanoes by geographic areas. While some 79 percent of all active volcanoes are in the Pacific area, their distribution is very irregular, with about 45 percent in the Western Pacific islands and only 17 percent in the Pacific coastal regions of North and South America. There are strikingly large gaps in the belt of volcanoes between Alaska and the

table 21–1   Worldwide Distribution of Active Volcanoes

area	percentage of active volcanoes	
Pacific		79
Western Pacific Islands	45	
North and South America	17	
Indonesian Islands	14	
Central Pacific Islands		
(Hawaii, Samoa)	3	
Indian Ocean Islands		1
Atlantic		13
Mediterranean and Asia Minor		4
Other Areas		_3_
		100

source: Data from A. Rittman, *Volcanoes and Their Activity*, pp. 153–57.

Cascade Mountains, and between the Cascades and northern Chile, but these regions contain numerous extinct volcanoes. The Indonesian islands are especially rich in active volcanoes (14 percent), while islands of the Central Pacific (Hawaii and Samoa) account for 3 percent.

The most active volcanoes in the populated areas of the United States are those in Hawaii. These include the Haleakala volcano on Maui and the Hualalai, Mauna Loa, and Kilauea volcanoes on Hawaii. Haleakala last erupted in 1750 and Hualalai around 1800, whereas Mauna Loa has erupted once every 3.6 years on the average since 1832, and Kilauea has been in constant activity with at least 32 cataloged eruptions since 1750.[10]

Most of the potentially dangerous volcanoes in the conterminous United States lie along the crest of the Cascade Range of Washington, Oregon, and California. At present, most of these volcanoes are inactive and do not appear to pose a threat to the surrounding countryside, but they are potentially dangerous. Geological investigations have identified layers of lava, ash, and other ejecta from these volcanoes throughout the coastal areas of the Pacific Northwest.

Probability

Study of volcano hazards on and near the slopes of Mount Rainier by USGS and others have documented a sequence of eruptive and noneruptive events that have taken place. All of them are typical of events that can be expected to occur in the future as a result of activities of Mount Rainier and, possibly, of all other volcanoes in the Cascade region.

The type of activity and possible frequency of occurrence at Mount Rainier are:

type of activity	frequency
Small debris flows not related to eruptions	one in 3 to 10 years
Large debris flows related to eruptions	one in 2000 years
Eruption of airborne pumice and ash	one in 2500 years
Eruption of large rocks and related avalanches	one in 5000 years
Eruption of lava flows	one in 10,000 years

VULNERABILITY

The people, property, economy, and ecology of the area surrounding the active volcanoes of Hawaii, the Pacific Northwest, and Alaska are endangered by the threat of future volcanic activity.

People and property in the immediate vicinity of the volcanoes could be endangered by lava flows, pyroclastic flows, debris flows, mud flows, and floods. People and property within a radius of 50 to 75 miles could be seriously affected by the fallout of airborne ash and flood-transported debris. The former could cause serious respiratory problems or even suffocate people, while both ash and debris could ruin crops and reduce productivity for several years. If the fallout were sufficiently great, buildings would collapse and people and animals would be entrapped.

In short, all life and property is endangered by volcanic eruptions, and the extent of the devastation is chiefly a function of the magnitude of the particular volcanic event.

COUNTERMEASURES: PREDICTION SYSTEMS

Sensors and Surveillance

The staff of USGS's Hawaiian Volcano Observatory is currently monitoring the active volcanoes Kilauea and Mauna Loa. Their theoretical and applied research has demonstrated that Kilauea displays characteristic patterns of surface deformation as it inflates prior to an eruption. Studies of earthquake patterns in relation to this inflation have added considerable knowledge of the overall functioning of Kilauea, and eruptions can now be predicted with a high degree of confidence. A similar, but less intensive program of deformation and seismic monitoring is currently underway on Kilauea's active neighbor volcano, Mauna Loa. The combined results of these investigations have greatly increased the capability to anticipate Hawaiian eruptions.

Surveillance of active volcanoes can be carried out with seismic event counters—instruments that count the number of earthquakes occurring in a particular area—and with aerial scanning of infrared anomalies.

Activities such as these can detect volcanoes that show suspicious changes in normal seismic or thermal characteristics, thereby providing preliminary indications of possible danger.

COUNTERMEASURES: PREVENTION SYSTEMS

Because of their nature, volcanic eruptions cannot be avoided. Furthermore, some degree of hazard will always exist in areas near active volcanoes. A program of volcano disaster prevention, therefore, becomes necessarily one that attempts to minimize the damage associated with the event. Two types of prevention measures appear feasible: risk mapping of areas likely to be affected by the lava and debris flows, and control over the uses of the land in such areas.

Areas in the vicinity of active volcanoes should be analyzed to determine the types of risks to which they would be subjected as a result of volcanic activity. This effort is similar to the one now being conducted to identify those areas that are susceptible to hurricane damage. On the basis of these risk maps, local governments could then pass ordinances to prevent further buildup of the susceptible areas or otherwise control their use.

Warning signs must be heeded and evacuation promptly carried out. Part of the tragedy of some past disasters is that the volcanoes gave ample warning that something was coming, yet little was done about it. The worst example was the Mt. Pelée eruption in 1902. For many years, the volcano had been dormant. Then in April 1902, smoke and ashes were discharged. On May 2, there were loud explosions and the people became alarmed. The governor of Martinique, with the help of a commission, reassured the people and told them there was no need to flee. Then on May 8, the main eruption took place, killing all but two inhabitants of the city of St. Pierre.

NOTES

[1]CLIFF OLLIER, *Volcanoes* (Cambridge, Mass., and London: The MIT Press, 1969), p. 154.

[2]A. RITTMAN, *Volcanoes and Their Activity*, trans. E. A. Vincent (New York: John Wiley & Sons, Inc., 1962), pp. 1–19.

[3]Ibid., pp. 196–97, 209–20.

[4]Ibid., p. 19.

[5]Ibid., pp. 30–33.

[6]OLLIER, *Volcanoes*, pp. 73–75.

[7]DWIGHT R. CRANDELL AND HOWARD H. WALDRON, "Volcanic Hazards in the Cascade Range," *Geologic Hazards and Public Problems*, Conference Proceedings, May 27–28, 1969, Office of Emergency Preparedness, Region Seven.

[8]Data from U.S. Geological Survey.

[9]The following information is taken from Ollier, *Volcanoes,* pp. 153–54.

[10]GORDON A. MACDONALD, *Catalogue of the Active Volcanoes of the World Including Solfatara Fields: Part III, Hawaiian Islands,* International Volcanological Association (Naples, Italy: Stabilimento Tipografico Francesco Giannini & Figli, 1956), pp. viii, 2, 7, 16–18, 26–27.

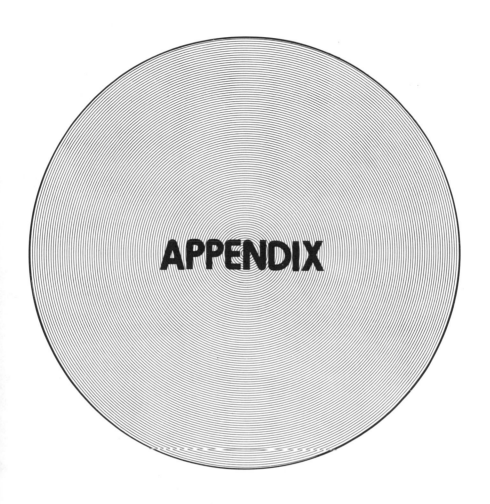

APPENDIX

table 1 *List of Alcohol Countermeasures*

1 Record in driver's record alcohol-related traffic convictions for court records.
2 Record in driver's record nontraffic alcohol-related convictions.
3 Record in driver's record all alcohol-related information from social health agency records.
4 Provide for flagging vehicle record for cars owned by problem drinkers.
5 Include alcohol safety questions in license examination and driver handbook.
6 Provide for certification by the license applicant regarding previous arrests and treatment for alcoholism.
7 Provide for including chemical test data in accident record.
8 Provide for chemical tests and specify concentrations.
9 Provide for implied consent for chemical tests.
10 Require license revocation if test is refused.
11 Set specifications and procedures for chemical tests.
12 Establish qualifications for alcohol safety personnel.
13 Provide for special enforcement of drinking-driving laws.
14 Provide for special training on breath testing equipment.
15 Determine locations and times of day of accidents involving drinking pedestrians.
16 Require presentence investigation of convicted drinking drivers.
17 Provide for referral of problem drinkers for treatment.
18 Establish medical advisory boards (MAB's) for licensing agency.
19 Provide for review of convicted DWI drivers by MAB prior to reinstating license.
20 Empower MAB to require physical exams on drivers whose records they review.
21 Provide for vehicle impounding for driving while license is revoked or for second DWI conviction within three years.
22 Provide for cancellation of collision insurance if insured driver has BAC above 0.10%.
23 Provide for special surveillance of revoked drivers.
24 Develop special pedestrian safety programs in areas of high accident risk or drinking, e.g., (1) better lighting, (2) reroute traffic, (3) reduce speed limits, (4) special caution signs.
25 Provide special patrols to assist intoxicated pedestrians.
26 Arrange for detoxification and treatment assistance for pedestrians.
27 Provide for suspension or revocation of license plates of vehicles owned by persons convicted of a drinking-driving offense.
28 Provide for special tags or registration certificates for vehicles owned by convicted drinking drivers.
29 Prohibit the transfer of vehicles with special registration certificates.
30 Develop mass media public education campaign on alcohol safety.*
31 Develop speakers bureau program on alcohol safety.
32 Augment alcohol safety sections of high school driver education programs.
33 Add sections on alcohol to primary safety courses and to appropriate secondary courses (family life courses).
34 Develop school driver improvement programs for special offenders.
35 Implement a driver assistance program in cooperation with social and health agencies.
36 Provide colored driver licenses for underage persons who might try to falsify entries on a license to purchase alcoholic beverages.

*Possible topics include: Extent of drinking driver problems, effects of alcohol on driving behavior, detail of laws, characteristics of the problem drinker driver, amount required to reach 0.10%, sources of help, public support for government and private agency efforts, penalties associated with DWI conviction, etc.

source: Gerald J. Driessen and Joseph A. Bryk, "Alcohol Countermeasures: Solid Rock and Shifting Sands," reprinted with permission from the *Journal of Safety Research,* a National Safety Council publication, Volume 5, Number 3 (September 1973), pp. 123–25.

37 Revoke driver's license for multiple convictions of drunkenness, even if unrelated to driving.

38 Establish more severe penalties for drinking and driving.

39 Provide insurance discounts for nondrinkers.

40 Advise taverns and public drinking places of identity of convicted DWI offenders and forbid sale of liquor to them (practical only in small towns).

41 Make temperproof, breath-meter control of car starting a mandatory device for all vehicles.

42 Control maximum speed according to BAC as indicated by breath-meter.

43 Place notices on liquor and beer bottles telling maximum legal blood alcohol.

44 Use twisting obstacle driving course on the road. Those who knock over cones or lights are tested for alcohol.

45 Take the convicted DWI offender out some distance on a road without buses and force him to walk home (used in Turkey).

46 Revoke licenses of teenagers who drive after drinking any amount.

47 Provide for prosecution of an individual who can prevent an intoxicated person from driving but doesn't.

48 Provide for driver self-testing by commercially available breath-screening tests.

49 Revoke license for lifetime after three convictions for DWI.

50 Establish 50 milligrams percent alcohol as legal limit for those under 21.

51 Use state commission to contact DWI offenders who may be alcoholics for purposes of attempted rehabilitation.

52 Establish national prohibition effectively enforced. (Do special studies to determine why earlier law failed.)

53 Establish crisis intervention centers similar to suicide prevention centers.

54 Promote the adoption of *per se* laws and strong implied consent laws.

55 Establish selective licensing limitation on time or place of permitted driving.

56 Distribute portable breath tester devices to bars.

57 Establish blockades at the roadside.

58 Request high school principals to announce publicly the names of students killed or injured in alcohol-related accidents.

59 Establish measures to increase probability that prosecution for DWI will take place for actual DWI.

60 Establish measures to increase awareness of an increased probability that conviction will follow guilt.

61 Arrange for free mass transit on high-drinking holidays.

62 Pass a law stating that to purchase liquor one's BAC must be less than 0.10%.

63 Show color sound films of DWI suspects to lawyers and court.

64 Make penalties less severe, but more likely, e.g., all DWI's are fined two weeks' pay and required to work for local government for two weeks.

65 Provide "state-dependent" training, i.e., teach persons while they are intoxicated to drive safely.

66 Educate businesses (for example, promotion of liquorless parties or provision to transport people home without driving, in case drinking does take place).

67 Offer free coffee (mostly to delay driving long enough to reduce alcohol level somewhat).

68 Pay for taxis to take people home.

69 Sponsor the availability of individual nondrinkers at parties.

70 Create a youth driving corps, first for holiday driving such as at Christmas and New Years, and then use such a youth driving corps for every weekend (night?) in the year.

71 Provide for imprinting by manufacturers of liquor bottles warning of the dangers above certain levels.

72 Have cab companies with two-man teams of drivers available; a cabbie to drive a drinker home and his companion to drive the drinker's car home.

73 Educate as to methods of diminishing alcohol effects.

74 Search for counterchemicals to antagonize alcohol effect, e.g., a sober-up pill that rapidly oxidizes alcohol in the body.

75 Change opinions of peers. This might be especially effective in high school and early college age groups. The drinker would now be a member of an out-group, not an in-group.

76 Change the self-image of the drinking driver. For example, show sound color films or photographs of himself under the influence of alcohol *to him* rather than to the lawyers or jury for legal purposes.

77 Change the self-image of the driver by having drinking drivers referred to a psychiatrist, psychologist, or "mental health counselor. . . ."

78 Use publicity in regard to those convicted of driving while intoxicated.

79 Put person on an alcoholic ward over a weekend after first DWI conviction so he sees and talks with late-stage alcoholics.

80 Teach young drivers how to stay awake while driving at night: Shoes off, window open, sing, loud radio, short nap at roadside, etc.

81 Bring "peer pressure" to bear on the *buyer* of alcohol for underage drinkers.

82 Use telephone "hot lines": For drinker assistance, 24-hour information and referral, or for direct access to previous driver record.

83 Reduce time and red-tape requirements for arresting officers.

84 Use mobile breath-testing vehicles that move directly to scene of arrest or accident.

85 Organize and utilize local volunteers for public education efforts.

86 Make convicted DWI offenders who are at fault for an accident responsible for all associated financial losses, up to a level of 50% of their total net worth.

87 Have judges and police officers drink, in a protected environment, until their BAC reaches 0.10%.

88 Form a union of nondrinking drivers to lobby for legislation, reduced insurance rates, etc. . . .

89 Publicize the place at which the driver or pedestrian had been drinking as part of the accident report in alcohol-related accidents (especially fatals).

90 Use alcohol-related trigger films for group discussions.

91 Enhance social tolerance for alcohol abstinence.

92 Encourage employers to use the threat of job loss as a lever to move problem drinkers to obtain treatment.

93 Focus on early detection of problem drinking (alcoholism, like cancer, can be controlled if detected early enough).

94 Improve host behavior, e.g., serve fewer drinks, serve less potent drinks, serve food, provide sober drivers for heavy drinkers.

95 Publicize widely the stages of alcoholism and, especially, the symptoms associated with early stages.

96 Encourage public to drive less during high-risk hours for alcohol-related accidents.

97 Teach alcoholic drinkers (gulping pattern, several drinks in short time period) to become social drinkers (sipping pattern, fewer drinks over same period of time). . . .

98 Have police officers randomly sample BAC's in bars and issue warning to those with BAC's at or above 0.10% that they cannot drive.

99 Double the taxes on alcohol and devote increased revenue to countermeasures against alcohol-related traffic accidents.

100 Encourage the idea that even small amounts of alcohol may be deleterious to health.

101 Establish a new bar tax to which exemptions are granted on the basis of proximity of the customer's residence to the bar. . . .

102 Make technical literature and samples of previous alcohol-oriented public information campaigns available free to persons who request it. . . .

103 Standardize the closing time of all drinking establishments and increase substantially the enforcement shortly before and after that time. . . .

104 Promote the adoption of pre-arrest breath testing similar to that used in Great Britain.

105 Develop, validate, and apply paper-and-pencil tests to identify potentially dangerous drinker drivers. . . .

106 Identify community officials likely to be working with abusive drinkers and enlist their support in the planning and execution phases.

107 Reduce the frequency of "plea-downs," informal arrangements to plead guilty to a lesser offense, e.g., reckless driving rather than DWI.

table 2   *Index to the Driver Education Instructional Objectives*

subject	purpose
preparation	To enable the student to prepare the car and its occupants for a safe and comfortable trip.
starting	To enable the student to start the car.
accelerating	To enable the student to accelerate smoothly and safely from a standing position.
starting on grades	To enable the student to start a car on an upgrade and on a downgrade from a standing position.
steering — lane keeping	To enable the student to maintain proper position in required lane.
steering — turning	To enable the student to make a safe, comfortable turn.
speed control	To enable the student to adjust speed to existing traffic conditions to account for variations in traffic flow and legal speed limits.
downshifting	To enable the student to downshift to maintain speed or reduce speed, before starting down a hill, in heavy, slow-moving traffic, or in emergency situations.
stopping	To enable the student to come to a normal safe stop on level roadways and on hills and to make required rapid stops.
backing	To enable the student to back up safely and smoothly.
skid control	To enable the student to prevent and stop a skid.
surveillance	To enable the student to maintain a complete and accurate understanding of the driving environment and to identify any critical changes that might affect his driving.
urban driving	To enable the student to drive safely in an urban area and react appropriately to pedestrians and to other traffic.
highway driving	To enable the student to drive in a safe, efficient manner in open country and mountainous terrain.
freeway driving	To enable the student to safely enter, drive on, and exit from a freeway.
car following	To enable the student to maintain an adequate separation between the car and the vehicle ahead.
passing	To enable the student to make sound passing decisions and to complete passes safely without interference to other road users.
entering traffic	To enable the student to enter traffic without interfering with other vehicles.
leaving traffic	To enable the student to leave the line of traffic with minimal interference to the vehicles behind and to the side of the car.
lane changing	To enable the student to change lanes safely and without obstructing the flow of traffic.
parking	To enable the student to park the car safely and legally, and to exit from the car, with minimal interference with other vehicular or pedestrian traffic.
leaving a parking space	To enable the student to leave a parking space safely without obstructing other vehicular or pedestrian traffic.
pedestrians, cyclists, and animals	To enable the student to respond with safe and cautious actions when encountering pedestrians, cyclists, and animals.
emergency areas	To enable the student to drive safely through or by an attended emergency area, or to provide necessary assistance when he is the first to reach a severe accident.

source: Human Resource Research Organization.

subject	purpose
parked cars	To enable the student to drive safely alongside parked and parking vehicles.
being passed	To enable the student to accommodate a passing vehicle by adjusting the car's speed and/or position as necessary for the other vehicle to complete the pass quickly.
being followed	To enable the student to drive ahead of other vehicles with a minimum risk of rear-end collision.
oncoming cars	To enable the student to adjust his course as necessary when meeting oncoming vehicles, and to take evasive action when necessary to avoid a head-on collision.
overtaking	To enable the student to safely overtake a vehicle ahead and to avoid having to initiate emergency maneuvers.
special vehicles	To enable the student to act safely when in the vicinity of special vehicles, viz., school buses, police, fire, and other emergency vehicles.
intersections— approaching	To enable the student to approach an intersection and to react appropriately to other traffic and traffic controls.
intersections— through	To enable the student to proceed through an intersection prepared to react to changing traffic conditions.
intersections— right turn	To enable the student to safely make a right turn at an intersection.
intersections— left turn	To enable the student to safely make a left turn at an intersection.
traffic circles	To enable the student to negotiate traffic circles safely.
on-ramps	To enable the student to safely enter a main roadway from an entrance ramp with or without an acceleration lane.
off-ramps	To enable the student to exit safely from the main roadway.
hills	To enable the student to negotiate hills safely and effectively.
curves	To enable the student to negotiate highway curves safely and comfortably.
lane usage	To enable the student to select the appropriate lane for driving.
road surfaces	To enable the student to drive safely on different types of road surfaces; to enable the student to adjust his driving according to road surface conditions.
wet roads	To enable the student to drive safely on a wet surface.
road shoulders	To enable the student to deal effectively and safely with road shoulders.
obstructions	To enable the student to deal safely with roadway obstructions and barricades.
snow	To enable the student to drive, stop, and park safely on ice- and snow-covered roadways.
sand	To enable the student to drive safely on sand-covered roadways.
u-turns	To enable the student to perform a U-turn where legally permissible.
two- and three-point turns	To enable the student to turn around by means of a three-point turn, or a two-point turn using a driveway.
entering off-street areas	To enable the student to approach and enter off-street areas in a safe and efficient manner.
off-street driving	To enable the student to drive safely in and around off-street areas without impeding traffic flow.
railroad crossings	To enable the student to safely cross railroad crossings and to respond to possible dangers at such crossings.

subject	purpose
bridges and tunnels	To enable the student to enter, drive through or across , and leave a tunnel or bridge safely and expeditiously.
toll plazas	To enable the student to negotiate toll plazas in a safe and expeditious manner.
limited visibility	To enable the student to drive safely during weather conditions that limit visibility.
climate	To enable the student to drive safely and comfortably during extremely hot or extremely cold weather.
wind	To enable the student to maintain directional control during a high crosswind.
night driving	To enable the student to drive safely during darkness.
towing	To enable the student to adjust his driving behavior to compensate for the effects of towing a trailer.
hauling loads	To enable the student to adjust his driving behavior to compensate for the effects of hauling heavy loads within or on top of the car.
car emergencies	To enable the student to react safely when a car's malfunction endangers its occupants and other road users.
mechanical problems	To enable the student to respond appropriately to malfunction indications although the apparent malfunction may be unlikely to affect the safety of the driver or other road users.
disabled cars	To enable the student to deal safely with breakdowns that disable the car while on the road.
dealing with breakdowns	To educate the student to remedy various on-road emergency malfunctions.
pushing cars	To educate the student in the methods, procedures, and hazards involved when being pushed or pushing another vehicle.
trip planning	To educate the student in the planning and preparation which precede driving and in navigational activities.
loading	To enable the student to load objects securely in the passenger area, trunk, and on the roof.
trailers	To enable the student to attach a trailer to the car and load the trailer properly.
alcohol and drugs	To educate the student on the effects that drugs and alcohol have on driving safety and performance.
physical and emotional conditions	To enable the student to become aware of physical and emotional conditions that may affect driving ability and how to compensate for such conditions.
maintenance	To educate the student to maintain the car in sound operating condition through routine care and servicing.
inspection and servicing	To educate the student to have the car inspected and serviced in accordance with the recommendations of tne manufacturer.
repair	To educate the student to have the car repaired in response to breakdowns, symptoms of malfunctions, and deficiencies noted during inspection and servicing.
certification	To inform the student about driver and car certification.
accidents	To educate the student on the post-accident responsibilities of the driver.

table 3 Consumer Product Hazard Index, U. S. Consumer Product Safety Commission.[1] Hazards and Injuries Associated with Top 50 Products with Recommendations to Consumers to Minimize Risks of Injury.

product ranking	product name	projected annual[2] injuries treated in hospital emergency rooms during FY 1973	types of product-related injuries	hazard patterns	guide to consumer action
1	Bicycles and bicycle equipment including add-on features (baskets, horns, nonstandard seats, handbrakes)	372,000	Concussion, fractures, lacerations, amputations, broken teeth, bruises	Mechanical and Structural Brake failure Pedal broke Wheel loose or fell off Steering Foot caught in spokes Riding double Infant carrier caught in chain Loss of Control Struck obstruction Braking Riding double	Purchase bicycle appropriate to size and age of user with adequate lights, reflectors, and fenders. Riders must know and obey rules of the road. Maintain bicycle, especially brakes, in good working condition.

[1]The Consumer Product Hazard Index is based on the frequency and severity of injuries and gives double weight to injuries to children under 10 years old. This ranking was based on nation-wide estimates for consumer product related injuries treated in NEISS hospitals from July 1, 1972 to June 30, 1973.

Major hazard patterns revealed by analyses of injury reports in Commission files are included along with some recommendations to assist consumers to reduce risks of injury at home, at school, and at play.

[2]The Projected Annual Injuries Treated in Hospital Emergency Rooms was estimated by multiplying the number of product-related injuries reported by each NEISS hospital during FY 1973 by a numerical factor assigned to each of the hospitals. This factor is different for each hospital, and depends upon the number and nature of other similar hospital emergency rooms across the country. The values obtained from each of the multiplications were then added, resulting in the projected injury estimates for the United States.

product ranking	product name	projected annual injuries treated in hospital emergency rooms during FY 1973	types of product-related injuries	hazard patterns	guide to consumer action
				Stunting Skidded Turning Struck or struck by automobile	
2	Stairs, ramps, and landings; indoors and outdoors	356,000	Lacerations, contusions/abrasions, fractures, dislocations, strain/sprains, hematomas	Falls Slippery-tread surface, footwear Tripped—single riser, footwear, miscellaneous objects Slipped over nosing (narrow treads) Inadequate lighting Miscellaneous—hurrying, physical impairment, age, fainting, intoxication	Secure railings, keep firmly attached; evenly spaced steps; firmly attached rugs, treads; use nonslippery wax; repair broken places immediately; assure adequate lighting with easy to reach on-and-off switches (at both ends of stairway); keep free of clutter. Hold to banister, carry objects so steps can be seen.
3	Doors, other than glass doors, including folding, swinging, garage,	153,000	Lacerations, crushing, contusions/abrasions, fractures, strain/sprains,	Struck by or striking against door Opening into traffic flow	Keep hinges in good working condition; keep door entirely open or closed. Instruct children not to play with or around doors, especially overhead

No.	Item	Est. injuries	Injuries	Hazards/Accidents	Prevention
	and screen doors		hematomas	Fall or slip against Closing (falling) garage door Entrapment of body part Between garage door sections On latch and hinge sides Garage door pull ropes	garage doors; use locks to hold doors closed; keep objects out of way of swinging door. Open cautiously.
4	Cleaning agents caustic compounds	35,000	Chemical burns, poisonings, inhalation of dangerous fumes. Swallowing	Ingestion Storage accessible to children Storage in unmarked or improper containers Chemical burns Splashing Removal of drain or cleanout plug Using no protection (gloves) Hands to eye or face Inhalation Mixing cleaners Vapor explosion	Keep in original container; read and follow instructions; use properly marked safety closures; store in locked compartments out of reach of children and animals. Do not mix bleaches with caustic cleaners. Keep away from eyes and mouth. Use gloves and/or protective clothing. Keep phone numbers of emergency treatment facilities handy.
5	Tables, nonglass	137,000	Lacerations, contusion/abrasion, fractures, strains/sprains, hematomas	Sharp edges and corners Fell onto or ran into table	Position away from traffic lane through room; keep table in good repair, legs even to prevent tilting. Rough spots eliminated by covering or sanding. Supervise toddlers near tables.
6	Beds, including	100,000	Broken bones, cuts,	Fall from or against	Place out of line of traffic, away from

product ranking	product name	projected annual injuries treated in hospital emergency rooms during FY 1973	types of product-related injuries	hazard patterns	guide to consumer action
	springs, box springs, and frames		bruises, concussion, lacerations, contusions/abrasions, fractures, strain/ sprain, hematoma, burns	Fabric ignition of box springs	heaters or source of flame. Use nontoxic paint. Bunk beds should be well built, easy to climb into, have sturdy, secure ladders. Use adequate guard rails for upper bunk. Regular beds should be well constructed with rounded corners, easy to move and sturdy enough for users. Springs should be well covered; slats evenly spaced and placed to prevent bed from falling. Do not smoke in bed. Purchase flame-resistant bedding. Mandatory standard for mattress flammability went into effect for all mattresses introduced into Interstate Commerce on or after June 22, 1973.
7	Football activity and related equipment and apparel	230,000	Fractures, muscle and joint injuries, bruises, concussions, broken teeth, and other injuries	Unorganized activity No protective equipment Playing surface condition Organized activity Protective equipment not effective	Use complete outfits of proper fitting protective equipment designed for strong impact; keep in good repair; remove debris and dangerous objects from the surface and perimeter of playing area. CPSC has expressed intention to consider football activity for possible mandatory standards.
8	Swings, slides, seesaws, and	112,000	Concussion, fractures, bruises,	Pinch points, sharp edges, protruding	Keep playing surface free from holes, stones, broken glass, etc. Select equip-

#	Product	Number	Injuries	Hazards	Recommendations
	climbing apparatus		lacerations, amputations	bolts Falls (from ladders, bars, seats) Failures (collapse, supports, seats)	...ment in accord with size and age of users. Keep equipment in good repair. Anchor heavy equipment and eliminate sharp or rough edges by taping. Remove and replace open-end "S" hooks. Have separate areas for ball games. Provide instruction as to use of equipment and games. Supervise children at play. CPSC intends to develop regulations for both public and private playground equipment under the Federal Hazardous Substances Act.
9	Liquid fuels, kindling or illuminating (including gasoline, kerosene, lighter fluid, charcoal starter)	25,000	Swallowing, burns and explosions of fumes. First, second, and third degree burns, carbon monoxide poisoning	Vapor ignition Improper use of product Improper storage Ingestion Fabric ignition Refueling operations Adding product to heat source	Purchase only quantity needed and keep in original container; use according to instructions; store and use away from heat or pilot lights and out of reach of children; do not use in closed or unventilated room. Cautionary labeling and child-resistant packaging are required for these products.
10	Architectural glass including doors, tub enclosures, shower enclosures, windows	178,000	Punctures, severe lacerations	Breaking of glass Fall into (tripping) Run into Pushing on Slamming door Mistaken for opening Mistaken for open door Slipping in tub or shower	Use safety glass in large doors, windows and fixed panels which could be mistaken for means of ingress and egress and in tub and shower enclosures. Use decals to direct attention to the presence of large glass panels. Do not have scatter rugs close to glass doors, windows, and fixed panels. Do not allow children to run or play near glass doors, panels, or windows. The development of mandatory standards for architectural glass is now underway.

product ranking	product name	projected annual injuries treated in hospital emergency rooms during FY 1973	types of product-related injuries	hazard patterns	guide to consumer action
				Slipping on throw rugs	
11	Power lawn mowers, including rotary and reel, gas and electric; riding and nonriding	58,000	Amputations; broken bones, cuts, bruises, electric shock	Ejected objects containing blade (making adjustments, clearing grass chute, slipping under mower) Tipping over Reverse operation Malfunction (blade, starter, wheel, drive) Frayed and exposed wiring	Read instructions completely before use. Clear area of stones and debris. Do not adjust, clean out discharge chute, or leave machine without completely stopping motor. Be properly clothed — wear heavy shoes. Never allow a child to ride, use, or play near when mowing. Never add fuel unless mower is cool. Don't mow when grass is wet. Store in a special place away from line of traffic through yard or garage. The development of mandatory standards for power lawn mowers soon will be underway.
12	Baseball, activity, related equipment and apparel	191,000	Cuts, bruises, head and leg injuries, broken bones	Struck by bat Second party batter Self inflicted Struck by thrown ball Hit by pitch Tipped off glove Struck by batted ball	Select playing area away from street traffic and area with minimum hazards (litter and debris). Provide gloves, protective headgear, and footwear. Instruct players in how to throw, catch, and bat safely. Separate the players and spectators. Stay clear of the batter.
13	Nails, carpet tacks, screws, and thumb	275,000	Puncture wounds, lacerations,	Stepped on nail, carpet tack	Eliminate protruding nail or screw ends; always keep such items out of mouth;

	Product	Injuries	Type of injury	Hazard	Precautions
	tacks		swallowing	Contacted exposed nail Ingestion	keep picked up and away from children.
14	Bath tub and shower structures other than doors and panels, including the tub, walls, hand-grips, etc.	41,000	Bruises, cuts, fractures from falls, scalds, electric shock	Slippery surface Falls Protrusion into tub Product or fixture failure Soap dish, towel bar, pulled out of wall Faucet breakage Hot water burns	Use nonskid rugs, decals, strips, etc., and provide hand-grips within easy reach. Use mixing faucet where possible to keep temperature even (always check temperature of water before entering tub or shower). Do not have electrical appliances near the tub or shower.
15	Space heaters and heating stove	22,000	Burn injuries, resulting from clothing ignition, explosion, and hot surfaces; carbon monoxide poisonings	Contact with hot surface or flame Contact with sharp edge Fabric ignition Explosion Carbon monoxide poisoning	Locate well away from flammable structures and materials; keep children away. Maintain in good operating condition with no fuel leaks; follow operating instructions carefully. Use extreme caution in operating, and do not leave completely unattended for long periods of time. Gas heaters must be vented to the outside. Try to avoid locating a space heater in normal traffic patterns. Be especially careful with long or flowing dresses, etc. Area should be as well ventilated as possible. Do not modify heater. Keep clean to prevent CO. CPSC has stated its intention to develop mandatory standards for space heaters.
16	Swimming pools and associated equipment, not	32,000	Drowning, fractures, bruises, cuts from falls	Diving Climbing ladder Slide board	Be sure pools are adequately fenced with self-closing/latching gates – latches 4 feet high. Be sure diving board is well

product ranking	product name	projected annual injuries treated in hospital emergency rooms during FY 1973	types of product-related injuries	hazard patterns	guide to consumer action
	including above ground pools			Accessory explosion Small child access Slipping	constructed and anchored. Teach family members to swim and always with a buddy. Post regulations on fence in regard to use of pool. Be sure a family member knows mouth-to-mouth resuscitation. Use slide in feet-first position only. No horseplay or running in pool area. Keep deck clear of clutter. Have rescue equipment (shepherd crook or life ring). Know the water depth before jumping or diving into a pool. The Commission is analyzing an offer to develop a standard for swimming pool water slides. CPSC may undertake further action for swimming pools in general.
17	Cooking ranges, ovens, and equipment	25,000	Burns, blisters, bruises, and scalds	Excessive temperature on noncooking surface Inability to distinguish whether or not surface unit was hot Unintentional control activation Accidental contact with cooking surface Explosion	Install according to directions and follow instructions as to use. Keep burners and oven completely turned off when not in use. Use extreme care when lighting a nonautomatic oven. Do not reach across burner while wearing loose sleeves or cuffs. Turn handles of pots and pans toward back of stove. Prevent children from playing on or near stoves. Use hot pads. Should not be installed by the consumer.

No.	Product	Number	Injury	Hazard Pattern	Recommendations
				Children contacting cooking surface Fabric ignition	
18	Basketball activity and related equipment and apparel	188,000	Bruises, fractures, primarily from fall, strains/sprains	Player contact Hit in nose with elbow Bumped heads Landing on another's foot. Knocked over Landed on foot badly – twisted foot/knee Hit by ball Ran into obstructions Playing surface condition	Playing surface should be smooth, nonslippery and free of tripping hazards. Use basketball footwear with nonskid, "gripping" qualities. Also use elbow and knee pads.
19	Nonupholstered chairs	68,000	Broken bones, bruises, punctures	Tipping (falling) over Leaning back Climbing on Fall from chair	Purchase sturdy chair, place on even floor. Repair split or broken furniture. Sand rough surfaces to prevent splinters. Place out of traffic lane in room. Sit properly, avoid tipping and leaning. Supervise toddlers playing near chairs. Do not use for climbing.
20	Storage furniture; including chests, buffets, book shelves, etc.	68,000	Broken bones, cuts, bruises	Sharp edges and corners Fell or ran into furniture Tipping over Climbing into drawers Reaching for upper drawers	Use step-ladder to place items on top shelf. Keep drawers closed. Teach children not to climb on cabinets and shelves. Store heavy or bulky, unmanageable items in lower drawers. Place frequently used articles at front of shelves. Make sure enclosure can be opened from inside.

product ranking	product name	projected annual injuries treated in hospital emergency rooms during FY 1973	types of product-related injuries	hazard patterns	guide to consumer action
21	Cutlery, unpowered kitchen knives	172,000	Cuts	Use Slicing or cutting Distraction Improper use Use as screw-driver, punch, playing, etc.	Use properly—do not use knife for such purposes as screwdriver, hole punch, etc. When using, hold by handle with sharp edge away from body. Repair cutlery handle if loose or discard. Keep sharp objects out of the reach of children. Use cutting board when preparing food.
22	Clothing, including day and night wear	6000	Burns from fabric flammability	Ignited fabric	Keep matches out of reach of children. Be aware of flammable characteristics of clothing. Buy flame-retardant sleepwear and other clothing whenever possible. Avoid decorations that might detach from infant clothing. Avoid frilly, baggy, loose-fitting clothing near flames or sources of heat. A flammability standard for children's sleepwear (sizes 0–6X) went into effect July 29, 1972. A standard for sleepwear (sizes 7–14) went into effect May 1, 1975.
23	Paints and solvents	14,000	Poisonings; chemical burns, burns from ignition of fumes	Ingestion Storage acces-sible to children Peeling paint (lead poisoning) Vapor ignition	Store in original containers out of reach of children and away from extreme heat and flame; follow label instructions and warning; use protective gloves or other clothing to avoid skin contact where recommended; use in well-ventilated areas. Federal law limits the maximum amount of lead permitted in household paints.

No.	Product	Count	Injury	Hazard	Prevention
24	Household chemical products, other than caustics, paints, waxes	11,000	Chemical burns	Ingestion; Bit into product's tube; Other ingestions; Flammable properties; Use near heat source (cigarette, stove, electrical); Irritant; Body part contact in use; Inhalation	Be knowledgeable of content of product and use in accord with instructions. Keep all chemicals away from children. Some household chemicals require warning labels and child-resistant packaging.
25	Coins and toy money, paper money	9000	Choking from swallowing	Ingestion	Watch children carefully when playing with play money. Keep coins and small objects from small children.
26	Floors and flooring material	53,000	Contusions, fractures, concussions from falls	Slippery surface; Slipped on wet floor; Footwear wet; Vinyl surface; Falling (other than slipping)	Repair uneven floors. Eliminate hazards such as protruding nails, splintering, missing boards. Repair torn carpets. Place nonslip material on back of small rugs. Use nonskid wax according to directions to reduce possibility of falling; clean up spills immediately.
27	Glass bottles and jars, including soft drink bottles	111,000	Cuts and lacerations	Breaking and broken glass; In use; Exposed; Explosion; Spontaneous; Handling; Propulsion of cap	Keep home premises and play areas free of glass; dispose of these items properly and promptly in durable and sealable waste containers; clean up breakage immediately. Buy safety containers where available. Do not agitate.
28	Washing machines with wringer	9000	Tearing and crushing injuries,	Body part caught in wringer	Keep hand free of wringer and clothes when operating; know how to use any

product ranking	product name	projected annual injuries treated in hospital emergency rooms during FY 1973	types of product-related injuries	hazard patterns	guide to consumer action
				Playing with wringer Feeding clothes into wringer Caught in exposed gear Electric shock	and all safety "release" features; do not permit children to play with or near the machine. Turn off wringer when not in use.
29	Matches	11,000	Burns	Failure in use Head fragmentation, sparking or flaring Spontaneous ignition Friction Children playing Fabric ignition Vapor ignition	Keep matches out of reach of children and ignition source; hot matches should be placed in suitable receptacle or tray posing no risk of secondary ignition. Strike matches away from body with cover closed. Provide large ashtrays in sufficient numbers. Don't strike near highly combustible materials (e.g., gasoline) as vapors could ignite. The Commission has commenced a proceeding for the development of a standard for bookmatches.
30	Ladders and step stools	57,000	Fractures and bruises from falls	Falls Over-extending Insecure footing	Do not "walk" the ladder along the wall while standing on it. Be sure the ladder or step stool is sturdy and will carry the weight of the user. Keep it in good condition. Avoid standing on the topmost step or paint rack. Be sure it is properly balanced before using. Make sure footing is secure and ladder is firmly planted.

31	Sun lamps and heat lamps	11,000	Burns	Exposure Falling asleep Too close Too long Contact with hot surface	*Sun:* Follow manufacturers' directions; cover eyes. Avoid use while drowsy. Remember: A sun lamp is intensified ultra-violet rays. It will work much faster and to a greater degree than the sun itself. *Heat:* Follow directions. Do not point toward combustible materials. Avoid touching lamp until cool. Use timer to turn off in case user goes to sleep.
32	Home workshop saws (electric)	37,000	Lacerations; electrical burns and shock; contusions from material being thrown by sawing operation; amputations	Contact with blade No blade guard Malfunction of blade guard Ineffective blade guard Kickback Hand placed in path of blade Reaching across or under blade Blade rotation after shut off	Saws should be carefully selected for particular task. Each should have a specific place for use and for storage and should be close to the outlet (eliminating long cords) and grounded. Instruction for use should be carefully read and followed. When electrical tool is not in use, it should be disconnected. Do not remove blade guard.
33	Fences, not electric, outdoor, all types (including posts)	55,000	Bruises, fractures, cuts from collisions and falls	Contact with sharp points, edges, corners Climbing, jumping, or vaulting fence Slipped or fell against fence, gate, or post	Fences should be kept in good repair, free of projecting nails, bolts, and wire ends. Posts and fences should be plainly visible.
34	Pens, pencils, and other desk supplies	33,000	Cuts, puncture wounds	Ingestion Sharp points	Teach children not to place pens and pencils in their mouths and ears, and not

product ranking	product name	projected annual injuries treated in hospital emergency rooms during FY 1973	types of product-related injuries	hazard patterns	guide to consumer action
35	Pins and needles	43,000	Cuts, puncture wounds, swallowing	Inadvertent stapling of body part Ingestion Contact with sharp point	to run with pointed objects. Have a specific place for staplers and sharp objects. Keep out of reach of small children. Use pin cushions and keep these out of the reach of children. Do not use pins or needles as medical instruments. Do not put pins and needles in mouth.
36	Cans, including self-openers and resealable closures	68,000	Cuts	Contact with sharp edge Opening can (self-contained openers) Removing lid from partially opened cans	Use can opener rather than knife or other sharp object and be cautious with sharp edges. Do not lick lids. Dispose of sharp-edged can lids properly.
37	Upholstered furniture	34,000	Burns, smoke inhalation from flammable fabrics ignition	Fabric ignition (cigarettes, matches)	Use care when smoking and always check for smoldering ashes. Be sure cigarette matches and ashes are placed in proper nonflammable receptacles and trays. Avoid smoking when sleepy. CPSC is developing a flammability standard for upholstered furniture.
38	Furnaces and floor furnaces	8000	Burns, including ignition of flammable materials	Explosions Not following instructions for	Be certain furnaces are installed according to building code regulations. Have the heaters regularly inspected (prior to the

No.	Item	Type of injury	Est. injuries	Hazards	Precautions
		and explosion		lighting pilot Safety valve malfunction Carbon monoxide poisoning Clogged vent pipe Rusted through vent pipe Asphyxiation Escaping gas Contact with hot floor grates	heating season). Do not force furnace to burn materials beyond its capacity (such as at holiday time). Keep children and flammable materials away from furnaces. Some floor furnaces are in hallways and difficult to skirt. If possible put a guard around floor furnaces (these are available) to protect children. Where they are not easily avoided, alert all persons in the home to the fact that the grate is hot.
39	Water heaters	Burns from explosion and hot surface temperatures; carbon monoxide	3000	Lighting pilot light Gas explosion or backfire Contact with hot surface Carbon monoxide poisoning Plugged vent	Be sure heaters are installed in accord with local codes and that gas water heaters are properly vented. Temperature and pressure relief valves should be set at proper level. Take special care when lighting pilot light or touching water heater surface. Keep in good repair and clean. Dirty burners cause CO emissions.
40	Porches, balconies, floor openings, and open-sided rooms	Lacerations, fractures, contusions/abrasions, strains/sprains	18,000	Falls Inadequate protection Railings too low Wide space between balusters Structural defects	Every opening should be equipped with railing or fence. Guard rails in good repair. Such devices should be durable, sturdy, and of adequate height with closely spaced balusters to protect children.
41	Baby cribs, gates, and playpens	Fractures, cuts, lacerations, etc., bruises, strangulation	12,000	Fall from crib Climbing out Leaning over side Tripped release Bounced out Product Failure	Infants' cribs should have slats close together, no sharp or rough edges. Place crib on carpet or rug out of line of traffic. Check hinges or folding points to be sure fingers could not be pinched. Be sure mattresses fit snugly. Use bumper pads

product ranking	product name	projected annual injuries treated in hospital emergency rooms during FY 1973	types of product-related injuries	hazard patterns	guide to consumer action
				Locking mechanism released Mattress support Hitting against crib part (outside) Entrapment Between side and springs Between side and headboard Between slats and metal guide rod Between headboard and mattress Head between slats	to prevent babies from slipping through slats. Remove child from playpen when he can climb out. Keep crib in good condition to avoid spaces which could lead to entrapment. Full-size baby cribs introduced into interstate commerce on or after February 1, 1974, that do not comply with Commission regulations (16 CFR 1508) are banned under the Federal Hazardous Substances Act.
42	Roller skates, scooters, and skateboards	55,000	Fractures, concussions, abrasions, lacerations, punctures	Falls Lost balance Struck uneven surface Turning Collision	Use should be restricted to play areas which are smooth, free of collision and tripping hazards, and away from heavy pedestrian and vehicular traffic. Use should be away from steps.
43	Pots and pans (including lids)	10,000	Burns	Contact with hot liquid Splattering,	Arrange pots and pans on stove with handles facing away from front to prevent knocking over. Use pot holders. Check

	Product	Est.	Injury	Cause	Prevention
				splashing, and pouring Spills, tipping, dropping, knocked over Product failure, handles Ignition of cooking oil Contact with hot surface	handles periodically to be sure they are secure. Keep toddlers away from area when hot pots and pans are in use. Don't leave oil or grease unattended on lighted burner.
44	Fishing equipment (poles, lines, hooks, fishing knives, scalers, tackle box, etc.)	44,000	Punctures and lacerations	Cut by hook Casting Handling equipment	Keep hooks, knives, and other equipment in proper containers when not in use; exercise extreme caution in casting and in transporting fishing equipment.
45	Jewelry, watches, keys, and key rings	11,000	Swallowing, cuts	Ingestion Inserting in body orifice Caught on object	Keep jewelry away from small children. When working around equipment or machinery with moving parts, remove jewelry to avoid entanglement.
46	Hockey equipment and apparel	30,000	Lacerations, fractures, concussions, contusions/abrasions	Hit by puck Hit by stick Cut by skate Checked or fell into sideboard	Keep play areas free from debris; wear complete outfits of protection equipment and pads. These problems are common to street hockey as well as ice hockey.
47	Irons	7000	Burns	Contact with hot surface Pulled on cord or jolted iron, causing it to fall Hot water Overflow Iron fell	Read instructions before use (steam, spray, regular). Be sure to set at proper heat control for material being ironed. Never leave hot side down on fabric or flammable materials. Do not allow children to play near the ironing board. Never leave a hot iron untended. Do not unplug by pulling cord.

product ranking	product name	projected annual injuries treated in hospital emergency rooms during FY 1973	types of product-related injuries	hazard patterns	guide to consumer action
48	Outside structures (including retaining walls, patios, terraces)	23,000	Concussions, fractures, lacerations, abrasions, sprains/strains	Falls Slips Trips Wet surfaces Uneven surfaces Inadequate lighting	Retaining walls should have secure railings and fences, or other barriers to prevent falls; maintain adequate lighting around patios and terraces. Patios should have slip-resistant surfaces.
49	Wagons and other ride-on toys (not including bicycles and tricycles)	15,000	Broken bones, bruises, cuts	Fall from toy Tipped over Struck obstruction Lost balance Sharp edges Pinch points	Keep in good repair. Have place to store when not in use. Check stability before purchasing. Check for sharp edges and pinch points. Teach children where, when, and how to ride.
50	Minibikes	26,000	Fractures, lacerations, hematoma, concussion, contusion/abrasion, puncture, burn, strain/sprain, amputation, cerebral hemorrhage, severed artery	Mechanical and Structural Brake failure Sticking throttle Chain breaking or coming off Handlebars separating or locking Fork broke Body part caught in chain drive Loss of control	Do not ride in public thoroughfares (streets). In areas provided for minibike riding, remove "pot holes," low tree limbs, rocks, loose gravel, etc. Keep in good repair; check for broken, loose parts. When purchasing, check for adequate guards on moving parts (chain, pulleys, etc.). Do not ride "double."

Collision with
other vehicles
Accidently acceler-
ating rather than
braking
Contact with hot
surfaces

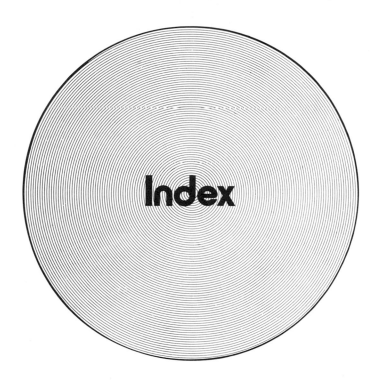

Index